Urine Formed Elements

Lei Zheng • Lizhi Yan • Shimin Zhang
Editors

Urine Formed Elements

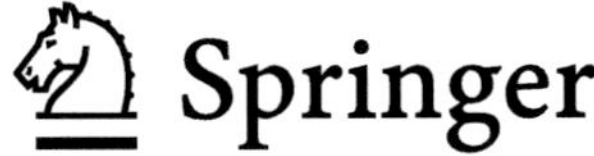

Editors
Lei Zheng
Department of Laboratory Medicine
Nanfang Hospital, Southern Medical University
Guangzhou, China

Lizhi Yan
Department of Laboratory Medicine
Nanfang Hospital, Southern Medical University
Guangzhou, China

Shimin Zhang
Department of Clinical Laboratory
Peking Union Medical College Hospital, Peking Union Medical College
Beijing, China

ISBN 978-981-99-7741-3 ISBN 978-981-99-7739-0 (eBook)
https://doi.org/10.1007/978-981-99-7739-0

This Springer imprint is published by the registered company Springer Nature Singapore Pte Ltd.
The registered company address is: 152 Beach Road, #21-01/04 Gateway East, Singapore 189721, Singapore

Paper in this product is recyclable

Foreword 1

I am greatly honored to write the preface for this pioneering atlas, *Urine Formed Elements*. The examination of urinary formed elements is a widely used, noninvasive testing method. By observing cells, crystals, casts, and other formed elements in urine, we can gain insights into the health condition of the human body and obtain crucial diagnostic evidence. Whether for early disease screening or complex disease diagnosis, urinary formed element tests hold significant clinical value. They are especially critical in providing crucial diagnostic evidence in areas such as kidney diseases, urinary system inflammation, tumors, and more. Although advanced instruments are increasingly used in urine testing, manual microscopy remains the gold standard for distinguishing urinary formed elements.

Professor Lei Zheng of Southern Hospital, Southern Medical University, is a well-known Chinese laboratory medicine expert and the corresponding chief editor of this book. Under his leadership, a group of Chinese experts specializing in urinary morphology examination has been gathered, focusing on the writing of this book. Their rich experience and solid professional knowledge ensure the depth and breadth of the content of this book. China, as a populous country, possesses abundant clinical sample resources, providing us with a greater advantage of sample size, enabling more extensive and in-depth research and analysis. After careful study of this monograph, I found its chapters well-structured and content comprehensive, providing a detailed introduction to common cells, crystals, casts, and other formed elements in urine. The book is well-illustrated, featuring a wealth of types and many schematic diagrams, more intuitively reflecting the morphological characteristics of various formed elements, making it easier for readers to understand.

Urine Formed Elements is more than just a simple reference book, and it is an invaluable resource for learning. For medical professionals, whether practicing doctors or technicians, or medical students undergoing education, it can serve as a comprehensive and in-depth understanding tool of urinary formed elements test, improving capabilities and standards in diagnosis, treatment, research, etc. For researchers engaged in related research, this book is also a valuable reference resource. The detailed introduction of the types, morphology, and clinical significance of urinary formed elements in the book, and their role in disease diagnosis, will undoubtedly have a positive impact on their research, promoting a deeper exploration and understanding of the mechanisms of human health and disease hidden behind the changes in urinary morphology. What impresses me even more is that this book presents not only knowledge but, more importantly, the professional spirit and pursuit of excellence it conveys. I firmly believe that no matter who you are or where you are, as long as you are interested in this field and eager to learn and improve, this book will bring you great gains and inspiration.

Writing the foreword for this book is an extreme honor for me. I firmly believe that this book will become a valuable, practical tool. I trust that during the process of reading this book, you will deeply perceive the authors' professional spirit and dedication to the field of urinary formed elements examination. On the journey ahead, I sincerely hope that *Urine Formed Elements* will accompany you, providing invaluable assistance for your learning and research.

Department of Laboratory Medicine
Chinese PLA General Hospital
Beijing, China
Yulong Cong
July 2023

Foreword 2

Recently, I had the pleasure of reading *Urine Formed Elements*, compiled by the team led by Professor Lei Zheng. I felt both delighted and reassured. It is my honor and pleasure to write a foreword for this book. On reading through it, I was deeply impressed by the comprehensive content, clear and representative images, as well as the detailed introduction of common cells, crystals, casts, and various other morphological features of urine formed elements. It also highlights their diagnostic significance and clinical implications.

Urine is a clinical sample that is easy to obtain and collected noninvasively. Urinalysis is one of the three routine clinical tests, and the analysis of urine formed elements is a crucial part of urinalysis. It provides valuable diagnostic information in the diagnosis and monitoring of urinary system diseases, the assessment of the course and treatment outcomes of kidney diseases, and the screening for tumor cells. Moreover, the examination of urine formed elements not only has significant clinical diagnostic value but also intersects with other disciplines. It plays a crucial role in understanding the pathogenesis of diseases, researching new biomarkers and diagnostic methods, guiding drug development and individualized treatment, and predicting disease progression.

Due to these unique features of urine samples, Professor Lei Zheng assembled several experts and scholars with abundant clinical experience in this field. They all shared a profound understanding of urine formed elements and years of research experience. Considering the characteristics of samples in our country, the current development status of domestic laboratories, and the latest research progress, they worked together to complete the compilation of this atlas.

The book is comprehensive, and all images and cases are clinically representative. It aligns with the practical needs of the clinic, enhancing the usability and operability of the atlas content. I believe the publication of this book will not only promote the development of urine formed element testing both domestically and internationally, but it will also actively contribute to improving the level of clinical diagnosis and treatment. This book is set to become an important reference in this field.

As I write this foreword, I would like to extend my sincere blessings to Professor Zheng Lei and his team and thank them for their hard work in this field. I hope *Urine Formed Elements* can be widely disseminated, benefit more medical colleagues, promote the development of laboratory medicine, and contribute more to the cause of human health.

Department of Laboratory Medicine
Zhujiang Hospital, Southern Medical University
Guangzhou, China
July 2023

Qian Wang

Preface

Urine is a clinical sample that is relatively easy to obtain. Urine tests are non-invasive, fast, accurate, and cost-effective, making them an important component of clinical examinations. Despite the application of advanced automation and intelligent technologies to urine tests, manual microscopic examination remains irreplaceable for identifying important and hard-to-distinguish formed elements. The array of information is crucial for disease diagnosis, prognostication, therapeutic monitoring, and scientific research. To further promote the worldwide clinical application of urinary sediment morphology testing, in response to our country's "Belt and Road" initiative, and to deepen the implementation of the concept of a shared future for mankind, we aim to provide Chinese wisdom and solutions for global health management and disease treatment. This is achieved through an in-depth introduction to China's technical advantages and research progress in the field of urinary sediment morphology testing, leading us to compile an English atlas on urinary sediment examination titled *Urine Formed Elements*.

Urine Formed Elements comprises five chapters, detailing the morphological features of cells, casts, crystals, and other urinary sediments in urine. With various staining techniques and microscopic methods, it explores the characteristics of various urinary sediments, focusing on their clinical significance and valuable contribution to clinical diagnosis and treatment. The book's authoring team consists of scholars who have made notable contributions in this field and experts with extensive clinical experience in China. Their deep research, summarization of experience, and perfect integration of theoretical knowledge with clinical practice have undoubtedly made this book unique. Additionally, in view of China's unique geography, environment, and population characteristics, the incidence of certain kidney and urinary system diseases is relatively high, providing a large number of rich instances for the study of urinary sediments. We have collected numerous cases and pictures based on China's sample advantage and disease characteristics, making this atlas another key feature of the book.

The book is primarily aimed at clinicians, laboratory physicians (technicians), medical students, and related medical researchers. Whether you are seeking better diagnostic methods in clinical practice or investigating the scientific problems behind the formation of urinary sediments in academic research, you can find useful information or clues in this book. We hope this book can serve as your practical reference and tool book, helping you achieve new breakthroughs in the field of clinical medicine.

Lastly, we hope that this book will attract the attention of a wide range of readers. We welcome all criticisms and suggestions. Only through continuous feedback and improvement can we better serve our readers and the medical community. We look forward to this book contributing a unique force to the study and application of urinary sediments. We hope that our efforts can bring new insights to you and contribute new strength to the development and application of world medicine.

Guangzhou, China
June 2023

Lei Zheng

Acknowledgments

There's an old Chinese proverb: "It's hard for one person to carry a thousand catties, but many people can move mountains." This quote deeply illustrates the importance of teamwork. Only when we unite and work together can we accomplish significant tasks. The writing of this book has followed the same principle. We took the bold step to create our first entirely English book. It was a huge challenge, but with the team's combined effort and dedication, we achieved our goal successfully. I wish to express my deepest gratitude to our team here. Their professional knowledge and infinite creativity made this work possible.

I sincerely express my gratitude to Professor Yulong Cong and Professor Qian Wang for their professional guidance, valuable suggestions, and for providing the foreword to this book. Your support is truly appreciated!

Simultaneously, I want to extend my most sincere thanks to the domestic medical experts. Their valuable advice and selfless help have greatly influenced our work. Their professional guidance has been irreplaceable in our endeavors.

Contents

Contributors

Yue An Clinical Laboratory, The Second Affiliated Hospital of Dalian Medical University, Dalian, China

Zhiliang Cai Department of Laboratory Medicine, Nanfang Hospital, Guangzhou, China

Ke Cao Department of Laboratory Medicine, Shenzhen Children's Hospital, Shenzhen, China

Nannan Cao Department of Laboratory Medicine, The Second Affiliated Hospital of Guangzhou University of Chinese Medicine, Guangzhou, Guangdong, China

Yu Cao Department of Laboratory Medicine, Affiliated Hospital of Zunyi Medical University, Zunyi, Guizhou, China

Zhixin Chen Department of Laboratory Medicine, Fujian Medical University Affiliated Union Hospital, Fuzhou, Fujian, China

Yingying Diao Department of Laboratory Medicine, The First Hospital of China Medical University, Shenyang, Liaoning, China

Aijun Duan Department of Laboratory Medicine, Henan Xinhe Hospital, Xinyang, Henan, China

Chongchong Feng Department of Laboratory Medicine, The Second Hospital of Jilin University, Changchun, China

Liang Fu Department of Laboratory Medicine, The Fifth Affiliated Hospital, Southern Medical University, Guangzhou, Guangdong, China

Xiufeng Gan Department of Laboratory Medicine, Nanfang Hospital, Southern Medical University, Guangzhou, Guangdong, China

Yang Gao Department of Pathology, Baotou Tumor Hospital, Baotou, China

Yulan Geng Department of Laboratory Medicine, The First Hospital of Hebei Medical University, Shijiazhuang, China

Yonghui Guo Department of Laboratory Medicine, Zhujiang Hospital, Southern Medical University, Guangzhou, China

Junjie Huang Department of Laboratory Medicine, Nanfang Hospital, Southern Medical University, Guangzhou, China

Ru Jia Department of Laboratory Medicine, Meihekou Central Hospital, Meihekou, China

Hong Kong Department of Laboratory Medicine, Shengjing Hospital of China Medical University, Liaoning Clinical Research Center for Laboratory Medicine, Shenyang, China

Ang Li Department of Laboratory Medicine, Peking University Third Hospital, Beijing, China

Haixia Li Department of Laboratory Medicine, Nanfang Hospital, Southern Medical University, Guangzhou, China

Jingfang Li Department of Clinical Laboratory, The Third Affiliated Hospital of Kunming Medical University, Kunming, China

Mianyang Li Department of Laboratory Medicine, Chinese PLA General Hospital, Beijing, China

Rui Li Department of Laboratory Medicine, Shenyang Fifth People's Hospital, Shenyang, Liaoning, China

Shengjun Liao Department of Clinical Laboratory, Zhongnan Hospital of Wuhan University, Wuhan, Hubei, China

Wanying Lin Department of Laboratory Medicine, Nanfang Hospital, Southern Medical University, Guangzhou, China

Xiaoqing Liu Department of Laboratory Medicine, The Eighth Affiliated Hospital of Sun Yat-sen University, Shenzhen, China

Huixian Luo Department of Laboratory Medicine, Zhujiang Hospital, Southern Medical University, Guangzhou, China

Yuhong Luo Department of Laboratory Medicine, Nanfang Hospital, Southern Medical University, Guangzhou, Guangdong, China

Yajuan Shen Department of Clinical Laboratory, Shandong Provincial Hospital Affiliated to Shandong First Medical University, Jinan, China

Bo Situ Department of Laboratory Medicine, Nanfang Hospital, Southern Medical University, Guangzhou, Guangdong, China

Dehua Sun Department of Laboratory Medicine, Nanfang Hospital, Southern Medical University, Guangzhou, Guangdong, China

Yi Tian Department of Neurosurgery, The First Affiliated Hospital of Zhengzhou University, Zhengzhou, Henan, China

Lixin Wang Center of Laboratory Medicine, General Hospital of Ningxia Medical University, Yinchuan, China

Yinfeng Wang Department of Clinical Laboratory, Ningxia Medical University General Hospital, Yinchuan, Ningxia, China

Rongzhang Xie Department of Laboratory Medicine, YunFu People's Hospital, Yunfu, Guangdong, China

Jiancheng Xu Department of Laboratory Medicine, First Hospital of Jilin University, Changchun, China

Lizhi Yan Department of Laboratory Medicine, Nanfang Hospital, Southern Medical University, Guangzhou, China

Wei Yang Department of Laboratory Diagnostics, The First Affiliated Hospital of Harbin Medical University, Harbin, Heilongjiang, China

Jinlong Yao Department of Clinical Laboratory, Jiangkou County Hospital of Traditional Chinese Medicine, Jiangkou, Guizhou, China

Qiangwu Zeng Department of Clinical Laboratory, The Second People's Hospital of Guiyang, Guiyang, Guizhou, China

Hui Zhang Department of Laboratory Medicine, The First Hospital of Jilin University, Changchun, China

Lixia Zhang Department of Laboratory Medicine, The First Affiliated Hospital of Nanjing Medical University, Nanjing, China

Shimin Zhang Department of Clinical Laboratory, Peking Union Medical College Hospital, Peking Union Medical College, Beijing, China

Xiaohe Zhang Department of Laboratory Medicine, Nanfang Hospital, Southern Medical University, Guangzhou, Guangdong, China

Hongying Zhao Department of Laboratory Medicine, Guangxi District People's Hospital, Nanning, China

Lei Zheng Department of Laboratory Medicine, Nanfang Hospital, Southern Medical University, Guangzhou, China

Fuxian Zhou Department of Laboratory Medicine, Yanbian University Hospital, Yanji, China

1 Analysis of Urine-Formed Elements: Overview

Lei Zheng, Mianyang Li, Haixia Li, Fuxian Zhou, Rongzhang Xie, Ang Li, and Wanying Lin

1.1 Anatomy of the Kidneys and Urinary Tract System

1.1.1 Anatomy and Function of the Urinary System

The urinary system consists of the kidneys, ureters, bladder, urethra (Fig. 1.1). Its main function is to expel waste and excess water produced during the body's metabolic process, maintaining the balance and stability of the body's internal environment. The kidneys generate urine, which is transported through the ureters to the bladder for storage and then expelled from the body through the urethra [2].

L. Zheng (✉) · H. Li · W. Lin
Department of Laboratory Medicine, Nanfang Hospital, Southern Medical University, Guangzhou, China
e-mail: nfyyzhenglei@smu.edu.cn

M. Li
Department of Laboratory Medicine, Chinese PLA General Hospital, Beijing, China

F. Zhou
Department of Laboratory Medicine, Yanbian University Hospital, Yanji, China

R. Xie
Department of Laboratory Medicine, YunFu People's Hospital, Yunfu, Guangdong, China

A. Li
Department of Laboratory Medicine, Peking University Third Hospital, Beijing, China

1.1.2 Location and Structure of the Kidneys

The kidneys are substantial organs, located on both sides of the spine, within the retroperitoneal space.

1.1.2.1 Renal Parenchyma

The renal parenchyma is divided into the renal cortex and renal medulla (Fig. 1.2). The renal cortex, which primarily lies in the superficial part of the renal parenchyma, is rich in blood vessels and is made up of nephrons and renal tubules. The nephron includes the glomerulus and Bowman's capsule, and the term "glomerulus" is commonly used to refer to the entire nephron. Nephrons and renal tubules together form the basic structural and functional units of the kidney, known as renal units [4].

The renal medulla is located in the deeper part of the renal parenchyma and is composed of several cone-shaped renal pyramids. The portions of the renal cortex that extend between the renal pyramids are called renal columns. The renal pyramids have many darker, radiating stripes, called medullary rays, formed by parallel arrays of straight tubules and blood vessels (Fig. 1.3). The space between the medullary rays is a continuation of the cortex, known as cortical labyrinth. The base of the renal pyramid faces the cortex, and the blunt tip, called the renal papilla, faces the renal sinus. Sometimes, two to three renal pyramids merge to form one renal

L. Zheng et al. (eds.), *Urine Formed Elements*, https://doi.org/10.1007/978-981-99-7739-0_1

papilla. The final urine flows through the renal papillary hole into the minor calyx, then into the major calyx, and finally into the renal pelvis. The renal pelvis leaves the renal hilum, bends downward, gradually narrows, and transitions into the ureter [7].

1.1.2.2 Renal Interstitium

The renal interstitium is defined as the intertubular, extraglomerular, extravascular space of the kidney, and the renal interstitium comprises a small amount of the connective tissue, blood vessels, and nerves. Renal interstitial cells can synthesize fibers and matrix within the interstitium and produce prostaglandins. Prostaglandins can dilate blood vessels, promote blood flow in the surrounding vessels, accelerate the transportation of reabsorbed water, and thus facilitate urine concentration. Additionally, interstitial cells also produce erythropoietin, stimulating the production of in the bone marrow [8].

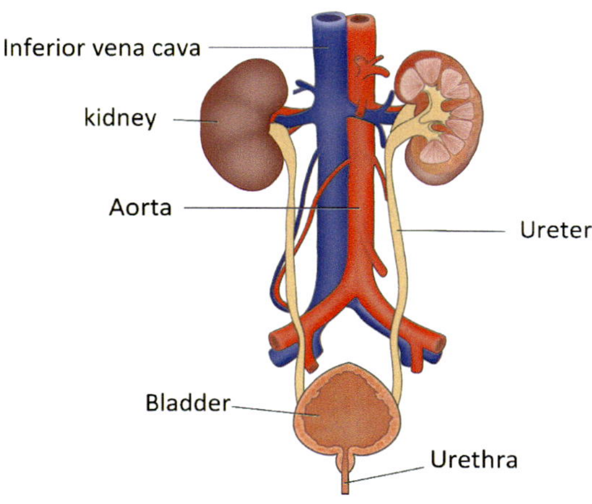

Fig. 1.1 Diagram of the urinary system [1]

1.1.3 Location and Structure of the Ureter

The ureters are narrow and muscular tubes that transport urine from the kidneys to the bladder [9]. Each ureter is about 25 cm long in adults. The average diameter of the ureter is 0.5–1.0 cm. There are three narrow points along its length, where the narrowest point is only 0.2–0.3 cm in diameter. The upper half of the ureter lies in the abdomen, and the lower half in the pelvic area. One end of each ureter connects to the renal pelvis, which collects urine from the kidney, and the other end connects to the bladder, where urine is stored until being excreted from the body.

1.1.4 Location and Structure of the Bladder

The bladder is the organ responsible for storing urine. This triangle-shaped and hollow organ is

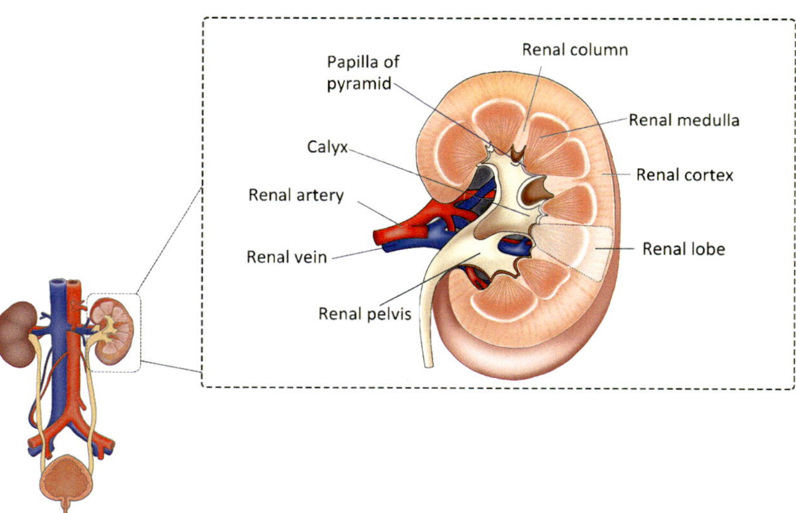

Fig. 1.2 Anatomical structure of the kidney [1, 3]

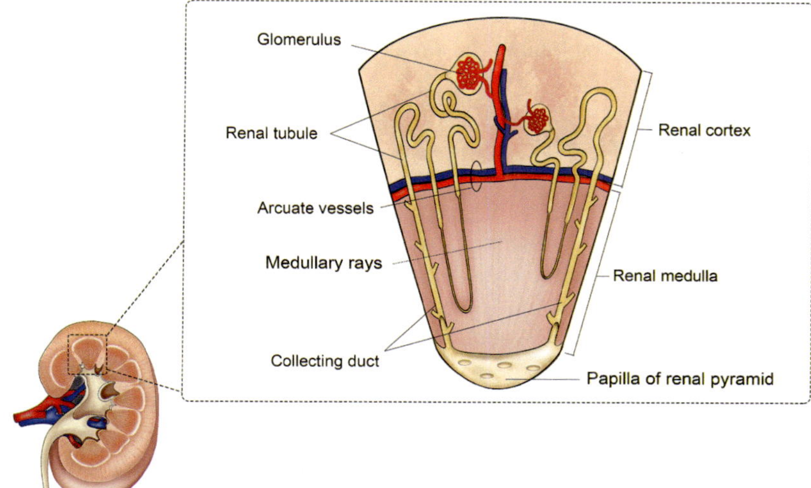

Fig. 1.3 Diagram of the renal cortex and renal medulla [5, 6]

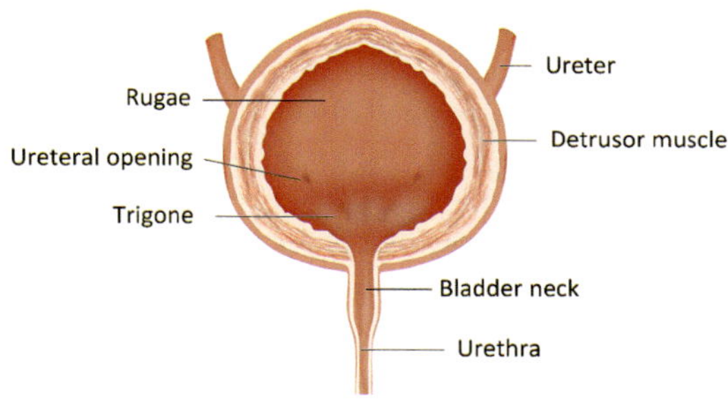

Fig. 1.4 Anatomical structure of the bladder [10, 11]

located in the lower abdomen (Fig. 1.4). It is held in place by ligaments that are attached to other organs and the pelvic bones. The bladder's walls relax and expand to store urine, and then contract and flatten to empty urine through the urethra. Its shape, size, position, and wall thickness vary depending on the degree of urine filling, age, and gender. Usually, the average bladder capacity of a normal adult is between 350 and 500 mL [12].

When the bladder is empty, its shape is like a tetrahedron. On the inner surface of the bladder base, there is a triangular area located between the left and right ureter openings and the internal opening of the urethra, known as the trigone of the bladder. The bladder mucosa and muscle layer are closely connected at this site, lacking the submucosal layer. Regardless of whether the bladder is filled or empty, the mucosa always remains smooth. The trigone of the bladder is a common site for tumors, tuberculosis, and inflammation and should be given special attention during cystoscopic examinations [13].

1.1.5 Location and Structure of the Urethra

The male urethra has the function of ejaculation and urination, beginning from the internal urethral orifice of the bladder and ending at the external urethral orifice at the tip of the penis. The male urethra is 16–22 cm long with an average diameter of 0.5–0.7 cm, which is divided into three parts: prostatic, membranous, and spongy. The male urethra has three narrowings, three enlargements, and two bends. The three narrow points are the internal urethral orifice, membranous urethra, and external urethral orifice, where urethral stones are prone to get stuck. The three enlargements are the prostatic urethra, bulbar urethra, and navicular fossa, where stones are likely to settle, and the two bends are the subpubic curve and the prepubic curve [14].

The female urethra is 3–5 cm long with an average diameter of 0.6 cm, which is shorter, wider, and straighter than that of the male urethra. The internal urethral orifice is approximately at the center or lower part behind the pubic symphysis. Its course runs forward and downward, passing through the urogenital diaphragm, and opens at the external urethral orifice in the anterior vestibule of the vagina [15].

1.1.6 Epithelial Cells from the Urinary System

Epithelial cells in the urine originate from the renal tubules, renal calyx, renal pelvis, ureters, bladder, and urethra, among other places. The epithelial cells of the renal tubules are cuboidal. Urothelial cells (also known as transitional epithelial cells) are divided into superficial cells, intermediate cells, and basal cells. The characteristic of the urothelium is that the shape and number of cell layers can change according to the empty or distended state of the organ. For example, when the bladder is empty, the epithelium becomes thicker, the number of cell layers increases, and the superficial cells are large and cuboidal; when the bladder is distended, the epithelium becomes thinner, the number of cell layers decreases, and the superficial cells are flattened. In addition, columnar epithelial cells shed from the male prostate and mid-urethra, as well as squamous epithelial cells from the female vaginal surface, can also appear in the urine [16].

1.2 Composition and Function of the Nephron

The nephron is the structural and functional unit of the kidney, composed of the renal corpuscle and the renal tubule connected to it. Each kidney contains approximately 1.5 million nephrons, which together with the collecting ducts perform the function of urine formation. The kidney cannot regenerate new nephrons, and the number of nephrons will gradually decrease under conditions of kidney damage, disease, or normal aging [17].

1.2.1 Renal Corpuscle

The renal corpuscle is spherical in shape, with a diameter of about 200 μm, composed of the glomerulus and the Bowman's capsule (Fig. 1.5).

1.2.1.1 Glomerulus

The glomerulus is a cluster of twisted capillaries located between the afferent arteriole and the efferent arteriole. It consists of endothelial cells, basement membrane, and epithelial cells [19]. The cells of the free surface of the capillary endothelium are rich in negatively charged sialoprotein. The endothelial layer is dotted with pores of different sizes, with diameters ranging from 50 to 100 nm, most without a diaphragm, forming a pore diameter barrier that selectively filters out substances in the blood. The basement membrane is present everywhere on the basal surface of the endothelium, except for the parts in contact with the vascular endothelium [20].

The basement membrane of the glomerular capillaries is relatively thick, mainly composed of type IV collagen, laminin, and proteoglycans (the glycosaminoglycans are primarily negatively charged heparin). Type IV collagen forms a network structure, connecting with other glycoproteins, together forming a molecular sieve with a pore diameter of 4–8 nm, forming a filtration barrier and playing a key role in blood substance filtration [21].

The efferent arteriole and the glomerular capillary cluster are smaller than the afferent arteriole, resulting in high pressure within the capillary cluster. The resulting hydrostatic pressure enhances the filtration function of the glomerulus.

1.2.1.2 Bowman's Capsule

Bowman's capsule is a cup-shaped double-layered epithelial pouch formed by the enlargement and invagination of the initial end of the renal tubule during embryonic development. Its outer layer (or wall layer) is a single layer of flat epithelial cells, which is continuous with the epithelium of the proximal convoluted tubule at the urinary pole of the renal corpuscle. At the vascular pole, it folds back to become the inner layer (or visceral layer) of Bowman's capsule, with the narrow space between the two epithelial layers being Bowman's capsule space, which is connected to the lumen of the proximal convoluted tubule. The cells of the inner layer are called podocytes, which have large cell bodies

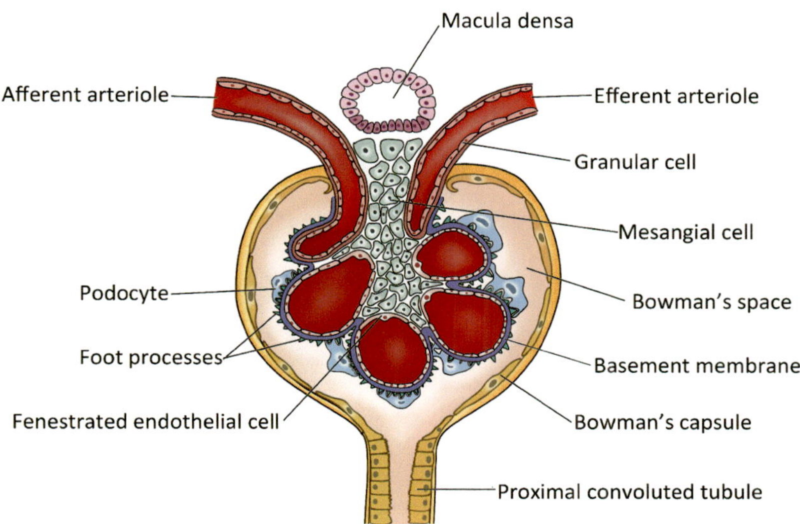

Fig. 1.5 A schematic overview of a glomerulus [3, 18]

and many finger-like secondary protrusions that interlock with each other in a lattice shape, closely attached to the outside of the capillary basement membrane, their surfaces covered with a layer of negatively charged sialoprotein [22]. There are slits about 25 nm wide between the secondary protrusions, called slit pores, covered with a thin membrane 4–6 nm thick, i.e., the slit diaphragm [23].

1.2.1.3 Filtration Membrane

The renal corpuscle acts like a filter. When the blood flows through the capillaries of the glomerulus, the blood pressure inside the capillaries is high, and some substances in the plasma are filtered into Bowman's capsule through the three-layer structure of the fenestrated endothelium, basement membrane, and slit diaphragm of the podocytes, collectively referred to as the filtration membrane. Under normal circumstances, substances with a molecular weight of below 70 kDa and a diameter of below 4 nm can pass through the filtration membrane, among which positively charged substances are easier to pass through, such as glucose, peptides, urea, electrolytes, and water. The filtrate that enters Bowman's capsule is called primary urine, which, except for not containing large molecular proteins, is similar in composition to plasma [24]. If the filtration membrane is damaged (such as in glomerulonephritis), even large molecular proteins and blood cells can leak out through the filtration membrane, resulting in proteinuria or hematuria.

1.2.2 Renal Tubules

The renal tubule is a continuation of the renal glomerulus, consisting of the proximal tubule, loop of Henle, and distal tubule (Fig. 1.6). The renal tubule walls are composed of single-layer cuboidal epithelium, with cells appearing hexagonal or polygonal when observed from the epithelial surface. In a vertical section, the cells appear cubic with a round, central nucleus. The renal tubule epithelial cells have the function of reabsorbing original urine components and excretion.

1.2.2.1 Proximal Tubule

The proximal tubule is the longest and thickest section of the renal tubule, with a diameter of 50–60 μm and an irregular lumen. The epithelial cells are cuboidal or pyramidal with a large cell body and eosinophilic cytoplasm. The nucleus is round and located near the base. The apical surface of the epithelial cells has a brush border. This structural feature of the proximal tubule gives it a good absorption function, making it the main site for reabsorption of original urine com-

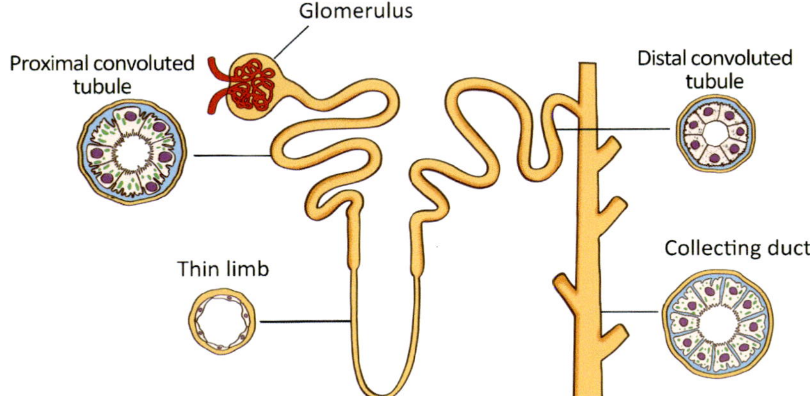

Fig. 1.6 The cross-sections of various tubular segments [18]

ponents. Nearly all glucose, amino acids, proteins, and a large part of water, ions, and urea in the primary urine are reabsorbed here [25].

1.2.2.2 Loop of Henle

The tubule is thin with a diameter of 10–15 μm. The tubular wall is a single layer of the flat epithelium, with an oval nucleus. The nucleated part protrudes into the lumen, and the cytoplasm is lightly stained and lacks a brush border. The thin epithelium of the loop of Henle is advantageous for the permeability of water and ions.

1.2.2.3 Distal Tubule

The tubule lumen is larger and more regular, with a diameter of 30–45 μm. The epithelial cells are cuboidal and smaller than the proximal tubule cells. The nucleus is located centrally or near the lumen. The cytoplasm is less stained than the proximal tubule, and the free surface lacks a brush border. The distal tubule cells have the function of absorbing water and Na+ and excreting K+, H+, and NH3. It's an important site for ion exchange and plays a crucial role in maintaining body fluid acid-base balance.

1.2.2.4 Collecting Duct

The collecting duct is not part of the nephron and is 20–38 mm long. Each collecting duct is connected to multiple distal tubules, collecting the urine transported from them and finally entering the renal calyx. The collecting duct is divided into arcuate collecting duct, straight collecting duct, and papillary duct [26]. Many arcuate collecting ducts merge into the straight collecting duct as it descends in the medullary rays. The diameter of the straight collecting duct changes from thin (40 μm) to thick (200–300 μm). The epithelium of the tubular wall changes from a single layer of cuboidal cells to a single layer of columnar cells, becoming high columnar at the papillary duct. The boundaries of the collecting duct epithelial cells are clear, with a round or oval nucleus located centrally or eccentrically. The cytoplasm is lighter stained than the distal tubule and even clear. The collecting duct further reabsorbs water and exchanges ions, playing a key role in urine concentration and maintaining internal acid-base balance [27].

1.3 Urine Formation

Urine formation is the primary excretory function of the kidneys. Urine formation involves three processes: plasma filtration at the glomeruli, followed by the reabsorption and secretion of selective components by the renal tubules. Through these processes, the kidneys play a critical role in eliminating metabolic waste, regulating water and electrolytes (such as sodium and chloride), and maintaining the body's acid-base balance, serving as a regulator for the body [28].

1.3.1 Glomerular Filtration

Glomerular filtration refers to the process where, as blood flows through the capillaries of the glomerulus, all components of the plasma, except for proteins, can be filtered into Bowman's capsule to form an ultrafiltrate (also known as primary urine). The composition of the fluid inside Bowman's capsule, except for proteins, is very similar to the plasma in terms of the concentrations of other components such as glucose, chloride, inorganic phosphates, urea, uric acid, and creatinine. Its osmotic pressure and pH are also very similar to plasma [29].

The volume of ultrafiltrate produced by both kidneys per unit of time (per minute) is called the glomerular filtration rate (GFR). The glomerular filtration rate is approximately 125 mL/min, and for a normal adult, the total volume of plasma filtered by the glomeruli of both kidneys in 24 h averages 180 L (ranging between 150 and 200 L). Factors such as physical activity, emotional excitement, diet, age, pregnancy, and circadian rhythm can affect glomerular filtration rate [30]. Any diseases that change the blood flow to the glomerulus, the hydrostatic pressure passing through the glomerular filtration barrier, the osmotic pressure, or the structural integrity of the glomerulus can impact the glomerular filtration rate and thus the urine output.

1.3.2 Reabsorption and Secretion by the Renal Tubules and Collecting Ducts

Once the ultrafiltrate enters the renal tubules, the majority of the water, nutrients, and inorganic salts are reabsorbed back into the blood, and some ions also undergo exchange at this stage (Fig. 1.7). The epithelial cells of the renal tubules also excrete some of the body's metabolic waste. This results in the formation of concentrated final urine. The volume and quality of the final urine

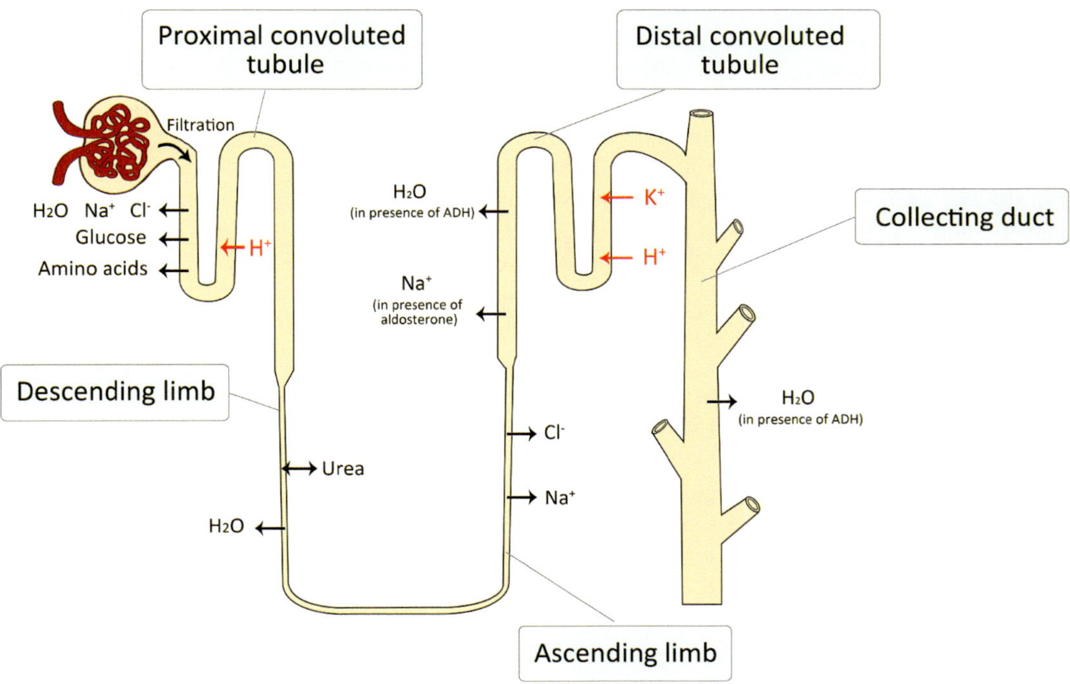

Fig. 1.7 Tubular reabsorption of solutes and water in various segments of the nephron

vary greatly compared to the tubular fluid. The volume of the final urine is only about 1.5–2 L per day, which is approximately 1% of the primary urine. The epithelial cells of the renal tubules and collecting ducts perform highly selective reabsorption and active secretion or excretion of various substances in the tubular fluid [31].

1.3.3 Concentration and Dilution of Urine

The concentration and dilution of urine is relative to the osmotic pressure of plasma. The osmotic pressure of urine can change significantly with changes in the body's fluid volume. When the body is dehydrated, urine is concentrated, and the osmotic pressure of the excreted urine is significantly higher than that of plasma, resulting in hypertonic urine. When the body's fluid volume is excessive, urine is diluted, and the osmotic pressure of the excreted urine is lower than that of plasma, resulting in hypotonic urine. The osmotic pressure of urine in a healthy person fluctuates between 50 and 1200 mOsm/(kg·H_2O), indicating that the kidneys have a strong capacity to concentrate and dilute urine. The kidney's ability to concentrate and dilute urine plays a crucial role in maintaining the body's fluid balance and osmotic stability. Depending on whether the body is dehydrated, the normal adult's 24-h urine volume varies between 1.5 and 2.5 L [32].

1.3.3.1 Concentration of Urine

The concentration of urine occurs due to the reabsorption of water from the tubular fluid, while the solutes remain. Two essential factors contribute to this: (1) The permeability of the renal tubules, especially the collecting ducts, to water. The antidiuretic hormone (ADH) can increase the expression of water channel proteins on the apical membrane of the epithelial cells of the kidney's collecting ducts, promoting the kidney's reabsorption of water. (2) The interstitial fluid of the renal medulla forms a high osmotic concentration gradient, further promoting the reabsorption of water [7].

1.3.3.2 Dilution of Urine

The dilution of urine primarily occurs in the collecting ducts. If the body has excess water, leading to a decrease in the crystalloid osmotic pressure of plasma, the release of the antidiuretic hormone can be suppressed. The permeability of the collecting ducts to water is very low, and water cannot be reabsorbed, while NaCl in the tubular fluid continues to be actively reabsorbed. This reabsorption of solutes significantly surpasses the reabsorption of water, causing a further decrease in the osmotic concentration of the tubular fluid.

1.3.4 Urine Composition

Urine consists of urea and other organic and inorganic chemicals dissolved in water. Urine is normally 95% water and 5% solutes. The concentration of these solutes in urine can be influenced by a range of factors, such as dietary intake, body metabolism, physical activity, endocrine functions, and even body position [33].

The organic substances primarily include urea, creatinine, and uric acid in urine. Urea, a metabolic waste product, is created in the liver from the breakdown of proteins and amino acids, and it accounts for nearly half of the total dissolved solids in urine. As for inorganic substances, chloride is the most prevalent, followed by sodium and potassium. Additionally, urine includes trace amounts of various other inorganic chemicals [34].

Other substances found in urine include hormones, vitamins, and medications. In disease conditions, urine may also include formed elements such as cells, casts, crystals, mucus, and bacteria. The presence of these substances holds different clinical implications, and they are the main focus of this book.

1.3.5 The Clinical Significance of Testing for Urine-Formed Elements

Microscopic examination of urine sediment still plays an important role in early diagnosis of kidney diseases, assisting in the diagnosis of urinary system disorders, and in screening for tumor cells, among other applications [35].

The urinary sediment examination is an analysis of certain solid materials or formed elements in urine. These elements include cells, crystals, casts, and other organic or inorganic substances. This test is a common and integral part of urinalysis as well as a routine examination of urine. The examination can provide valuable information about kidney and urinary tract health. It can help detect infections, kidney disease, metabolic disorders or the presence of urinary tract stones [36]. For example, red blood cells in the urine (hematuria) could indicate bleeding in the urinary tract, while white blood cells (pyuria) could suggest an infection. In terms of kidney disease, casts in the urine can provide clues about the type of kidney disorder. For instance, red blood cell casts might be seen in glomerulonephritis, while white blood cell casts might be seen in pyelonephritis. Moreover, urinary sediment can be used to screen for tumor cells, helping in the early detection of bladder or urinary tract cancers [37].

The combined approach of urine sediment examination and urinalysis (urine dry chemical analysis) still plays a significant role in diagnosing urinary system diseases. It can provide a valuable reference for diagnosis, prognosis, treatment evaluation, and disease monitoring of various conditions.

1.4 Collection and Testing of Urine Specimens

1.4.1 Specimen Collection

The laboratory should have a comprehensive standard operating procedure (SOP) for sample collection, transportation and reception. A requisition form must accompany the specimens delivered to the laboratory. The information on the form must correspond with the information on the specimen label. Additional information on the form can include the method of collection, the type of specimen, possible interfering medications, and the patient's clinical information.

Table 1.1 Acceptable and unacceptable urine samples

The acceptable sample	• Indicate the patient's name and identification number • Correctly note the date and time of collection • State the patient's age • Labels must be clearly attached to the container • The sample volume meets the requirements • The collected container complies with the requirements
The unacceptable sample	• Specimens with incomplete patient information • Specimens in unlabeled containers • Nonmatching labels and requisition forms • Specimens contaminated with feces or toilet paper • Containers with contaminated exteriors • Specimens of insufficient quantity

The time when the specimen is received in the laboratory should be documented on the form.

Acceptable samples received should be promptly tested. Any unacceptable samples should be rejected, and the relevant clinical teams should be contacted to request a re-sampling (Table 1.1). The tests should be completed within the timeframe specified by the institutional protocol. Any samples that are not tested in a timely manner should be stored in the refrigerator, and the clinical team should be notified of the specific reason for the delay.

Urine is classified as a biohazardous specimen. Therefore, gloves should be worn at all times when handling or coming into contact with the specimen to ensure safety.

1.4.2 Containers for Urine Specimen

Containers for urine specimen collections must be clean, dry, and made of disposable material such as plastic or glass. These containers should be clear or translucent to facilitate observation of urine transparency and color. If the urine sample remains untested for more than 2 h or is intended for microbial testing, it is advisable to store it in

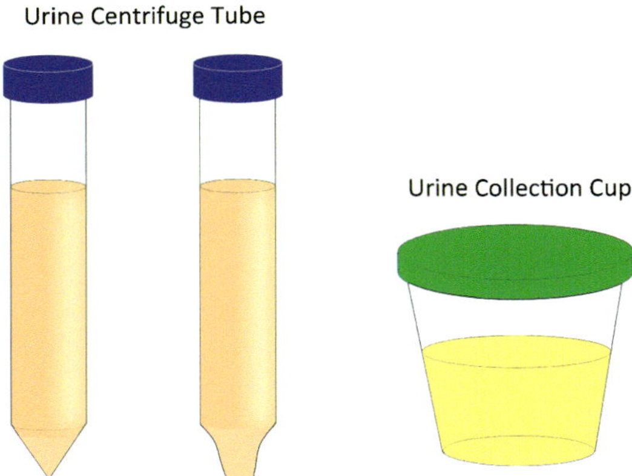

Fig. 1.8 Containers for urine specimen

a sterile container. They should be fitted with a lid and must be leak-proof sealed for ease of transportation (Fig. 1.8).

1.4.3 Specimen Volume

Routine urinalysis typically requires 10–15 mL of urine. The specimen volume may be increased if necessary for additional or repeat testing. In special cases, such as pediatric patients or those with difficulty urinating, the urine volume can be appropriately reduced. If these specimens are used for testing, it should be noted in the report. Whenever the actual volume used to prepare the sediment for the microscopic examination is less than that routinely required, it should also be noted in the report.

1.4.4 Reporting Formats of Urine Microscopic Examination

Manual microscopic examination is used to assess or enumerate urine components and remains an important method in clinical practice for diagnosing and monitoring renal and urinary tract diseases, despite the emergence of automated systems.

Larger substances and casts in urine are observed using a low-power field during a manual microscopic examination. At least 20 low-power fields (LPF) should be inspected to ensure a comprehensive examination [35]. Cell components are then identified using a high-power field. At least ten high-power fields (HPF) should be examined, and both the lowest and highest values for the number of cells seen under the microscope should be recorded.

RBCs, WBCs and casts are enumerated as a range of formed elements present (e.g., 0–2, 2–5, 5–10). The quantity of mucus, crystals, and bacteria is qualitatively assessed per field of view (FOV) in either descriptive or numeric terms (e.g., 1+, present but hard to find or one present in almost every FOV. 2+, easy to find or number present in FOV varies. 3+, large number present in all FOVs. 4+, FOV is crowded or overwhelmed with the elements).

1.4.5 Centrifugation of Specimens

After well-mixed urine is poured into a centrifuge tube, cover it with a lid and centrifuge at 400–450 g for 5 min [38]. This centrifugation speed allows for the appropriate concentration of sediment without damaging fragile-formed elements such as cells and casts and without causing leukocyte aggregation. After centrifugation, decant the supernatant urine, or remove it using a disposable pipette, leaving 1 mL of sediment at the bottom for microscopic examination.

1.4.6 Choose an Appropriate Microscopic Examination Method

Brightfield microscopy is a commonly used and convenient method. Mix the sediment at the bottom of the tube. Transfer a small amount of the well-mixed sediment onto a glass microscope slide using a pipette or transfer pipette. Place a coverslip over the sample, making sure there are no air bubbles. Observe the formed elements under low-power (10×) and high-power (40×) objectives. Make note of the quantity, morphology, and any abnormalities observed.

Some components of formed elements, such as casts and cells, may appear unclear when observed under brightfield microscope. To further clarify these components, appropriate staining methods can be used. SM staining or S staining can be chosen to identify different types of casts. Wright's stain can be selected to identify different cell types.

Other microscopic examination methods can be used to observe hyaline casts, lipid components, and some crystals in urine sediment. These include phase-contrast microscopy, darkfield microscopy, and polarized microscopy.

1.5 Staining Techniques

The purpose of staining is to color cells, casts and other components in urine. Their structure becomes clear after staining, making them easy to identify and leading to accurate test results. There are various staining methods available, and the appropriate one can be chosen based on the identifiable components in urine (Table 1.2).

Table 1.2 Urine sediment stain characteristics

Stain	Function
Sternheimer-Malbin (SM) or Sternheimer (S) stain	• Identifies WBCs, epithelial cells, and casts • Screens for tumor cells • Crystals and fat droplets are not stained • Living cells and fungi are not easily stained
Toluidine blue	• Differentiates WBCs and renal tubular epithelial (RTE) cells
Wright's stain	• Classifies white blood cells • Identifies epithelial cells • Differentiates tumor cells
Oil Red O and Sudan III stain	• Distinguishes free fat • Identifies oval fat bodies or fat granule cells • Differentiates fatty casts
Hansel stain	• Identifies urinary eosinophils
Gram stain	• Differentiates gram-positive and gram-negative bacteria
Prussian blue stain	• Identifies yellow-brown granules of hemosiderin • Identifies cells containing hemosiderin • Identifies hemosiderin casts
2% acetic acid	• Lyses RBCs and enhances nuclei of WBCs • Distinguishes RBCs from WBCs, yeast, oil droplets, and crystals

1.5.1 Supravital Stains

1.5.1.1 Sternheimer-Malbin (SM) Stain and Sternheimer (S) Stain

Supravital stains typically include SM stain and S stain. These stains enhance the identification of the formed elements by allowing more detailed viewing of internal structures, without altering the morphology of the components [39]. They effectively preserve their original structures and are often used to identify different types of epithelial cells, white blood cells and casts in urine. However, it should be noted that crystals and lipids cannot be stained, and living cells, bacteria, and fungi are not easily stained.

The colors of the casts are slightly different after supravital staining (Fig. 1.9). Cells can be divided into living cells and dead cells in urine, and supravital stains can distinguish between them. Dead cells appear pink in the cytoplasm, with deep purple nuclei and heavily stained nucleoli after SM staining. Living cells display a light blue color in both the cytoplasm and nucleus after SM staining. Cell structures become clearer after S staining, where dead cells show a purple-red cytoplasm and blue nuclei, while living cells' cytoplasm and nuclei are not easily stained (Fig. 1.10). The effect of supravital stains can be slightly affected by the pH of the urine.

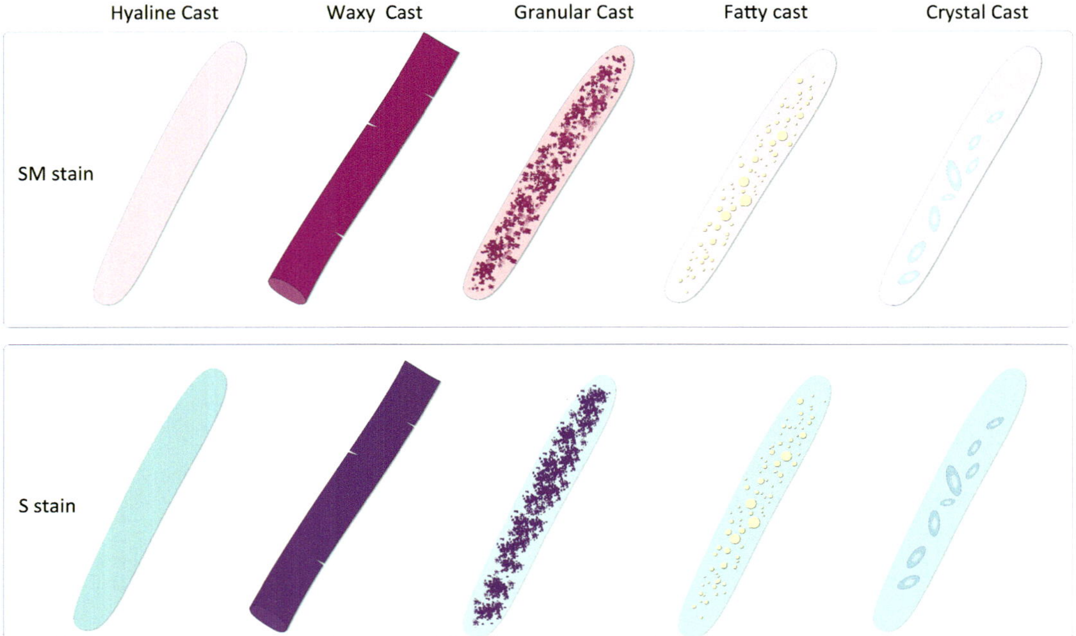

Fig. 1.9 Diagram of casts after SM stain and S stain

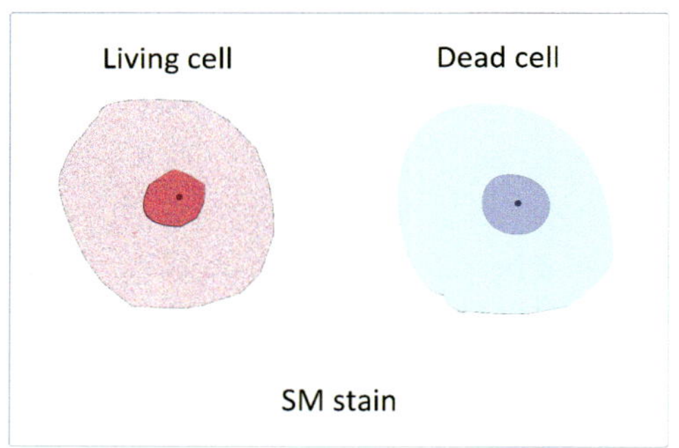

Fig. 1.10 Diagram of UTEs after SM stain and S stain

1.5.1.2 Toluidine Blue Stain

Toluidine blue stain is also an effective supravital stain for urine sediment. This metachromatic dye stains different cell components in unique ways, making the distinction between the nucleus and the cytoplasm more noticeable [40]. The toluidine blue stain aids in the specific identification of cells and facilitates differentiation between cells of similar size, such as leukocytes and renal collecting duct cells.

1.5.2 Wright's Stain

Wright's stain is commonly used to distinguish between bone marrow cells and peripheral blood cells. It can also be used for various cells in urine. (1) It can classify white blood cells. (2) It can identify urinary epithelial cells and renal tubular epithelial cells. (3) It can screen for abnormal cells and tumor cells. After staining, cell structures become clear, with a purple-red cytoplasm and deep blue nucleus.

1.5.3 Prussian Blue Stain

The Prussian blue stain can be used to identify hemosiderin in urine, which can be either free-floating or within epithelial cells and casts [41] (Fig. 1.11). Without staining, hemosiderin granules appear yellow or golden yellow, making them difficult to distinguish from other substances. Hemosiderin granules appear blue after Prussian blue staining. [42]. The prussian blue reaction is where ferric ions (Fe^{3+}) treated with hydrochloric acid are released from cells and react with potassium ferrocyanide to form ferrocyanide, an insoluble bright blue pigment [43].

1.5.4 Sudan III or Oil Red O Stain

The Sudan III stain or Oil Red O stains are typically used to confirm the presence of neutral fat or triglycerides during microscopic examination. These lipids stain orange or red after staining (Fig. 1.12). These methods can distinguish fat

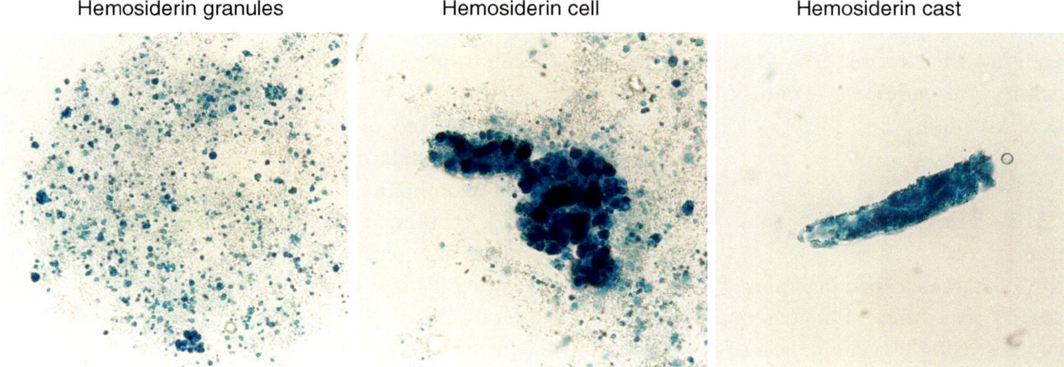

Fig. 1.11 Prussian Blue Reaction is positive, ×400

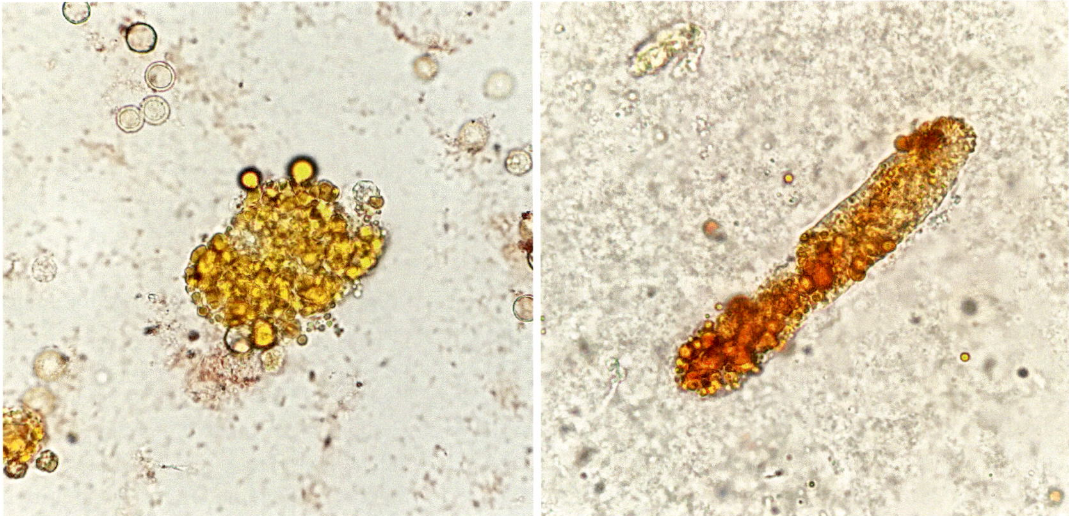

Fig. 1.12 Cell and cast after Oil Red O staining, ×1000

that is free-floating as droplets or globules and fat components within cells and identify fatty casts.

1.5.5 Gram Stain

The Gram stain is mainly used to identify bacteria in urine. It categorizes bacteria as either gram-negative or gram-positive. A slide is prepared and stained after being dried and fixed. Gram-negative bacteria appear pink, while gram-positive bacteria appear dark purple [44]. Due to the small size of bacteria, these substances are usually observed using a high-power oil immersion (×100) objective. The Gram stain can detect bacteria and differentiate their forms. If it's necessary to further identify the pathogen, it can be combined with bacterial culture.

1.5.6 Hansel Stain

Hansel stain is a specific staining method used to identify and differentiate eosinophils in urine. It involves using a combination of methylene blue and eosin-Y in methanol as the staining solution. The Hansel stain highlights the distinctive granules and cellular features of eosinophils, allowing for their accurate identification in the urine sediment [45]. It is a preferred method for eosinophil detection in the laboratory setting.

1.5.7 Adding Acetic Acid to Urine

Adding acetic acid to the urine sediment is indeed not for staining purposes, but for aiding in the identification of white blood cells. In certain situations, white blood cells may appear small, making their nuclei and granulation difficult to observe, especially in hypertonic urine. By adding one to two drops of a 2% solution of acetic acid, the nuclear pattern of white blood cells and epithelial cells becomes more accentuated. Red blood cells, on the other hand, are lysed, and certain phosphates dissolve rapidly.

1.6 Microscopy Techniques

Urine sediment microscopic examination is an essential part of routine urinalysis and has significant clinical relevance in the diagnosis of diseases. Enhancing the microscopic examination skills of personnel is a primary task, as it is necessary to understand the morphological characteristics of various urine-formed elements and their clinical significance. There are many types of microscopes for examination, each with its own structure and range of use. The brightfield microscope remains dominant in most laboratories and can observe most formed elements. However, sometimes the structures under the microscope are unclear, requiring the use of phase-contrast microscopes for observations, such as red blood cells, casts, etc. [46]. Some drug crystals may need polarizing microscopes for examination.

Obtaining a suitable microscope is paramount, but it is equally critical to undergo proper training on its use. Thorough maintenance and meticulous cleaning of the microscope are essential to ensure its optimal operation. Users must have a comprehensive understanding of each component of the microscope and its respective function, as well as proficiency in the proper adjustment and alignment procedures.

1.6.1 Brightfield Microscopy

Brightfield microscopy is the most common type used on microscopes. A brightfield microscope produces a magnified specimen image that appears dark against a brighter background. Compound brightfield microscopes predominate and consist of two lens systems (Fig. 1.13). The first lens system is the objective mounted in the nosepiece located closest to the specimen. The objective produces the primary image magnification and directs this image to the second lens system, the eyepiece. The eyepiece further magnifies the image received from the objective lens. The total magnification of a specimen is the product

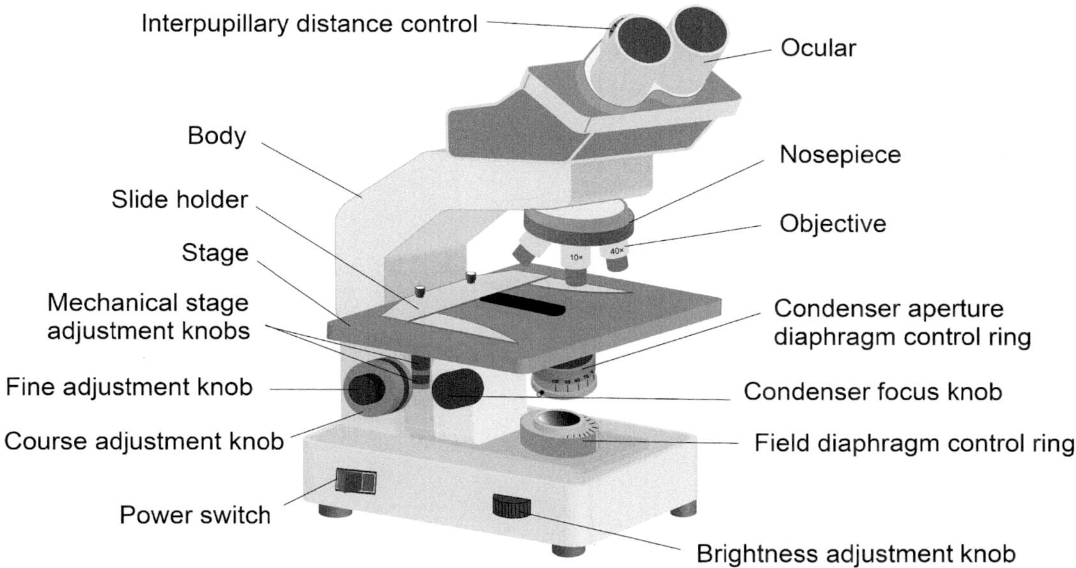

Fig. 1.13 Parts of the brightfield microscope

of these lens systems, which is obtained by multiplying the magnification of the objective lens by the magnification of the eyepiece lens. The eyepiece also determines the diameter of the FOV observed.

The eyepiece and objective of a microscope magnify an object sufficiently for viewing with maximum resolution. Resolution, or resolving power, describes the ability of the lens system to reveal fine detail. Stated another way, resolution is the smallest distance between two points or lines at which they are distinguished as two separate entities. Resolving power (R) depends on the wavelength (λ) of light used and the numerical aperture (NA) of the objective lens [47].

The composition of urinary sediments is complex and diverse, with notable variations in volume. When using brightfield microscopy, it's crucial to select an appropriate objective lens. For larger-volume cells, crystals, and casts, choosing a 10×, 20×, or 40× objective lens can yield satisfactory results. For smaller cells, fungi, and bacteria or when observing minute cellular structures, an oil immersion lens can be utilized. When studying urinary sediments, we frequently use brightfield microscopy. All images in the book have noted magnification for readers' reference. Besides, when observing unstained urinary sediments, adjusting the Condenser Lens is extremely necessary. By adjusting the position of the condenser, the angle and intensity of the light can be controlled, allowing the user to optimize the illumination of the sample. In addition to focusing the light, the condenser also helps control the amount of light that reaches the objective lens.

1.6.2 Phase-Contrast Microscopy

Phase-contrast microscopy is based on the phenomenon of phase difference when light passes through transparent materials. In traditional brightfield microscopy, transparent specimens often lack noticeable contrast because light only undergoes transmission or refraction without significant phase differences. Phase-contrast microscopy introduces additional optical path differences using a phase plate and an annular diaphragm to amplify the subtle phase differences within the sample. It is particularly useful for examining transparent or semi-transparent specimens that are nearly colorless or lack color, which would not be visible with brightfield microscopy.

Phase-contrast microscopy plays a crucial role in the examination of urine sediment. It enables the identification and differentiation of various components present in urine samples, including cellular elements such as RBCs and WBCs, epithelial cells (Fig. 1.14), crystals (Fig. 1.15), casts (Fig. 1.16), and microorganisms. Using phase-contrast microscopy, the formed elements in the urine can be accurately identified, providing valuable diagnostic evidence for clinical purposes.

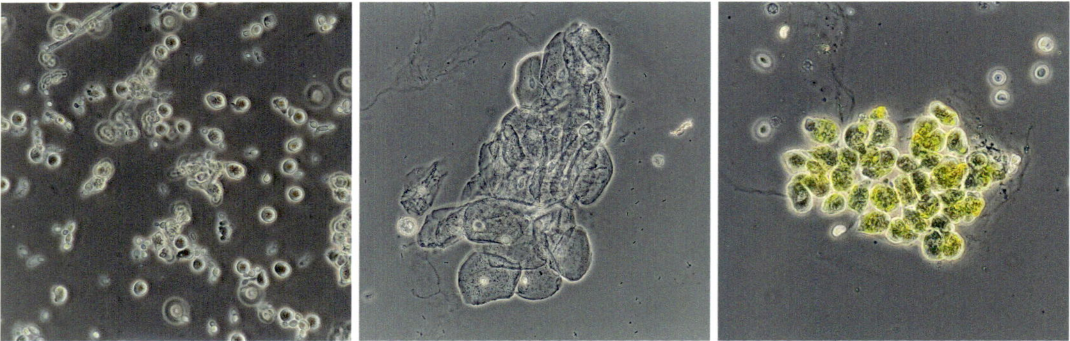

Fig. 1.14 Cells under darkfield microscopy, ×400

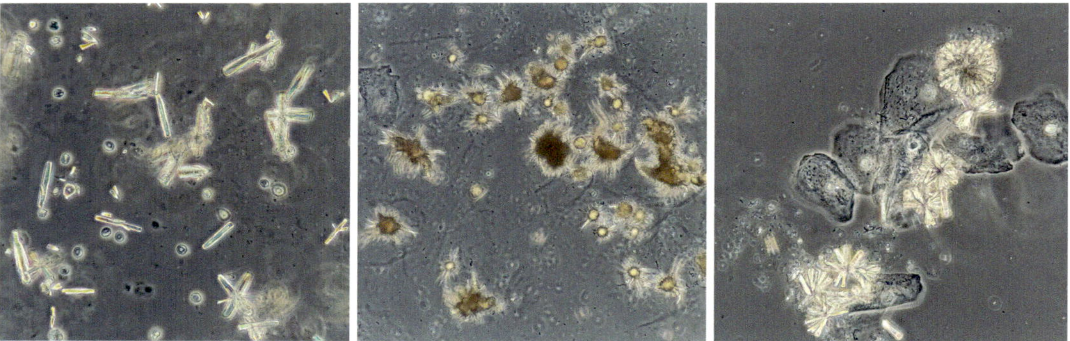

Fig. 1.15 Crystals under darkfield microscopy, ×400

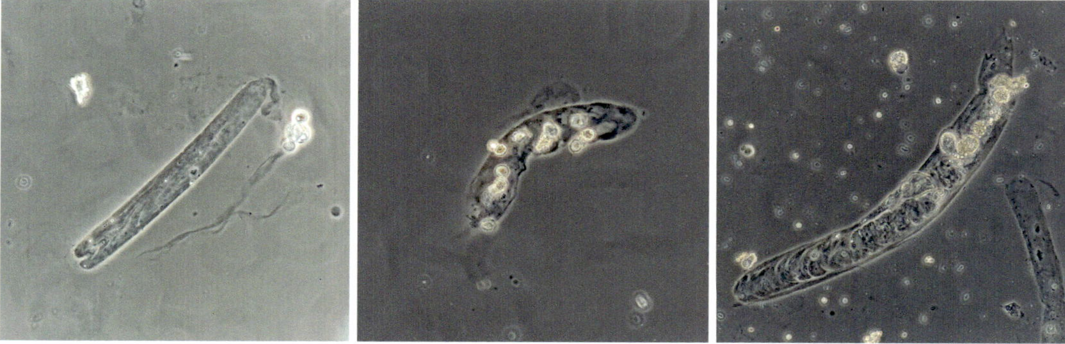

Fig. 1.16 Casts under darkfield microscopy, ×400

1.6.3 Interference Contrast Microscopy

In clinical practice, there are two commonly used types of interference microscopes: differential interference contrast (DIC) microscopy and modulated contrast microscopy. DIC microscopy is a technique that enhances contrast in unstained and transparent specimens. It is particularly beneficial for examining specimens with minimal color or refractive index changes, just like phase-contrast microscopy. When applied to urinalysis, DIC microscopy offers several advantages [48]:

1. Enhanced visualization: DIC enhances the contrast between different parts of the sample, making it easier to discern the intricate structures within urine-formed elements, like cells, crystals, or casts.
2. Three-dimensional appearance: One of the most notable advantages of DIC microscopy is that it imparts a pseudo three-dimensional (3D) appearance to the sample. This is particularly useful when trying to distinguish between similar looking structures in urine.
3. No requirement for staining: DIC microscopy doesn't require staining. This not only simplifies the sample preparation process, but it also preserves the original state of the sample, allowing for more accurate observations. DIC allows for the examination of living cells without killing them through fixation or staining.
4. It's important to note that DIC microscopy is not commonly used in routine urinalysis due to its relatively high cost and complexity. However, it offers substantial advantages in research settings or in cases where a high degree of detail is required.

1.6.4 Darkfield Microscopy

Darkfield microscopy is an optical microscopy technique that allows for the observation of elements that are nearly invisible under brightfield microscopy. When a light source illuminates a specimen, most of the light bypasses the specimen and is blocked; only the light scattered or refracted by the specimen can enter the eyepiece, creating an image of a bright specimen against a dark background (Fig. 1.17). The advantage of this method is that it allows visibility of specimens not discernable under normal illumination. However, its drawback is that it is less effective on specimens that absorb light, such as stained cells.

Darkfield microscopy is commonly used in the observation of formed elements in urine. Its high contrast enables the clear visibility of tiny particles or bacteria that are difficult to see under brightfield microscopy [49]. Darkfield

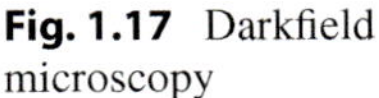
Fig. 1.17 Darkfield microscopy

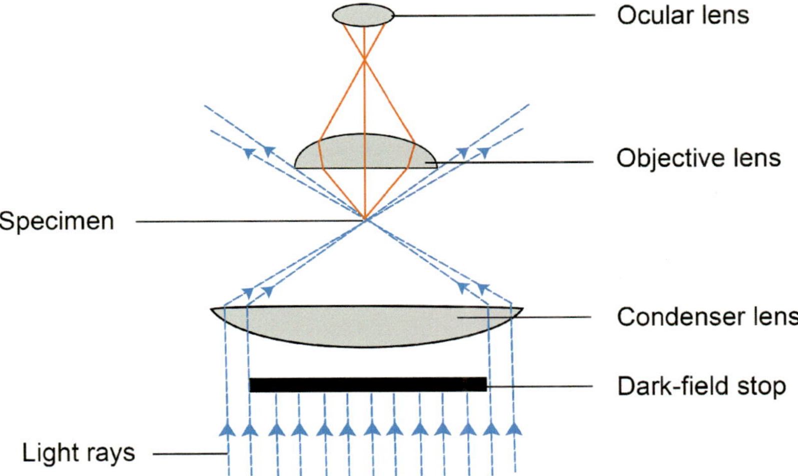

microscopy can detect active microorganisms in urine, such as trichomonas. Furthermore, substances with poor refractivity, such as casts, crystals, and mucous threads, can be easily identified using darkfield microscopy (Fig. 1.18).

1.6.5 Polarizing Microscopy

Polarizing microscopy is a technique widely used in various fields. It is used to identify birefringent materials, such as crystals (Fig. 1.19), fibers, bones, and minerals [50], based on their effects on plane-polarized light. Birefringent materials have two optical axes and refract plane-polarized light into two rays, known as the slow and fast rays, vibrating at 90° to each other. To observe birefringent materials under polarizing microscopy, the polarizer is initially rotated to achieve maximum extinction, resulting in the darkest background. When a birefringent object is present, the incident polarized light is refracted by the object, generating two rays that pass through the analyzer and reach the eyepiece. The birefringent object appears bright white against the dark background.

In the clinical laboratory, polarizing microscopy is primarily used in urine and synovial fluid examinations. In urinalysis, it helps confirm the

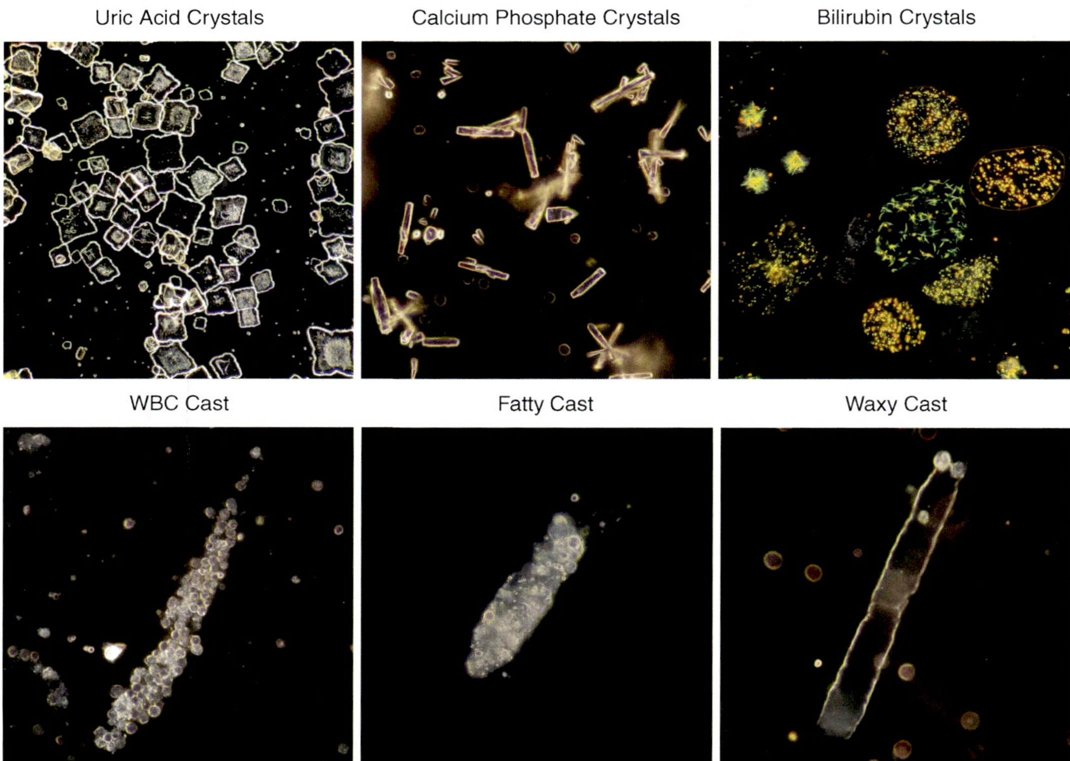

Fig. 1.18 Some urine-formed elements under darkfield microscopy, ×400

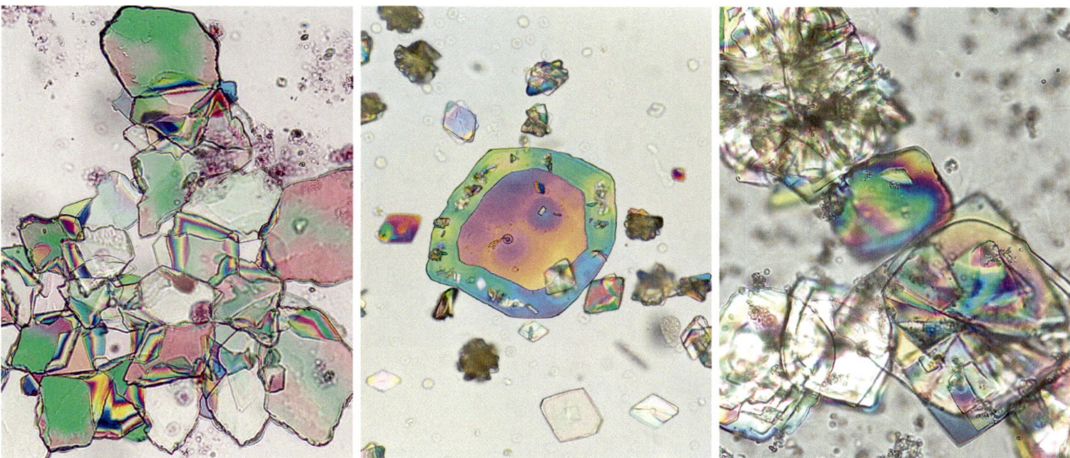

Fig. 1.19 Uric acid crystals under polarizing microscopy, ×400

presence of urinary fat, particularly cholesterol, by observing its characteristic Maltese cross pattern. Cholesterol droplets, which are birefringent, produce the Maltese cross pattern when viewed under polarized light [51]. Other neutral fats, such as fatty acids and triglycerides, cannot be identified using polarizing microscopy because they do not exhibit optical activity.

It is important to note that not all crystals are birefringent, and other birefringent substances like drugs, dyes, starch and contaminants can be encountered in urine and other body fluids. Proper adjustments of the microscope, including lighting optimization, are necessary to detect and evaluate birefringent crystals effectively. Expertise and training are crucial to ensure proper microscope adjustment and accurate identification of birefringent objects.

1.6.6 Fluorescence Microscopy

Fluorescence microscopy is based on the properties of fluorescent dyes. In fluorescence microscopy, the sample is first illuminated with an excitation light source. The energy from the excitation light causes the fluorescent molecules to transition from the ground state to the excited state. When returning to the ground state, the fluorescent molecules emit light, known as fluorescence emission. The fluorescence can be selectively captured through the use of filters and can be observed and recorded using an eyepiece or a camera [52]. This enables the visualization and study of the spatial distribution of specific molecules or structures within the sample. Fluorescence microscopy has wide applications in biology, biomedical research, drug discovery, and cellular imaging, allowing for the exploration of cellular functions, disease mechanisms, and dynamic processes in living organisms.

Fluorescence microscope is widely used to detect components in urinary sediment. It is capable of identifying and differentiating various cellular elements such as white blood cells, epithelial cells, and tumor cells. It aids in the detection of microorganisms [53], including bacteria, fungi (Fig. 1.20), and parasites. Cells can

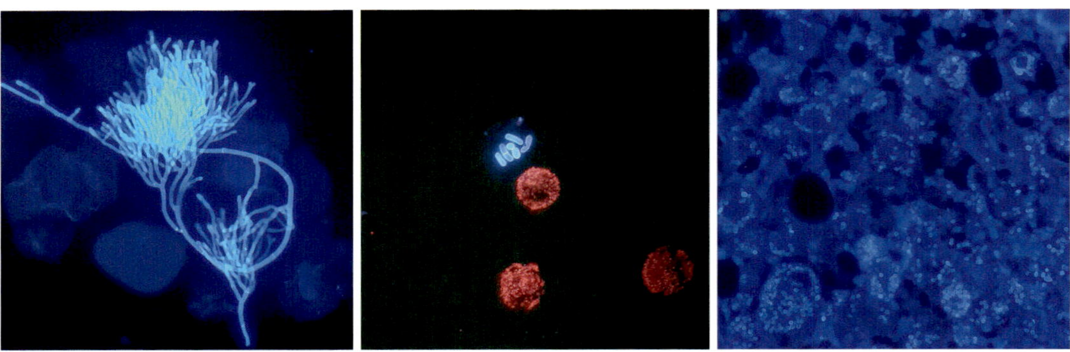

Fig. 1.20 Fungi under fluorescence microscope, ×400

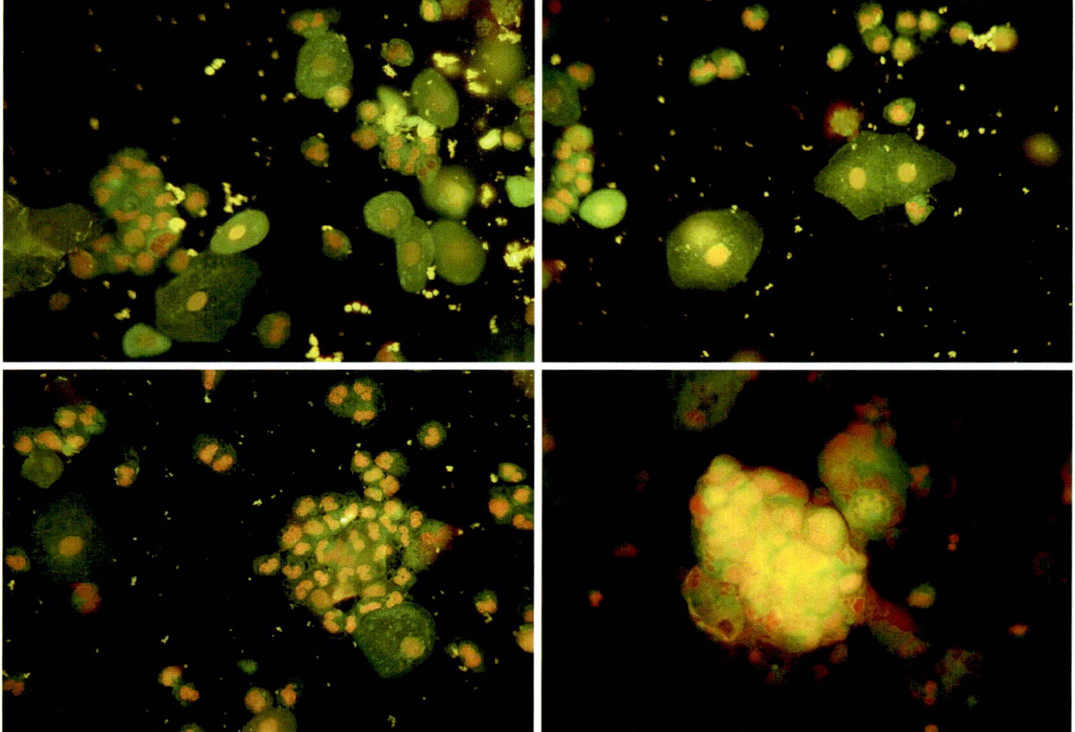

Fig. 1.21 Cells exhibit varying fluorescence intensities and colors under fluorescence microscope, ×400

bind with specific fluorescent dyes, resulting in different fluorescence intensities and colors in urine (Fig. 1.21). Some crystals can also exhibit spontaneous fluorescence under a fluorescence microscope in urine without the addition of any fluorescent dyes (Fig. 1.22). Overall, the fluorescence microscope is a valuable tool in the analysis of urinary sediment, providing accurate identification, enhanced sensitivity, and the ability to detect and differentiate various components.

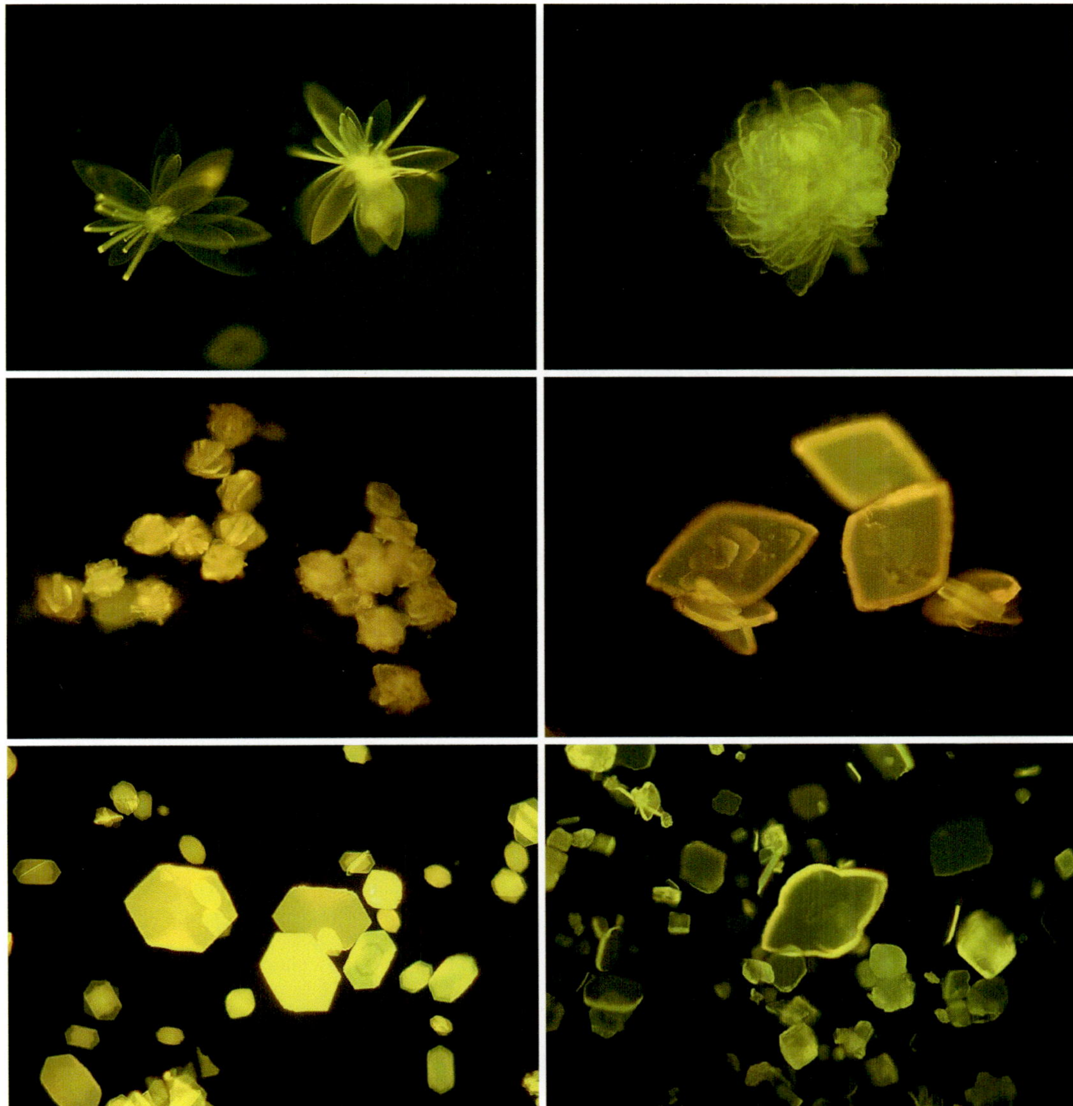

Fig. 1.22 Spontaneous fluorescence of uric acid crystals under fluorescence microscope, ×400

References

1. Netter FH. Netter atlas of human anatomy: a systems approach. 8th ed. Paperback + eBook. Elsevier Health Sciences; 2022.
2. Wallace MA. Anatomy and physiology of the kidney. AORN J. 1998;68(5):800, 803–16, 819–20; quiz 821–04.
3. Gilbert SF, Weiner DE, editors. National kidney foundation primer on kidney diseases, E-book. Elsevier Health Sciences; 2022.
4. Fogo AB, Kon V. The glomerulus—a view from the inside—the endothelial cell. Int J Biochem Cell Biol. 2010;42(9):1388–97.
5. Drake R, Vogl AW, Mitchell AW. Gray's anatomy for students E-book. Elsevier Health Sciences; 2009.

6. Moore KL, Dalley AF, Agur AM. Clinically oriented anatomy. Lippincott Williams & Wilkins; 2013.
7. Nawata CM, Pannabecker TL. Mammalian urine concentration: a review of renal medullary architecture and membrane transporters. J Comp Physiol B. 2018;188(6):899–918.
8. Kurtz A. Endocrine functions of the renal interstitium. Pflugers Arch. 2017;469(7–8):869–76.
9. Petsepe DC, Kourkoulis SK, Papadodima SA, Sokolis DP. Regional and age-dependent residual strains, curvature, and dimensions of the human ureter. Proc Inst Mech Eng H. 2018;232(2):149–62.
10. Standring S. Gray's anatomy. 41st ed. Edinburgh: Elsevier Churchill Livingstone; 2016.
11. Netter F. Atlas of human anatomy. 7th ed. Philadelphia, PA: Saunders; 2019.
12. Sharma AK. An examination of regenerative medicine-based strategies for the urinary bladder. Regen Med. 2011;6(5):583–98.
13. Vahabi B, Drake MJ. Physiological and pathophysiological implications of micromotion activity in urinary bladder function. Acta Physiol (Oxf). 2015;213(2):360–70.
14. Galgano SJ, Sivils C, Selph JP, Sanyal R, Lockhart ME, Zarzour JG. The male urethra: imaging and surgical approach for common pathologies. Curr Probl Diagn Radiol. 2021;50(3):410–8.
15. Pomian A, Majkusiak W, Kociszewski J, Tomasik P, Horosz E, Zwierzchowska A, et al. Demographic features of female urethra length. Neurourol Urodyn. 2018;37(5):1751–6.
16. Jackson AR, Hoff ML, Li B, Ching CB, McHugh KM, Becknell B. Krt5(+) urothelial cells are developmental and tissue repair progenitors in the kidney. Am J Physiol Renal Physiol. 2019;317(3):F757–66.
17. Bertram JF, Hoy WE. Nephron loss in the ageing kidney—it's more than you think. Nat Rev Nephrol. 2016;12(10):585–6.
18. Brunzel NA. Fundamentals of urine and body fluid analysis. Elsevier Health Sciences; 2021.
19. Esselman AB, Patterson NH, Migas LG, Dufresne M, Djambazova KV, Colley ME, et al. Microscopy-directed imaging mass spectrometry for rapid high spatial resolution molecular imaging of glomeruli. J Am Soc Mass Spectrom. 2023;34(7):1305–14.
20. Pollak MR, Quaggin SE, Hoenig MP, Dworkin LD. The glomerulus: the sphere of influence. Clin J Am Soc Nephrol. 2014;9(8):1461–9.
21. Naylor RW, Morais M, Lennon R. Complexities of the glomerular basement membrane. Nat Rev Nephrol. 2021;17(2):112–27.
22. Miner JH. Glomerular basement membrane composition and the filtration barrier. Pediatr Nephrol. 2011;26(9):1413–7.
23. Duan T, Zhu X, Zhao Q, Xiao L, He L, Liu H, et al. Association of Bowman's capsule rupture with prognosis in patients with lupus nephritis. J Nephrol. 2022;35(4):1193–204.
24. Ndisang JF. Glomerular endothelium and its impact on glomerular filtration barrier in diabetes: are the gaps still illusive? Curr Med Chem. 2018;25(13):1525–9.
25. Fromm M, Piontek J, Rosenthal R, Günzel D, Krug SM. Tight junctions of the proximal tubule and their channel proteins. Pflugers Arch. 2017;469(7–8):877–87.
26. Tanigawa S, Nishinakamura R. Functional renal collecting ducts from human PSCs. Cell Stem Cell. 2022;29(11):1510–2.
27. Rao R, Bhalla V, Pastor-Soler NM. Intercalated cells of the kidney collecting duct in kidney physiology. Semin Nephrol. 2019;39(4):353–67.
28. Benzing T, Salant D. Insights into glomerular filtration and albuminuria. N Engl J Med. 2021;384(15):1437–46.
29. Holechek MJ. Glomerular filtration: an overview. Nephrol Nurs J. 2003;30(3):285–90; quiz 291–82.
30. Di Pino A, Scicali R, Marchisello S, Zanoli L, Ferrara V, Urbano F, et al. High glomerular filtration rate is associated with impaired arterial stiffness and subendocardial viability ratio in prediabetic subjects. Nutr Metab Cardiovasc Dis. 2021;31(12):3393–400.
31. McMahon RS, Penfold D, Bashir K. Anatomy, Abdomen and Pelvis: Kidney Collecting Ducts. In: StatPearls. Treasure Island (FL): StatPearls Publishing; July 24, 2023.
32. Gottschalk CW. Osmotic concentration and dilution of the urine. Am J Med. 1964;36(5):670–85.
33. Mozolowski W. Chemical composition of normal urine. Lancet. 1948;251(6498):423.
34. Wang P, Zhang H, Zhou J, Jin S, Liu C, Yang B, Cui L. Study of risk factor of urinary calculi according to the association between stone composition with urine component. Sci Rep. 2021;11(1):8723.
35. Cavanaugh C, Perazella MA. Urine sediment examination in the diagnosis and management of kidney disease: core curriculum 2019. Am J Kidney Dis. 2019;73(2):258–72.
36. Huussen J, Koene RA, Hilbrands LB. The (fixed) urinary sediment, a simple and useful diagnostic tool in patients with haematuria. Neth J Med. 2004;62(1):4–9.
37. Perazella MA. The urine sediment as a biomarker of kidney disease. Am J Kidney Dis. 2015;66(5):748–55.
38. Ko DH, Ji M, Kim S, Cho EJ, Lee W, Yun YM, Chun S, Min WK. An approach to standardization of urine sediment analysis via suggestion of a common manual protocol. Scand J Clin Lab Invest. 2016;76(3):256–63.
39. Yan L, Guo H, Han L, Huang H, Shen Y, He J, Liu J. Sternheimer-Malbin staining to detect decoy cells in urine of 213 kidney transplant patients. Transplant Proc. 2020;52(3):823–8.
40. European Confederation of Laboratory Medicine. European urinalysis guidelines. Scand J Clin Lab Invest Suppl. 2000;231:1–86.

41. Kiran M, Sonal S. Urine cytology in paroxysmal nocturnal hemoglobinuria. Diagn Cytopathol. 2012;40(9):804–5.
42. Taguchi S, Hidaka S, Yanai M, Ishioka K, Matsui K, Mochida Y, Moriya H, Ohtake T, Kobayashi S. Renal hemosiderosis presenting with acute kidney Injury and macroscopic hematuria in Immunoglobulin A nephropathy: a case report. BMC Nephrol. 2021;22(1):132.
43. Ghio AJ, Roggli VL. Perls' Prussian blue stains of lung tissue, bronchoalveolar lavage, and sputum. J Environ Pathol Toxicol Oncol. 2021;40(1):1–15.
44. O'Toole GA. Classic spotlight: how the gram stain works. J Bacteriol. 2016;198(23):3128.
45. Nolan CR 3rd, Anger MS, Kelleher SP. Eosinophiluria—a new method of detection and definition of the clinical spectrum. N Engl J Med. 1986;315(24):1516–9.
46. Becker GJ, Garigali G, Fogazzi GB. Advances in urine microscopy. Am J Kidney Dis. 2016;67(6):954–64.
47. Wolf DE. The optics of microscope image formation. Methods Cell Biol. 2013;114:11–42.
48. Haber MH. Interference contrast microscopy for identification of urinary sediments. Am J Clin Pathol. 1972;57(3):316–9.
49. Abe M, Furuichi M, Ishimitsu T, Tojo A. Analysis of purple urine bag syndrome by low vacuum scanning electron microscopy. Med Mol Morphol. 2022;55(2):123–30.
50. Oldenbourg R. Polarized light microscopy: principles and practice. Cold Spring Harb Protoc. 2013;2013(11):pdb.top078600.
51. Lee AJ, Yoo EH, Bae YC, Jung SB, Jeon CH. Differential identification of urine crystals with morphologic characteristics and solubility test. J Clin Lab Anal. 2022;36(11):e24707.
52. Lichtman JW, Conchello JA. Fluorescence microscopy. Nat Methods. 2005;2(12):910–9.
53. Sankaranarayanan R, Alagumaruthanayagam A, Sankaran K. A new fluorimetric method for the detection and quantification of siderophores using Calcein Blue, with potential as a bacterial detection tool. Appl Microbiol Biotechnol. 2015;99(5):2339–49.

2 Cells

Lizhi Yan, Lixin Wang, Yulan Geng, Ke Cao, Yu Cao, Yang Gao, Hui Zhang, Chongchong Feng, Yingying Diao, Ru Jia, and Yajuan Shen

2.1 Cells: Overview

A variety of cells can be found in urine, mainly including epithelial cells, leukocytes and RBCs (Table 2.1). These cells play important roles in the diagnosis of urinary system diseases. Additionally, in patients with urinary system tumors, various forms of tumor cells can be found in the urine. The detection and analysis of these cells are of significant importance for early screening, diagnosis, and monitoring of urinary system tumors.

Cells in urine are not only connected to diseases but are also influenced by the type of urine specimen, pH, osmotic pressure, and both the duration and method of urine sample preservation. Therefore, comprehensive analysis is required to avoid overdiagnosis when examining urinary cells. Staining methods play a crucial role in the identification of urinary cells,

L. Yan (✉)
Department of Laboratory Medicine, Nanfang Hospital, Southern Medical University, Guangzhou, China

L. Wang
Center of Laboratory Medicine, General Hospital of Ningxia Medical University, Yinchuan, China
e-mail: 13895630916@nyfy.com.cn

Y. Geng
Department of Laboratory Medicine, The First Hospital of Hebei Medical University, Shijiazhuang, China

K. Cao
Department of Laboratory Medicine, Shenzhen Children's Hospital, Shenzhen, China

Y. Cao
Department of Laboratory Medicine, Affiliated Hospital of Zunyi Medical University, Zunyi, Guizhou, China

Y. Gao
Department of Pathology, Baotou Tumor Hospital, Baotou, China

H. Zhang
Department of Laboratory Medicine, The First Hospital of Jilin University, Changchun, China

C. Feng
Department of Laboratory Medicine, The Second Hospital of Jilin University, Changchun, China
e-mail: fengcc@jlu.edu.cn

Y. Diao
Department of Laboratory Medicine, The First Hospital of China Medical University, Shenyang, Liaoning, China

R. Jia
Department of Laboratory Medicine, Meihekou Central Hospital, Meihekou, China

Y. Shen
Department of Clinical Laboratory, Shandong Provincial Hospital Affiliated to Shandong First Medical University, Jinan, China
e-mail: shenyajuan@sdfmu.edu.cn

L. Zheng et al. (eds.), *Urine Formed Elements*, https://doi.org/10.1007/978-981-99-7739-0_2

Table 2.1 Characteristics of common urinary cells

Name		Characteristics	Diagram
Red blood cells/erythrocytes		• Double concave disc-shaped • No cell nucleus	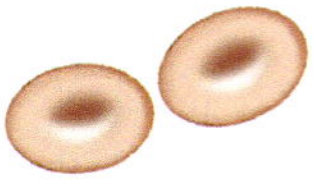
White blood cells/leucocytes		• Spheroid shape • Cytoplasmic granular appearance • Unstained cell nucleus with unclear structure	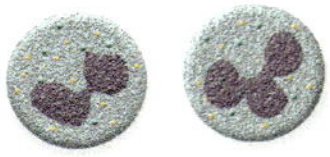
Squamous epithelial cells		• Polygonal shape • Abundant and thin cytoplasm • Small nucleus	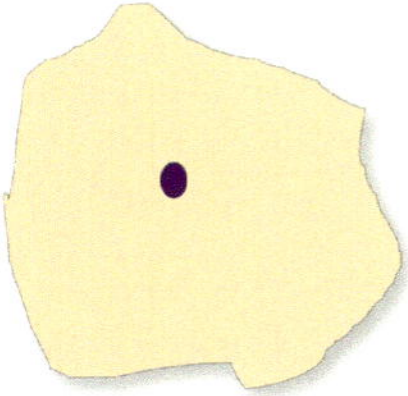
Urothelial cells	Superficial layer	• Large in size • Abundant cytoplasm with granules • Round nucleus, mostly centrally located • Visible small nucleoli	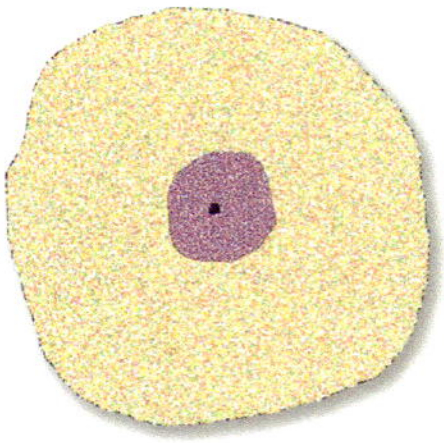
	Intermediate layer	• Spindle-shaped, fusiform, or round • Moderate cytoplasmic volume • Round nucleus • Visible small nucleoli	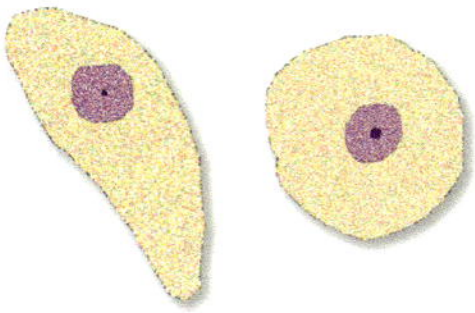
	Basal layer	• Small cell volume • High nuclear-cytoplasmic ratio • Round nucleus, centrally located • Visible small nucleoli	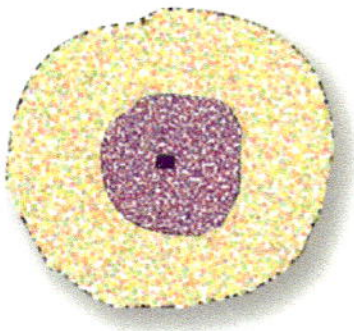
Renal tubular epithelial cells		• Polygonal shape • Slightly larger than white blood cells • Cytoplasmic granular appearance	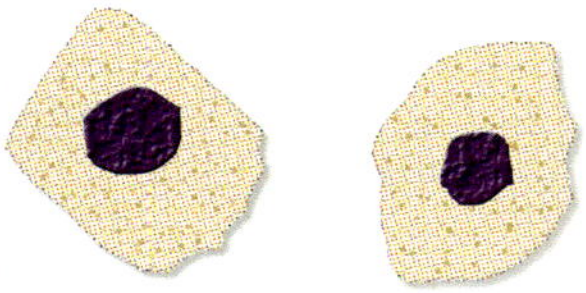
Macrophages/histiocytes		• Enormous in size • Frequently contain phagocytic material within the cytoplasm • Indistinct or absent nucleus	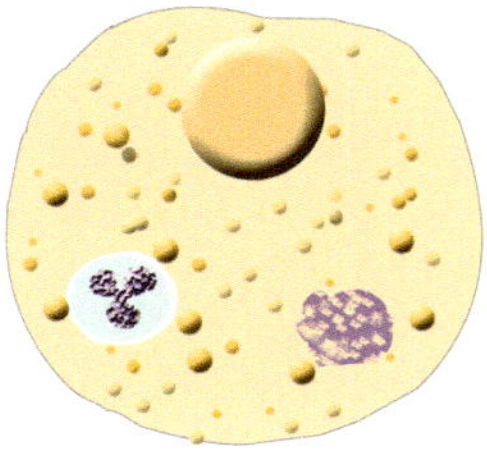

Table 2.1 (continued)

Name	Characteristics	Diagram
Oval fat bodies/lipid granule cells	• Pale yellow lipid droplets • Strong birefringence • Indistinct or absent cell nucleus	
Decoy cells	• Increased cell body size • Enlarged and vacuolated nucleus • Thickened nuclear membrane • Presence of nuclear inclusions	

and the appropriate staining method should be selected based on the specific cell types to be identified.

2.2 Red Blood Cells (RBCs)/Erythrocytes

2.2.1 Normal Red Blood Cells

RBCs are a common component formed in urine sediment. Under a conventional light microscope, normal RBCs appear as biconcave discs without a cell nucleus, with a diameter of approximately 7 μm, a depth of about 3 μm. The size or diameter of RBCs is affected by urine concentration (i.e., osmolality, specific gravity) [1] (Fig. 2.1). They can be observed using a high-power objective lens (×40) or an oil immersion lens. Phase contrast microscopy is particularly suitable for the observation of RBCs [2, 3].

Due to kidney diseases or the influence of urine pH, specific gravity, osmotic pressure and specimen storage time, the size and morphology of RBCs may vary [1]. Differentiating the morphology of RBCs is significant for distinguishing between non-glomerular and glomerular hematuria in the clinic.

2.2.2 Crenated Red Blood Cells

In concentrated urine (hypertonic urine) or acidic urine, the dehydration of RBCs leads to the shrinkage of their volume. The membrane surface of these cells exhibits evenly distributed short, jagged projections, resembling mulberries, starbursts, or irregular shapes (Fig. 2.2). This morphological change is reversible.

2.2.3 Ghost Cells

In hypotonic urine, when the extracellular fluid enters the RBC, they swell and rupture. The loss of intracellular hemoglobin results in the presence of ghost cells, which are colorless and hollow circular structures formed by the remaining cell membrane. These ghost cells are challenging to be observed under a conventional bright field microscope due to the absence of hemoglobin. They are more conveniently visualized using phase contrast microscopy or interference contrast microscopy (Fig. 2.3). They can also be observed in alkaline urine, as RBCs are prone to dissolution and destruction in alkaline conditions. They may also exist in aged urine and eventually decompose and disappear completely.

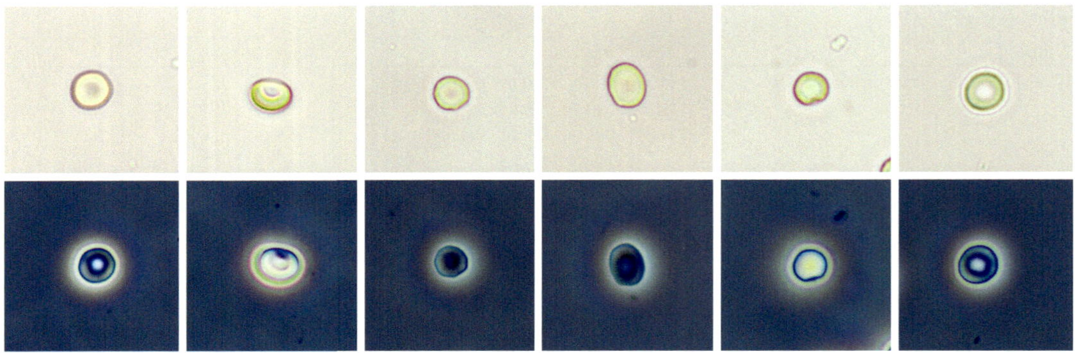

Fig. 2.1 RBCs, biconcave disc-shaped. Unstained, bright field, and phase contrast microscopy, ×1000

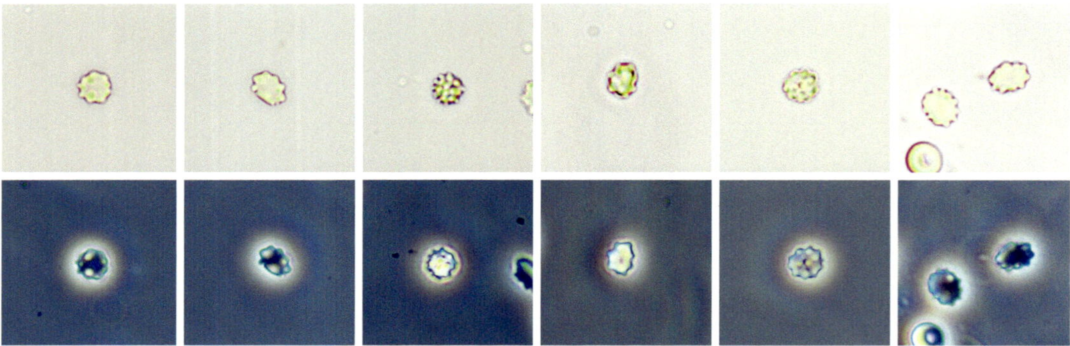

Fig. 2.2 Crenated RBCs. Unstained, bright field, and phase contrast microscopy, ×1000

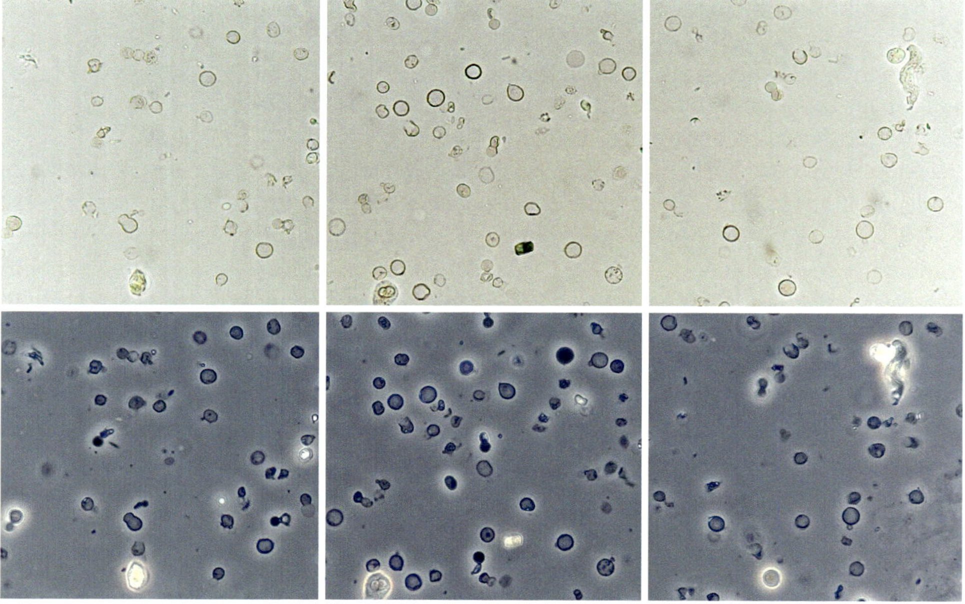

Fig. 2.3 Ghost cells do not exhibit birefringence and appear darker when observed under phase contrast microscopy. Normal RBCs exhibit birefringence. Unstained, ×400

2.2.4 Red Blood Cells with Knobby

RBCs are characterized by their variable size and the presence of small-rounded protrusions (spheroid-like) along the cell edges (Fig. 2.4). These protrusions can be single or multiple in number. Spherocytes are rich in hemoglobin, and there are no changes in the central pallor of the RBCs. They are commonly observed in non-glomerular hematuria, indicating a non-glomerular source of blood in the urine.

These RBCs are morphologically different from acanthocytes. Acanthocytes typically have an enlarged central pallor and are associated with renal hematuria.

2.2.5 Dysmorphic RBCs

Dysmorphic RBCs, also known as dysmorphic erythrocytes, exhibit various morphological changes due to compression damage when passing through the altered glomerular basement membrane in the kidneys. Subsequently, as they traverse different segments of the renal tubules, they are influenced by varying pH levels, fluctuating osmotic pressure, medium tension and various metabolic byproducts (such as fatty acids, hemolytic phospholipids, bile acids, etc.). These factors contribute to changes in red blood cell size, shape, and hemoglobin content. Common types of dysmorphic erythrocytes include acanthocytes, ring-shaped RBCs, target cells, saw-toothed and other renal RBCs.

2.2.5.1 Acanthocytes

Acanthocytes are RBCs characterized by the presence of one or multiple vesicle-shaped or bleb-like protrusions on the surface of the cell body, resembling a donut with spikes (Figs. 2.5 and 2.6). Some acanthocytes have a distinct appearance resembling "Mickey Mouse ears." It is important to note that acanthocytes are not caused by changes in urine pH or osmotic pressure but by damage to the glomerular basement membrane. Therefore, the presence of acantho-

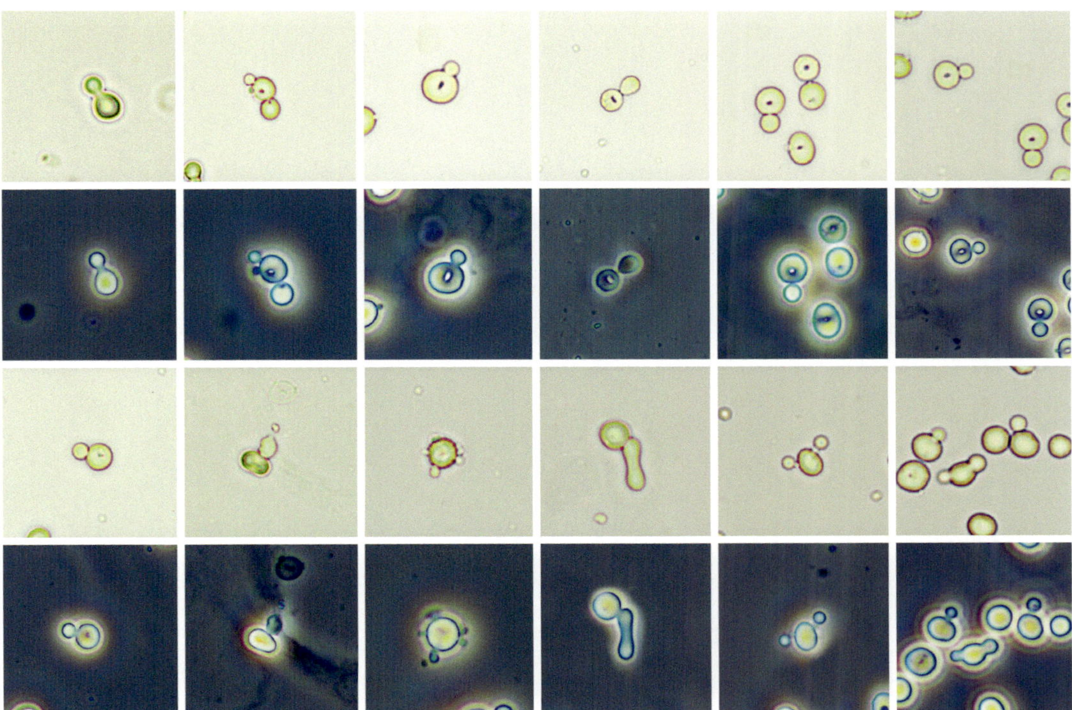

Fig. 2.4 RBCs with Knobby. Unstained, bright field, and phase contrast microscopy, ×1000

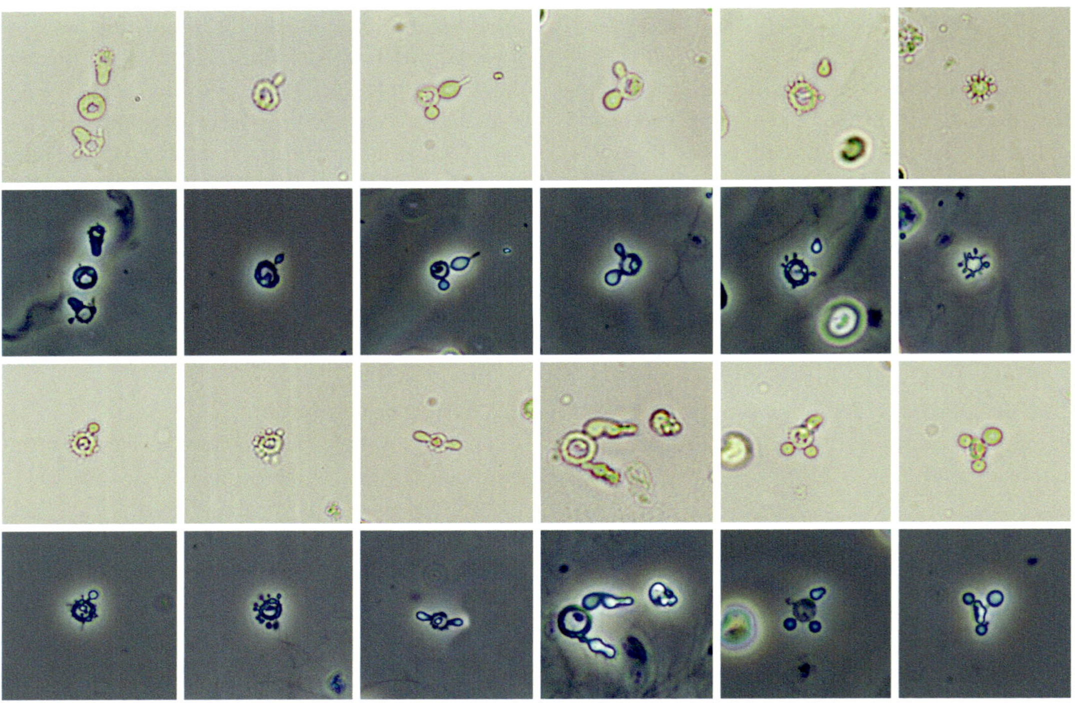

Fig. 2.5 Acanthocytes. Unstained, bright field and phase contrast microscopy, ×1000

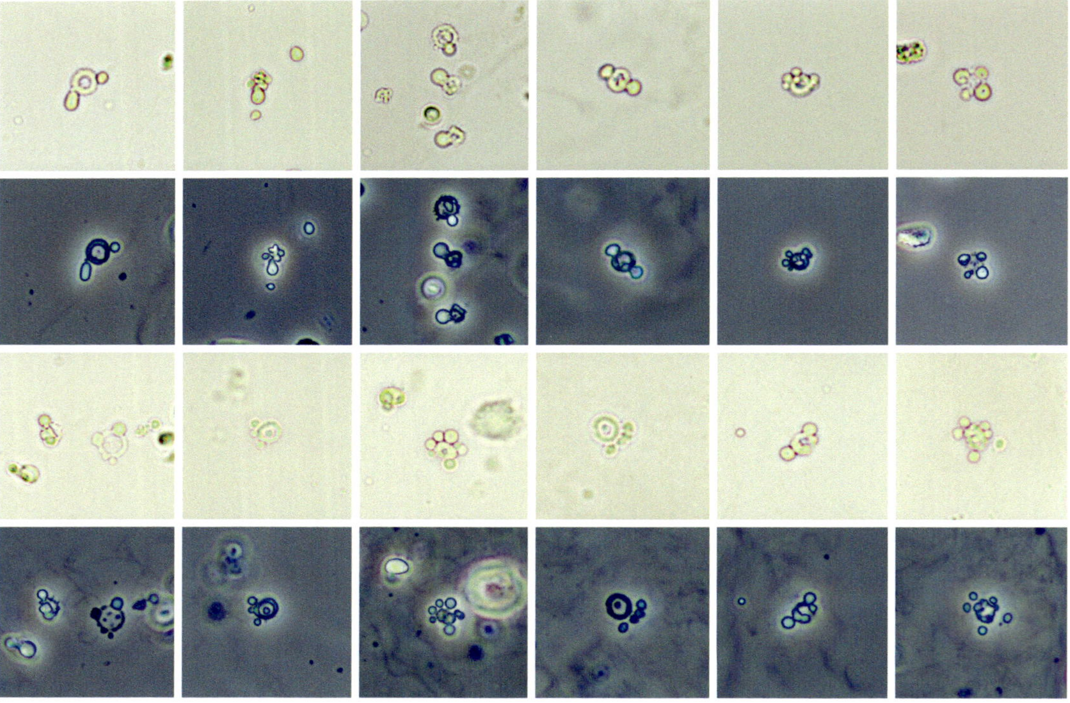

Fig. 2.6 Acanthocytes. Unstained, bright field, and phase contrast microscopy, ×1000

cytes in urine has a significant diagnostic value, and acanthocytes of ≥5% is a characteristic feature of glomerular hematuria [4].

2.2.5.2 Ring-Shaped RBCs

Ring-shaped RBCs, also known as ring erythrocytes, exhibit an expanded central pallor, resembling a donut-shaped structure (Fig. 2.7). The central area of these RBCs can take on various shapes, including triangular, cross-shaped, or irregular. Ring-shaped RBCs are commonly associated with glomerular diseases [5].

2.2.5.3 Target Cells

Target cells are ring-shaped RBCs that exhibit a central bullseye or peninsula-like appearance (Fig. 2.8). They have irregular shapes and are commonly associated with renal hematuria.

2.2.5.4 Saw-Toothed Cells

The characteristics of saw-toothed cells are an enlarged central pallor and irregular, saw-toothed, or wheel-like projections along the cell periphery (Fig. 2.9). They are commonly seen in glomerular diseases.

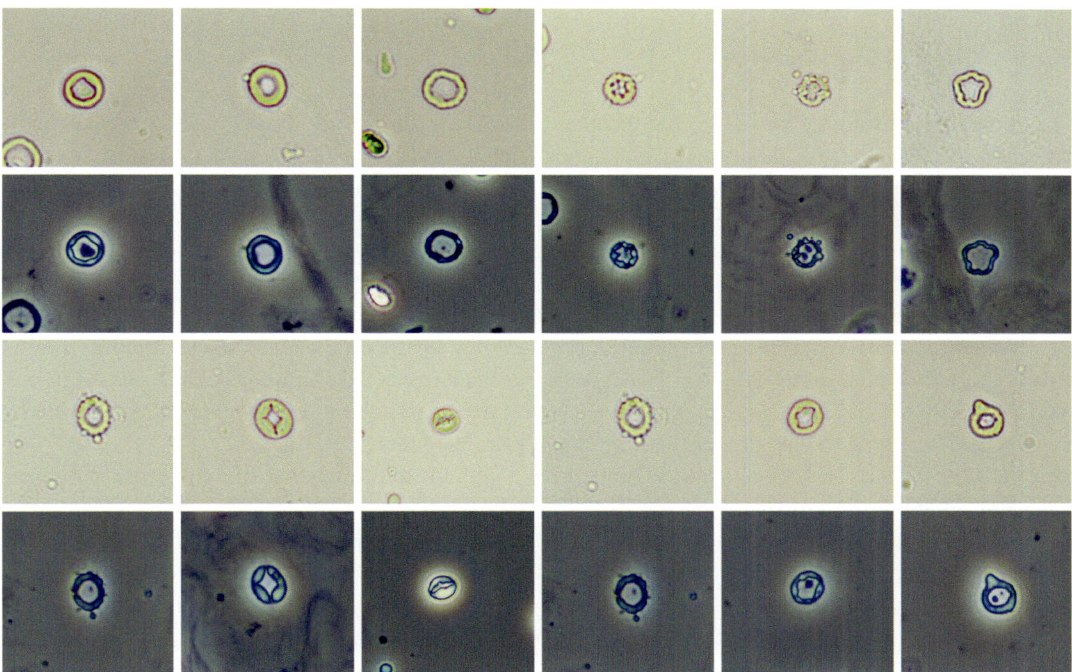

Fig. 2.7 Ring-shaped RBCs. Unstained, bright field, and phase contrast microscopy, ×1000

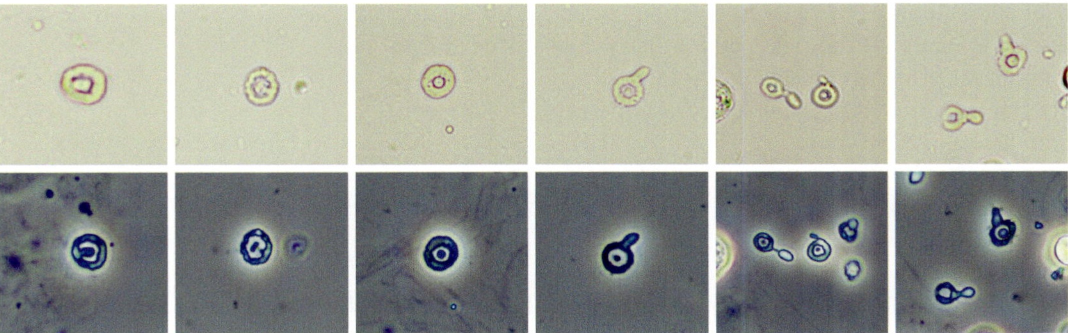

Fig. 2.8 Target cells. Unstained, bright field, and phase contrast microscopy, ×1000

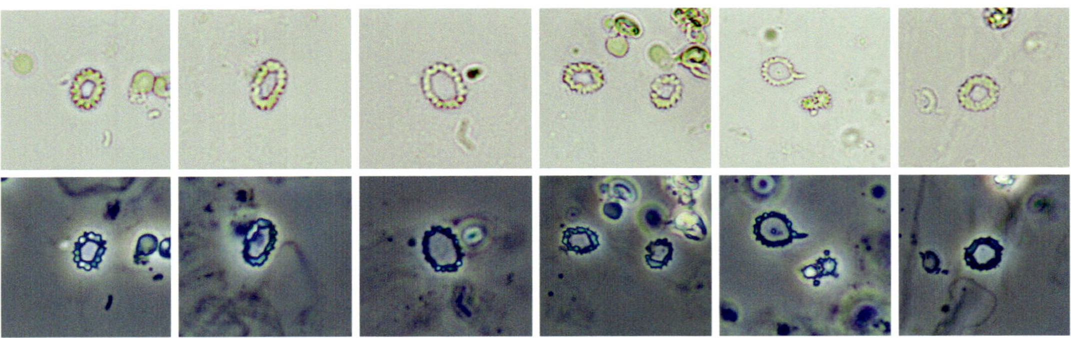

Fig. 2.9 Saw-toothed cells. Unstained, bright field, and phase contrast microscopy, ×1000

2.2.6 Clinical Significance

The glomerular filtration barrier in the kidneys prevents the passage of large molecules and blood cells under normal conditions, resulting in very few RBCs entering the urine [6]. In healthy individuals, occasional RBCs may be observed in the urinary sediment. Some literatures have reported a maximum of five RBCs per high-power field (≤5/HPF) [3], while other literatures have reported a maximum of three RBCs per high-power field (≤3/HPF) [1].

Hematuria refers to the presence of a certain amount of RBCs in the urine. When the blood volume in the urine is ≥1 mL/L, the urine appears pale red, which is referred to as gross hematuria. In case of significant bleeding, the urine can appear bright red or dark red with a cloudy appearance and may contain blood clots. When the visual changes in the urine are not evident, the presence of ≥3 RBCs per high-power field is considered microscopic hematuria upon centrifugation. Various structural or functional injuries to the urinary system can cause hematuria, and the morphological observation of RBCs under a microscope can help determine the source of the urinary RBCs [7].

When normal-shaped RBCs are predominant, the RBCs mostly originate from below the underside of the renal tubules and urinary tract, primarily from the ureter, bladder and urethra, indicating non-glomerular source of RBCs. This can be seen in urinary system diseases including inflammations, tumors, tuberculosis, stones and traumas, as well as systemic bleeding disorders such as idiopathic thrombocytopenic purpura, hemophilia, aplastic anemia, leukemia and disseminated intravascular coagulation (DIC). Other systemic diseases like hypertension, arteriosclerosis, high fever and systemic lupus erythematosus (SLE) can also cause non-glomerular hematuria. Transient hematuria, with relatively normal-shaped RBCs, can occur in normal individuals, especially in adolescents after vigorous exercise, marching, cold water baths, and heavy physical labor.

When abnormal-shaped RBCs are predominant and at least two or more types of morphological changes are observed, the RBCs are of glomerular origin. This is commonly seen in various primary and secondary glomerular diseases such as IgA nephropathy, mesangial proliferative glomerulonephritis, focal segmental glomerulosclerosis, nephrotic syndrome, lupus nephritis and purpuric nephritis. In case of glomerular hematuria, it is accompanied by proteinuria or the presence of RBC casts.

2.2.7 RBCs and Similar Substances

Many substances in urinary sediment have morphological characteristics and sizes similar to RBCs, such as calcium oxalate crystals, yeast cells, air bubbles, oil droplets, lipoid bodies, starch granules, and blastocystis hominis, among others (Table 2.2). These substances may inter-

Table 2.2 Similar substances to RBCs

Name	Characteristics	Diagram
RBCs	• Pale yellow in color • Biconcave disc-shaped • Weak refractive index • Susceptible to disruption by acetic acid • Positive for occult blood	
Yeast cells	• Colorless • Elliptical shape • Slightly stronger refractive index • Not disrupted by acetic acid • Negative for occult blood	
Calcium oxalate crystals	• Colorless, round, or oval in shape • Strong refractive properties • Soluble in HCl, insoluble in acetic acid	
Oil droplets/ lipid droplets	• Pale yellow in color, spherical in shape • Strong refractive properties • Positive staining with Sudan III or Oil Red O	
Starch granules	• Colorless, pebble-like, or irregular in shape • Weak refractive properties • Not destroyed by acetic acid • Stain blue-purple with iodine	
Blastocystis hominis	• Circular in shape. No central pallor • Slightly stronger refractive properties • Not destroyed by acetic acid • Identified by iodine staining or Giemsa staining	

fere with the accurate counting of RBCs [6]. Differentiation can be done based on the morphological characteristics, refractive index, the addition of acetic acid to the sediment, or a combination of other tests.

2.2.7.1 Circular Calcium Oxalate Crystals

Circular calcium oxalate crystals with a central depressed area are easily confused with RBCs, especially with certain instrumental methods that may mistake them for RBCs. Calcium oxalate crystals have strong refractive properties and vary in size under bright field microscopy (Fig. 2.10). They can appear alongside other forms of calcium oxalate crystals and are not destroyed by the addition of acetic acid.

2.2.7.2 Yeast Cells

Yeast cells are round or oval in shape with a diameter of 3–6 μm (Fig. 2.11). Occasionally, budding spores or pseudohyphae can be observed. After adding 1–2 drops of 10% KOH, components such as RBCs and WBCs dissolve and disintegrate, while spores and pseudohyphae remain clearly visible [1].

2.2.7.3 Air Bubbles

During the preparation of a urine sediment slide, air bubbles may be generated. They vary in size and are typically round in shape, exhibiting strong refractive properties (Fig. 2.12). When the slide is touched with an object, the air bubbles can move, and their size may change. Air bubbles can sometimes interfere with microscopic examination. To avoid the formation of air bubbles, it is recommended to slowly place the cover slip on one side of the slide at a 45° angle during slide preparation [1].

2.2.7.4 Lipid Droplets: Oil Droplets

Lipid droplets are variable in size, pale yellow, and with strong refractive properties (Fig. 2.13). They are not in the same focal plane as other formed elements in urine. Sudan III stain or Oil Red O stain results in an orange or red color. They are commonly observed in the urine of patients with conditions such as nephrotic syndrome, pregnancy, or hyperlipidemia. In addition, oil droplets can be seen in women of childbearing age after ultrasound or topical medications.

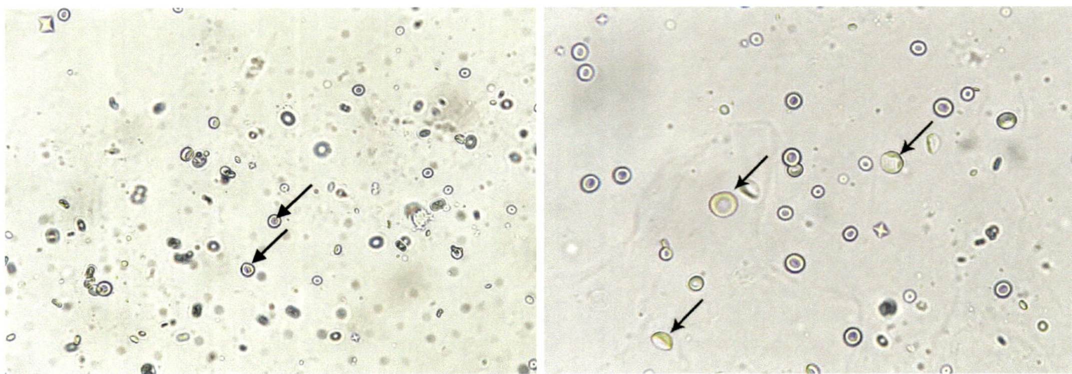

Fig. 2.10 Calcium oxalate crystals: circular, central depression, strong refractive index, similar to RBCs (↑), ×1000

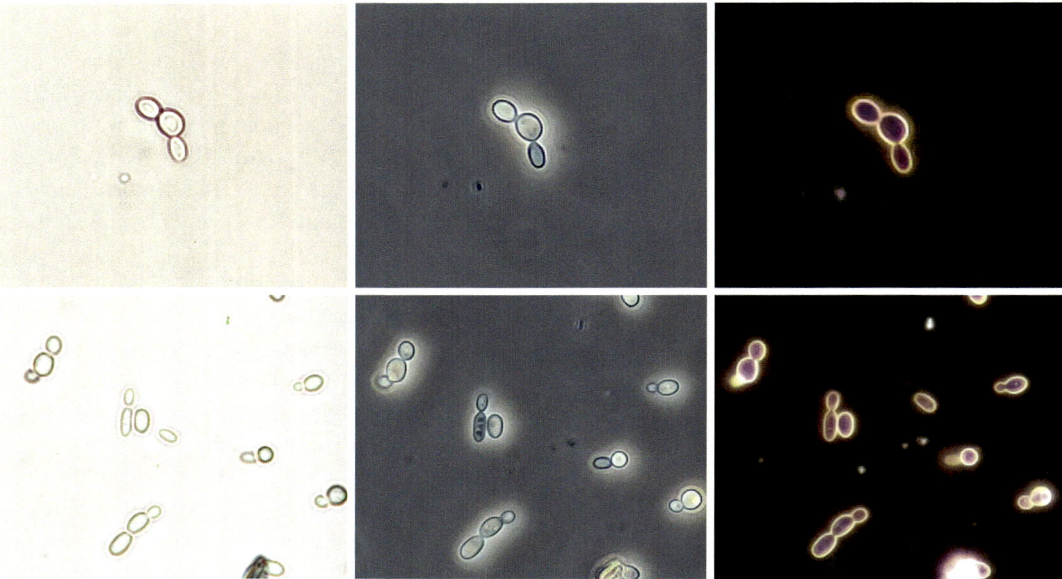

Fig. 2.11 Yeast cells. Unstained, ×1000

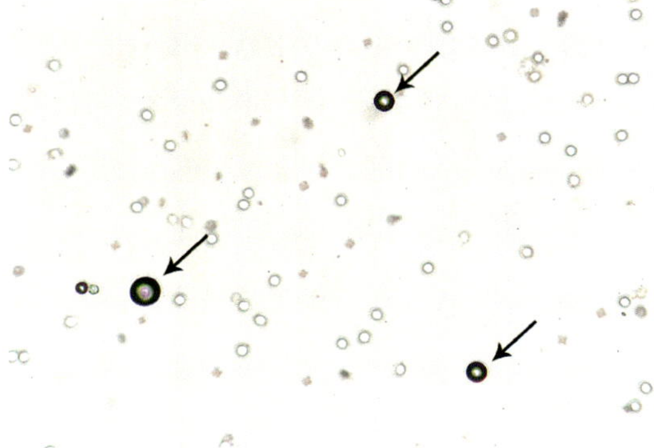

Fig. 2.12 Air bubbles. Unstained, ×400

2.2.7.5 Starch Granules

Starch granules have an irregular appearance, typically round or oval with a central depression (Fig. 2.14). They exhibit birefringence under polarized light microscopy and appear blue-purple after iodine staining. Starch granules are commonly encountered as contaminants in urine sediment.

2.2.7.6 Blastocystis Hominis

Blastocystis hominis organisms are round or oval-shaped vacuoles, typically ranging from 4 to 15 μm in size (Fig. 2.15). Moon-shaped notches are often observed at the edges of the vacuoles,

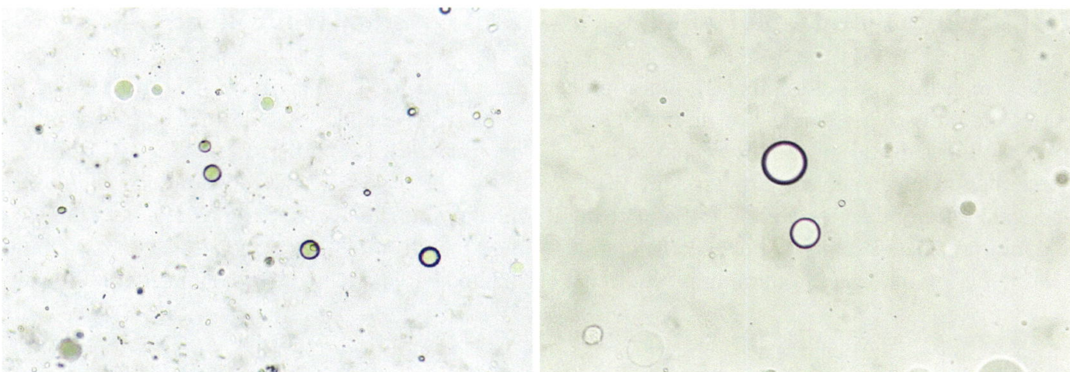

Fig. 2.13 Lipid droplets. Unstained, ×400

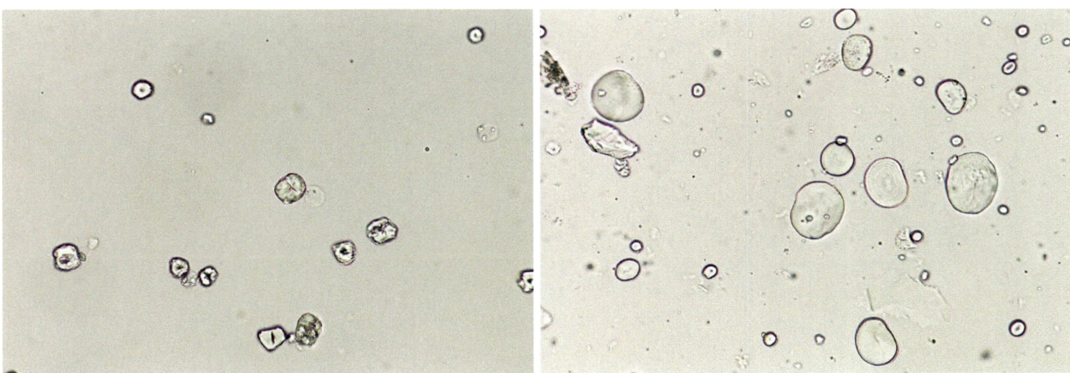

Fig. 2.14 Starch granules, two different morphological forms. Unstained, ×400

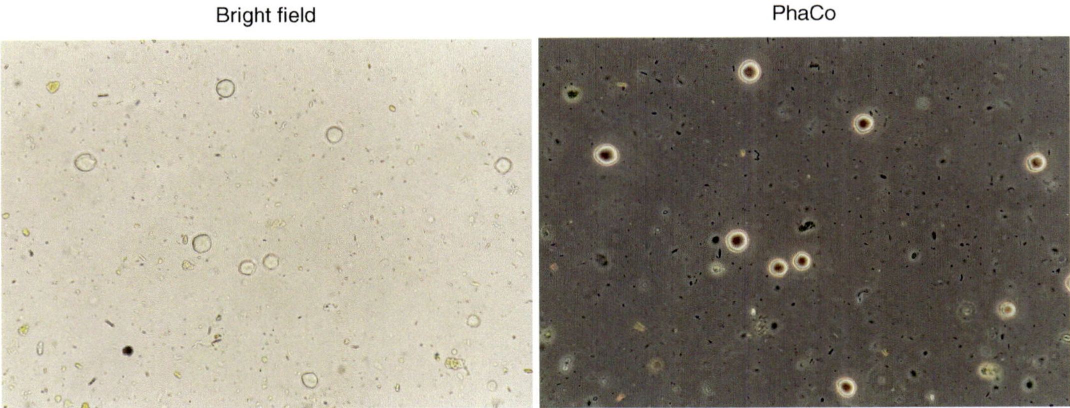

Fig. 2.15 Blastocystis hominis. Unstained, ×400

with one to four circular nuclei present at the edges [8]. Blastocystis hominis primarily parasitizes the human cecum and colon. Patients may experience symptoms such as diarrhea, abdominal pain, malaise and vomiting. Diagnosis can be confirmed through iodine staining or Giemsa staining. If fecal contamination occurs in the urine, it can be detected in the urine sample.

2.3 White Blood Cells (WBCs)

WBCs in urine are predominantly neutrophils, but eosinophils, lymphocytes, or monocytes can also be observed [2]. Specimens treated with acetic acid show clear nuclear structures of WBCs, and can differentiate between single-nucleated and multinucleated cells [9]. For specific classification, the use of Wright's staining is required.

2.3.1 Normal White Blood Cells

Unstained WBCs appear round or irregular in shape with granular cytoplasm. The clarity of the nuclear structure may vary in some cells (Fig. 2.16). WBCs in urine can be easily confused with renal tubular epithelial cells, but they can be differentiated based on cell size, morphology, or staining methods. Renal tubular epithelial cells are slightly

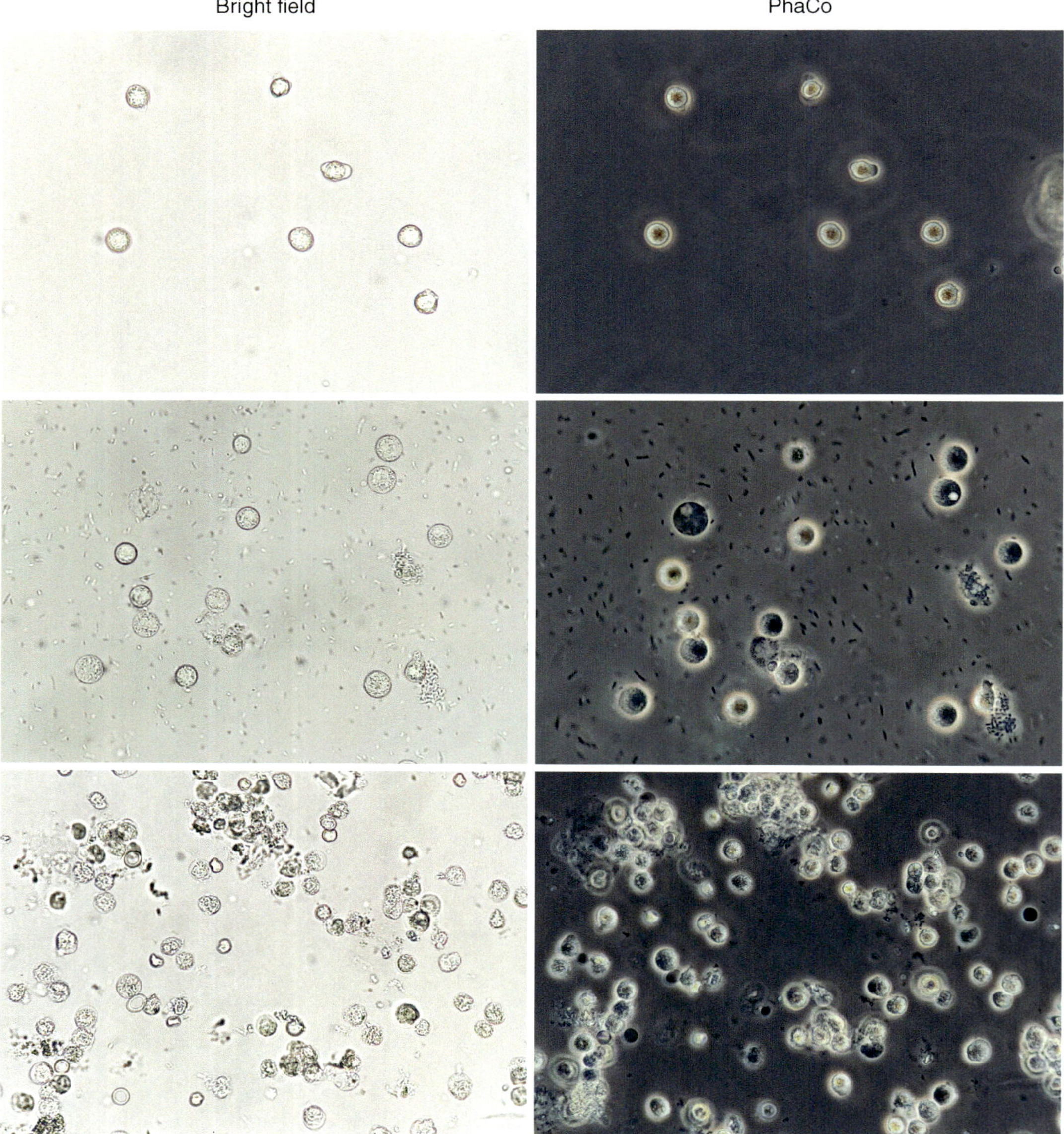

Fig. 2.16 The number of WBCs varies in different cases, and some cells may form clusters or groups. Unstained, ×400

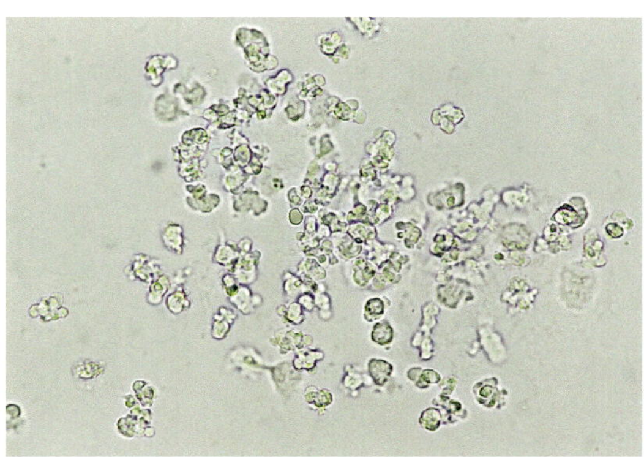

Fig. 2.17 Deformed WBCs. The cells are irregular and exhibit pseudopodia-like. Unstained, ×400

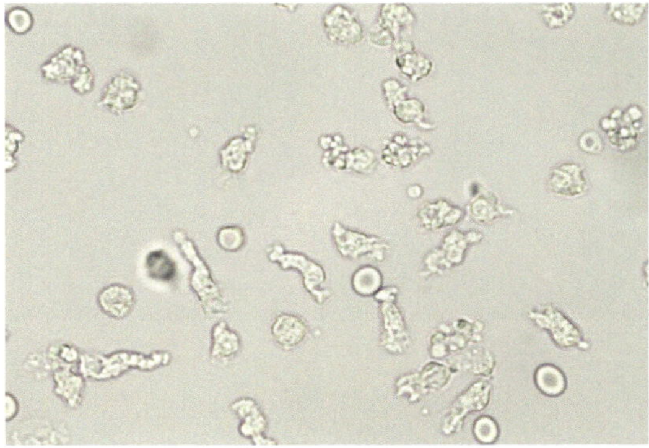

Fig. 2.18 Deformed WBCs. Spindle-shaped or irregular. Unstained, ×400

larger than WBCs and have irregular cell bodies, granular cytoplasm, and a single nucleus. WBCs have smaller volumes compared to renal tubular epithelial cells and are mostly round in shape, with unclear nuclear structures when unstained.

2.3.2 Deformed White Blood Cells

In some cases, WBCs can exhibit various morphological changes. They may have surface protrusions (Fig. 2.17) or appear spindle-shaped (Fig. 2.18).

2.3.3 White Blood Cell Clumps

In some purulent urine specimens, WBCs may have indistinct borders and aggregate into clusters (Fig. 2.19).

2.3.4 Old White Blood Cells

If the urine specimen is left for more than 2 h or it is alkaline in pH, significant morphological changes can occur in WBCs. Various types of old WBCs can be observed in such cases, including enlarged cell bodies, cytoplasmic degeneration with granules or vacuoles, nuclear dissolution, or nuclear condensation (Fig. 2.20).

2.3.5 Glitter Cells

The intracellular fluid of WBCs increases in hypotonic urine, resulting in an enlargement of cell volume (Fig. 2.21). The granules within the cytoplasm become coarser, and exhibit faster Brownian motion. These cells show faint sparkling phenomenon under dark field microscope (Fig. 2.22), referred to as "glitter cells" [10]. Glitter cells are most commonly associated with urinary tract infections or pyelonephritis, especially in conditions of low urine osmolality.

2.3.6 Wright's Stain

Wright's stain is a commonly used method for WBC classification. Prior to performing Wright's stain, the sample needs to be prepared as a smear and undergo staining procedures. WBCs are more easily classified after Wright's stain, including neutrophils (Fig. 2.23), eosinophils (Fig. 2.24), basophils, lymphocytes (Fig. 2.25) and monocyte (Fig. 2.26). In some cases, neutro-

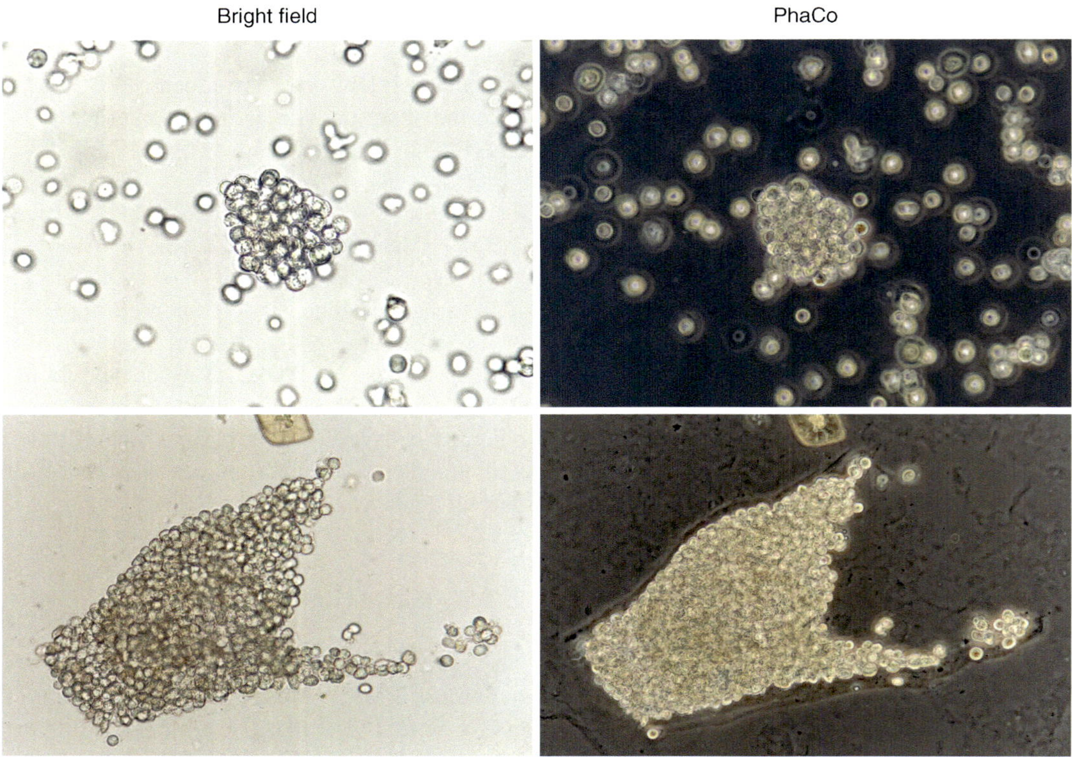

Fig. 2.19 White blood cell clumps. Unstained, ×400

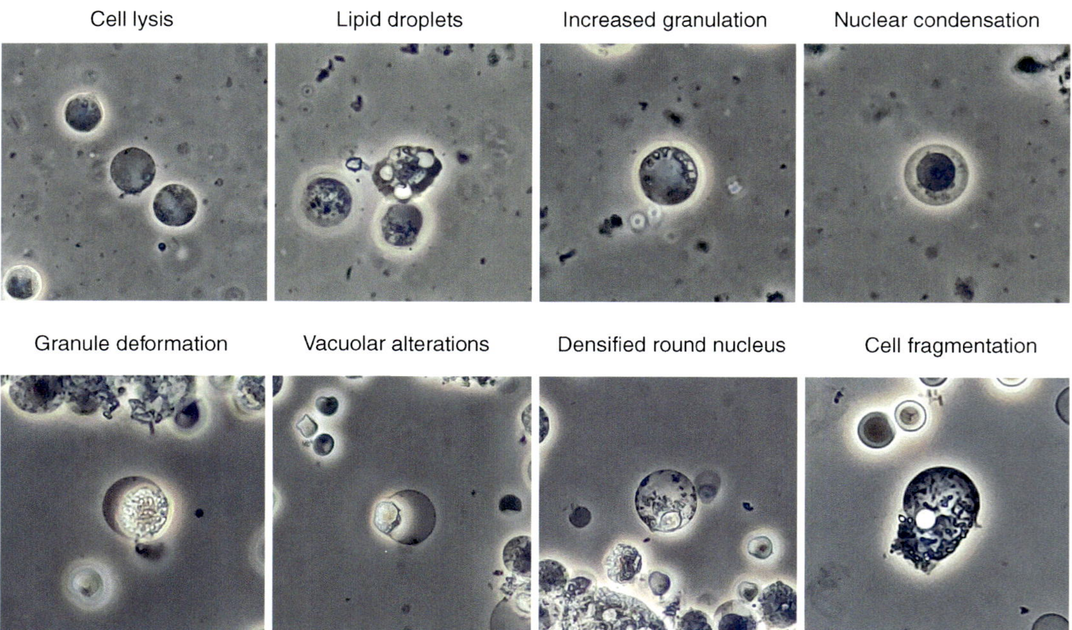

Fig. 2.20 Old WBCs. Unstained, phase contrast microscopy, ×400

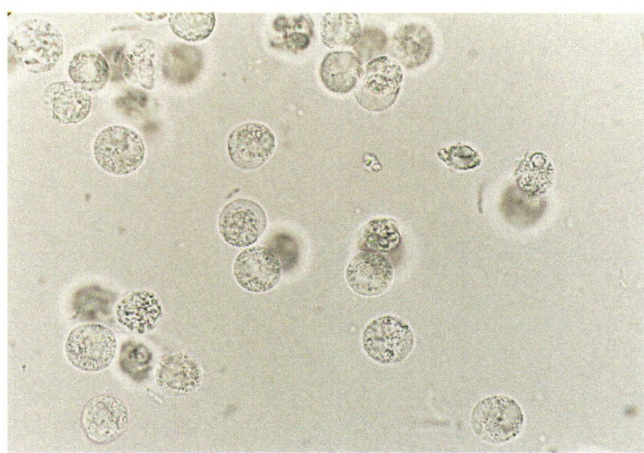

Fig. 2.21 Glitter cells. Unstained, bright field, ×1000

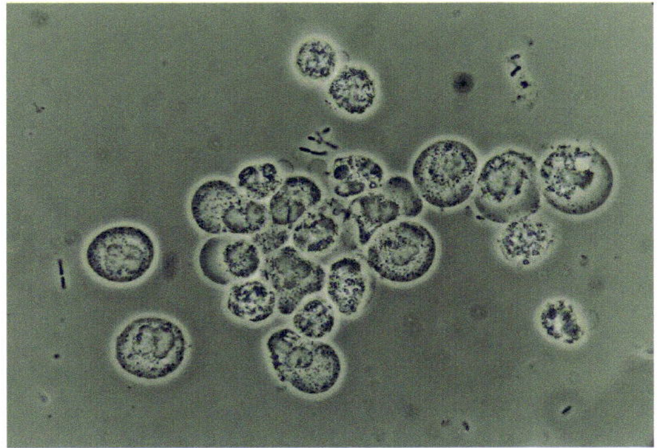

Fig. 2.22 Glitter cells. Unstained, phase contrast microscopy, ×1000

phils can phagocytize a large number of bacteria (Fig. 2.27). However, the morphology of cells may be influenced by the urine environment and collection time, leading to changes in the appearance of stained WBCs, such as irregular cell bodies, increased cytoplasmic granules, or the presence of vacuoles [11].

2.3.7 SM Stain or S Stain

SM stain is a method used to differentiate between living WBCs and dead WBCs. Living WBCs exhibit minimal cytoplasmic staining or appear pale blue (Fig. 2.28), while dead WBCs stain easily, with the cytoplasm appearing pink and the nuclei appearing deep red (Fig. 2.29). The principle of S stain is similar to SM stain, where the cytoplasm of dead WBCs appears purple-red and the nuclei appear blue (Fig. 2.30), while the cytoplasm of living cells appears pink (Fig. 2.31).

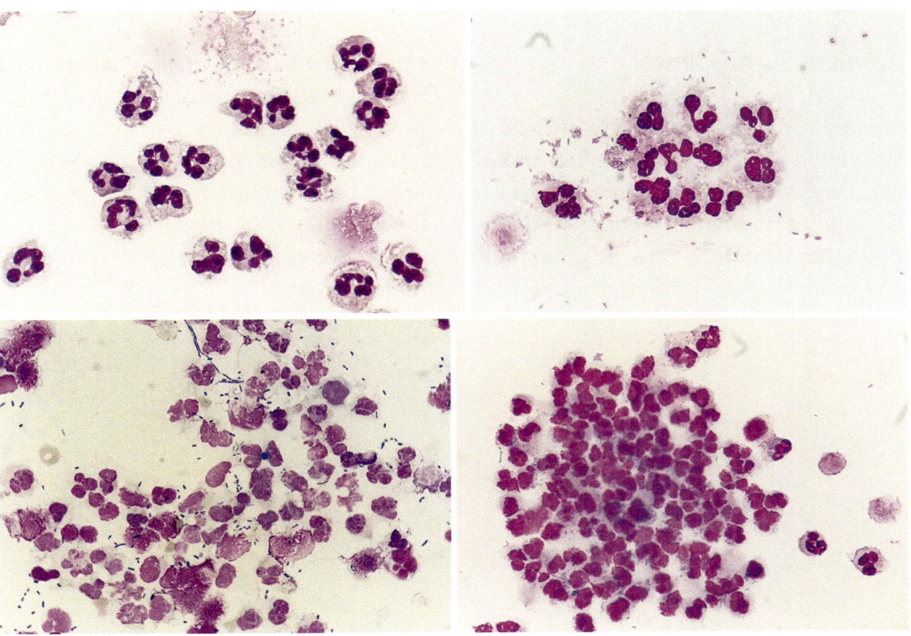

Fig. 2.23 Neutrophils. They are scattered or clustered together, and some cells are incomplete. Wright's stain, ×1000

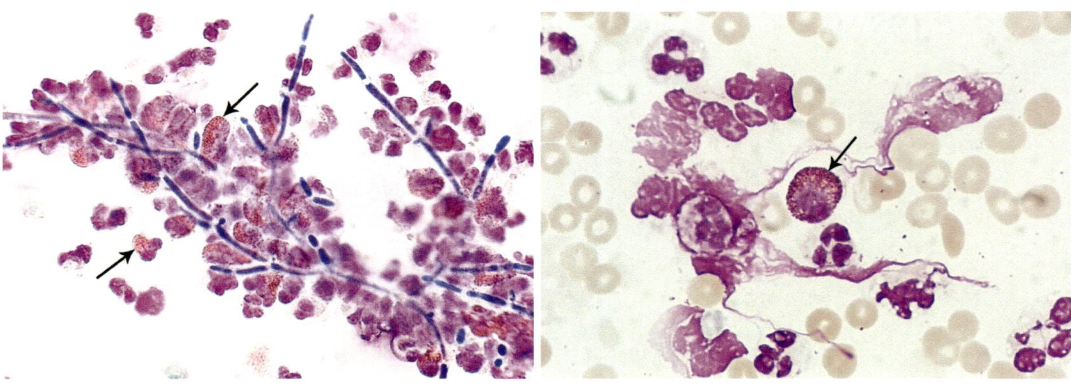

Fig. 2.24 Eosinophils (↑). Orange-red acidophilic granules can be seen inside the cells. Wright's stain, ×1000

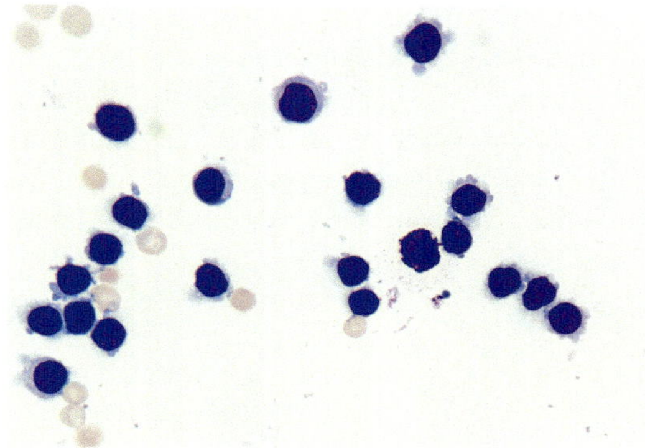

Fig. 2.25 Lymphocyte. They are small in size, with minimal cytoplasm. Wright's stain, ×1000

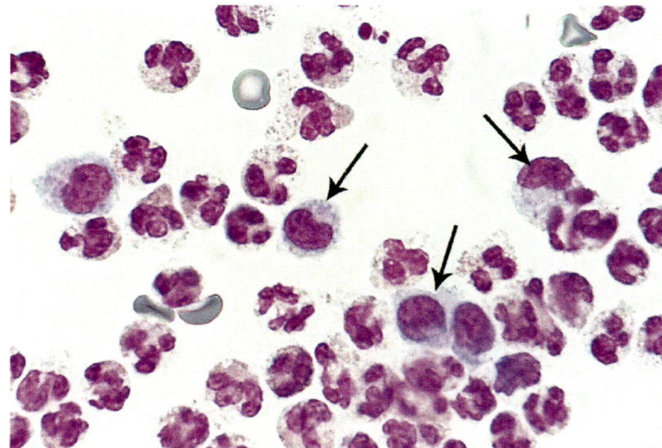

Fig. 2.26 Monocytes (↑). They have a single nucleus, and the nuclear shape is irregular. Wright's stain, ×1000

2.3.8 Clinical Significance

A small amount of white blood cells (<5 cells/HP) is considered normal. After intense physical activity, there may be a temporary increase in WBCs. In pathological conditions, an increased number of neutrophils are commonly observed in urinary system inflammations such as pyelonephritis, prostatitis and urethritis [12]. Increased lymphocyte count can be seen in conditions such as kidney transplant rejection and crescentic glomerulonephritis [13, 14]. An increase in eosinophils is associated with drug-induced interstitial nephritis, allergic reactions and hypersensitivity-related urinary system inflammations [15].

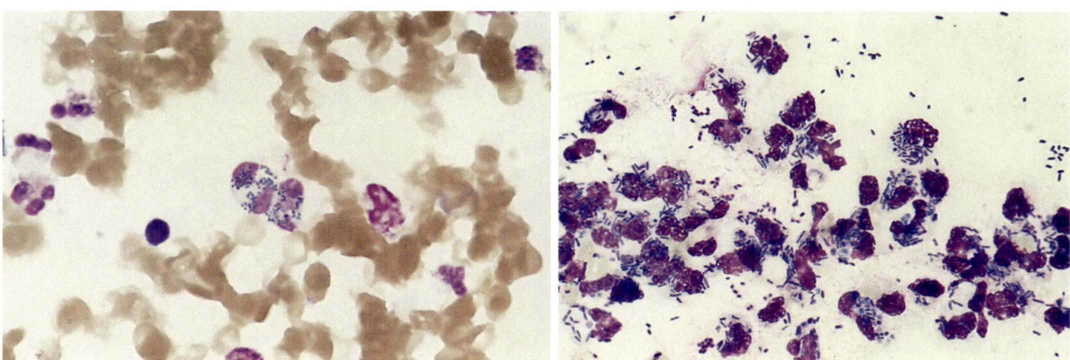

Fig. 2.27 A large number of spherical or bacillus that have been phagocytized can be seen inside the cells. Wright's stain, ×1000

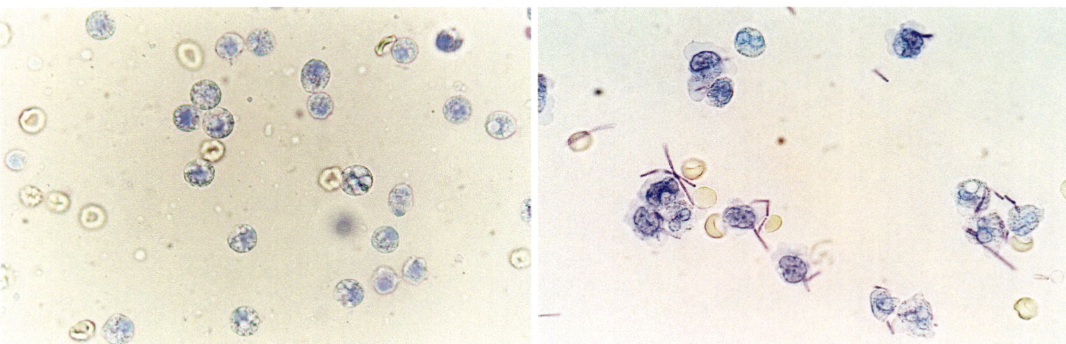

Fig. 2.28 Living WBCs. SM stain, ×1000

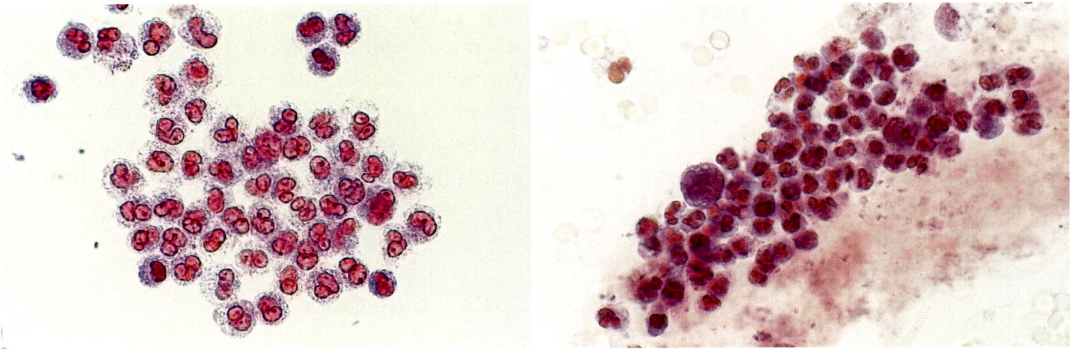

Fig. 2.29 Dead WBCs. The cytoplasm appears pink, and the nuclei appear deep red. SM stain, ×1000

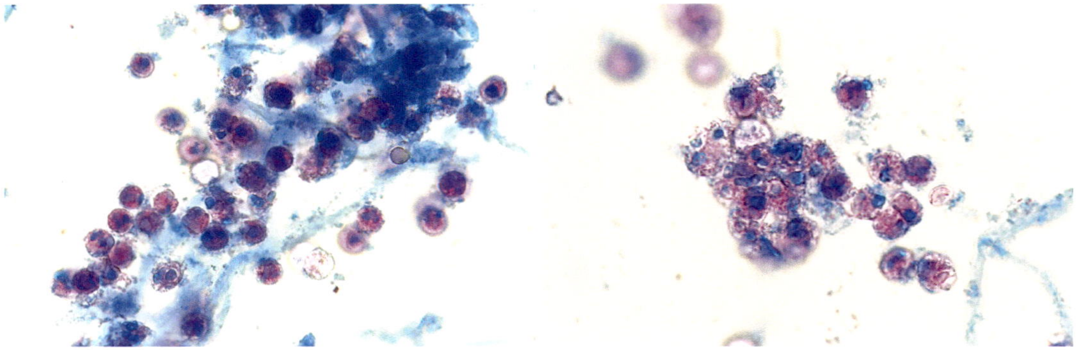

Fig. 2.30 Dead WBCs. The cytoplasm of the cells appears purple-red, and the nuclei stain blue. S stain, ×1000

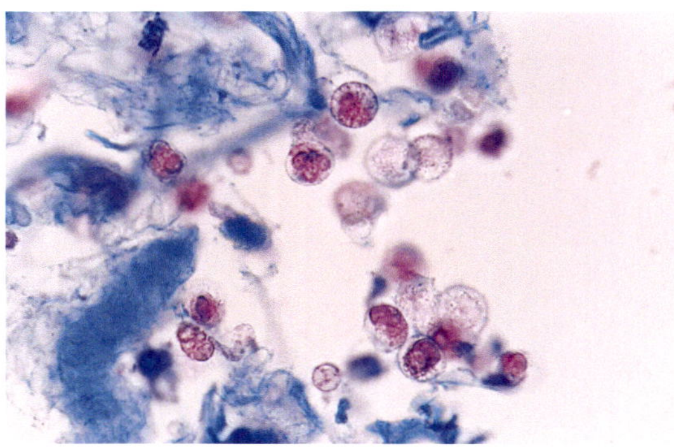

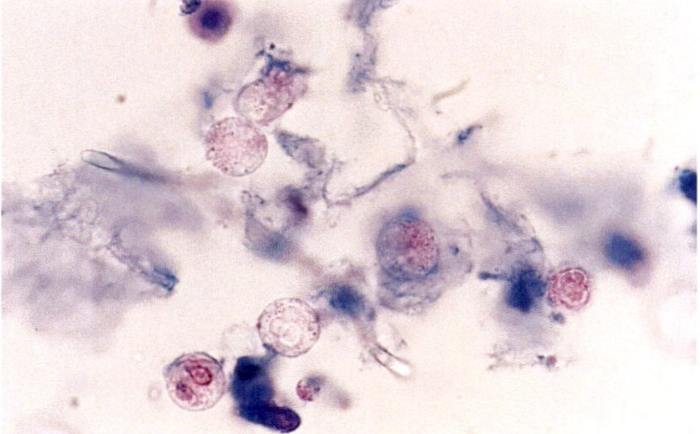

Fig. 2.31 Living WBCs. They appear pink, S stain, ×1000

2.4 Squamous Epithelial Cells (SECs)

2.4.1 Origin

Squamous epithelial cells (SECs) originate from the female vagina and urethra, as well as the distal part of the male urethra [16]. SECs from different layers vary in their size (Fig. 2.32).

2.4.2 Unstained

Unstained SECs are relatively large found in urine, which are quite common. The superficial layer cells are polygonal in shape, with folded edges and abundant cytoplasm, giving them a thin texture. They may contain a small number of granules, and their nuclei are relatively small (Fig. 2.33). The intermediate and basal layers of squamous epithelial cells have a similar cytoplasm thickness to the superficial layer. As you move closer to the basal layer, the cell volume decreases, and the nucleus-to-cytoplasm ratio gradually increases. The cellular bodies in these layers are mostly circular in shape.

2.4.3 Clue Cells

SECs have the ability to adhere to various substances. When a large number of short bacilli adhere to cells, they are referred to as "clue cells" (Fig. 2.34). The presence of clue cells during microscopic examination of urine can provide valuable clues to aid in the diagnosis and evaluation of urinary tract infections or other urethral-related diseases such as bacterial vaginosis.

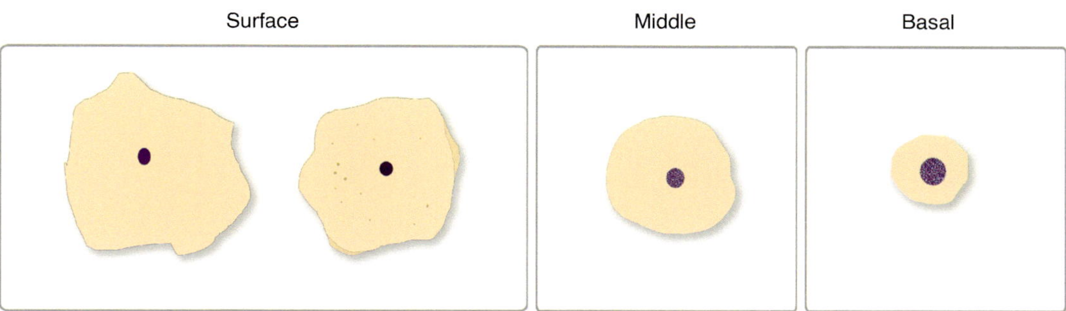

Fig. 2.32 Illustration of squamous epithelial cells

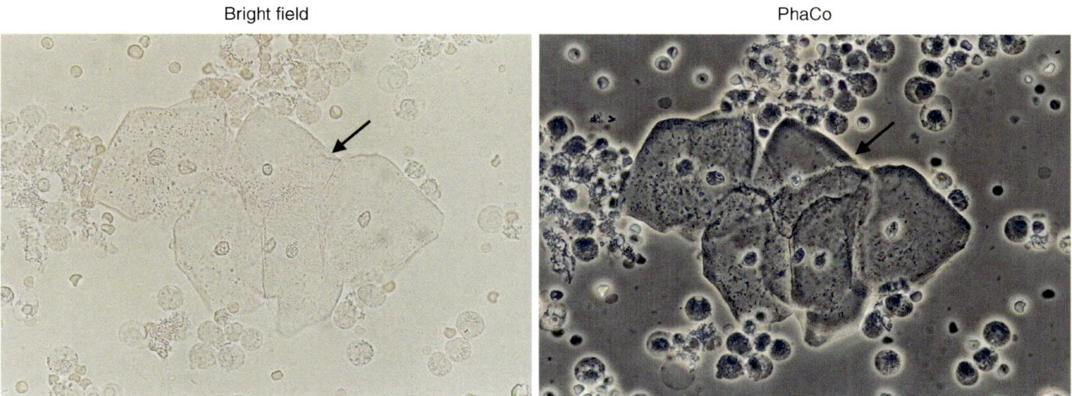

Fig. 2.33 Squamous epithelial cells (↑). Unstained, ×400

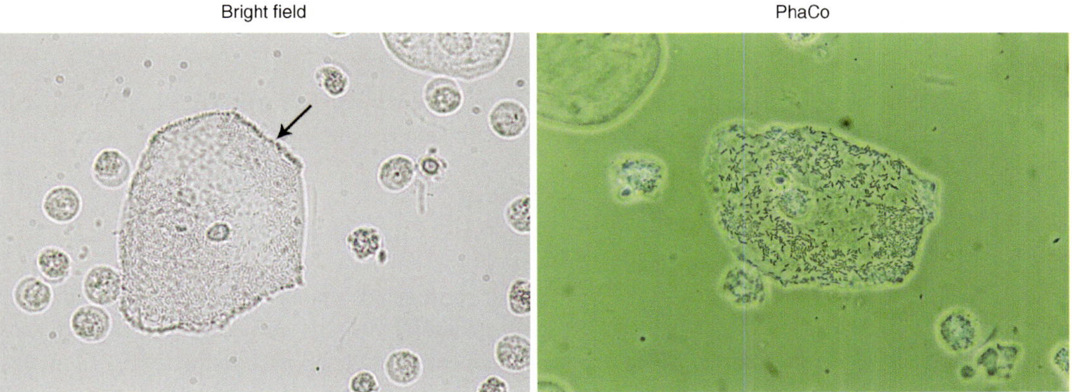

Fig. 2.34 Clue cells. A large number of bacilli adhere to the surface of SECs. Unstained, ×400

2.4.4 SM Stain and S Stain

The purpose of staining is primarily to differentiate SECs from urinary tract epithelial cells. The cytoplasm of SECs appears pale pink after SM staining (Fig. 2.35), with some cells showing few granules. The nuclei are small and appear deep red. Living SECs are not easily stained, and both the cytoplasm and nuclei appear pale blue. After S staining, the cytoplasm of SECs appears

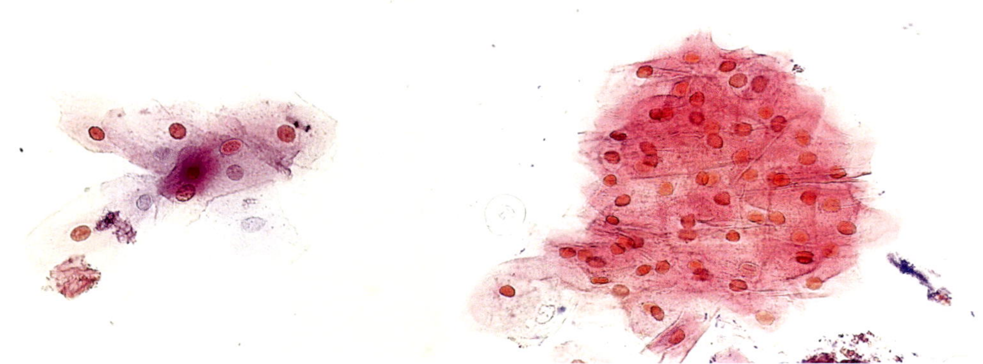

Fig. 2.35 SECs. The cytoplasm appears pink, while the nuclei are stained darker. SM stain, ×400

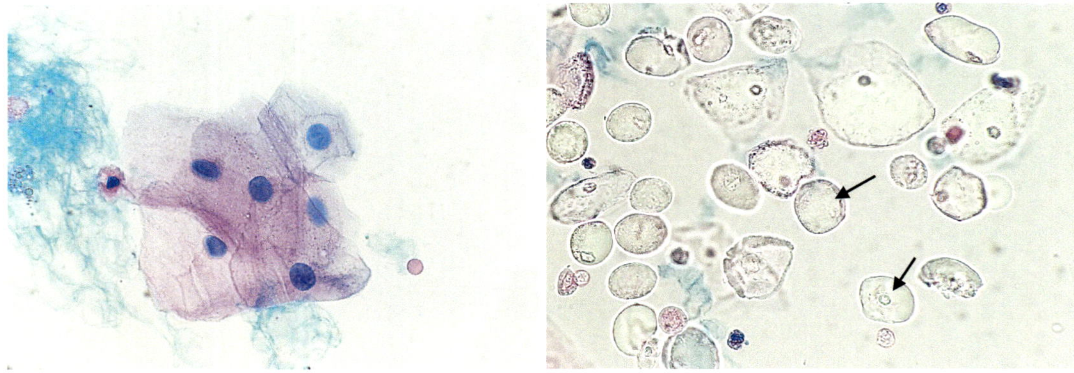

Fig. 2.36 SECs. The cytoplasm appears purplish-red, while the nuclei appear blue. Some cells are not easy to color (↑). S stain, ×400

purplish-red, and the nuclei appear blue. Some living cells may have nuclei that appear purple-red (Fig. 2.36).

2.4.5 Other Squamous Epithelial Cells

In some cases, SECs can adhere to some amorphous salts (Fig. 2.37). These cells generally have no clinical significance and are commonly observed in old urine specimens.

In some bilirubinuria samples, SECs may exhibit needle-like or granular bilirubin crystals within their cytoplasm (Fig. 2.38). The clinical significance is similar to bilirubin crystals.

2.4.6 Clinical Significance

The presence of a small number of SECs in urine is generally not clinically significant. They are more commonly observed in the urine of females and may be attributed to contamination from vaginal secretions. In urinary tract infections, the presence of clue cells in female urine often indicates a vaginal infection [17].

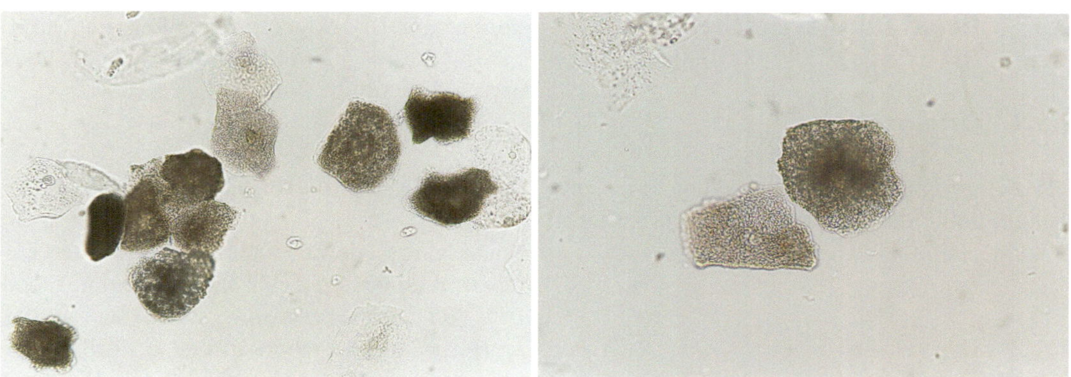

Fig. 2.37 SECs adhere to crystals, and they may appear dark brown. Unstained, ×400

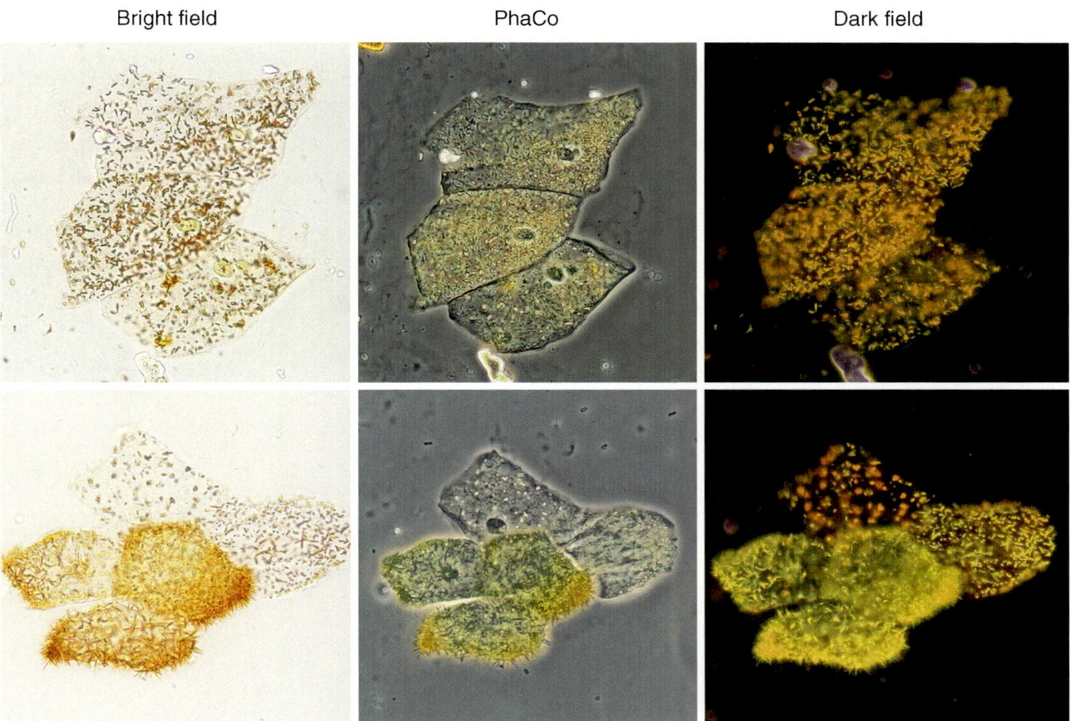

Fig. 2.38 Bilirubin crystals can be observed within the SECs. Unstained, ×400

2.5 Renal Tubular Epithelial Cells (RTE Cells)

2.5.1 Origin

RTE cells originate from the shedding of the epithelium lining the various segments of the renal tubules, exhibiting variable sizes and shapes.

2.5.2 Unstained

RTE cells detach in response to various stimuli, and their morphology is diverse and influenced by pH and osmotic pressure. They can exhibit cuboidal, polygonal, serrated, round, or oval shapes. The cytoplasm of RTE cells is granular, and the nucleus is typically round or oval in shape. In some cells, the nucleus may not be clearly visible. Unstained cytoplasm of RTE cells appears grayish-white or pale yellow (Fig. 2.39), but in cases of high bilirubinuria, the cells may appear dark yellow (Fig. 2.40).

2.5.3 SM Stain and S Stain

Staining methods are primarily used to differentiate basal urinary epithelial cells from white blood cells. RTE cells are readily stained and appear with a pale red cytoplasm and a deep purple nucleus after SM staining (Fig. 2.41). The cytoplasm appears purplish-red, and the nucleus appears blue after S staining (Fig. 2.42). The color may vary slightly due to the differences in urine pH.

In some cases of acute tubular necrosis, a large number of RTE cells are exfoliated. These cells exhibit increased cell volume, degeneration of intracytoplasmic granules, increased

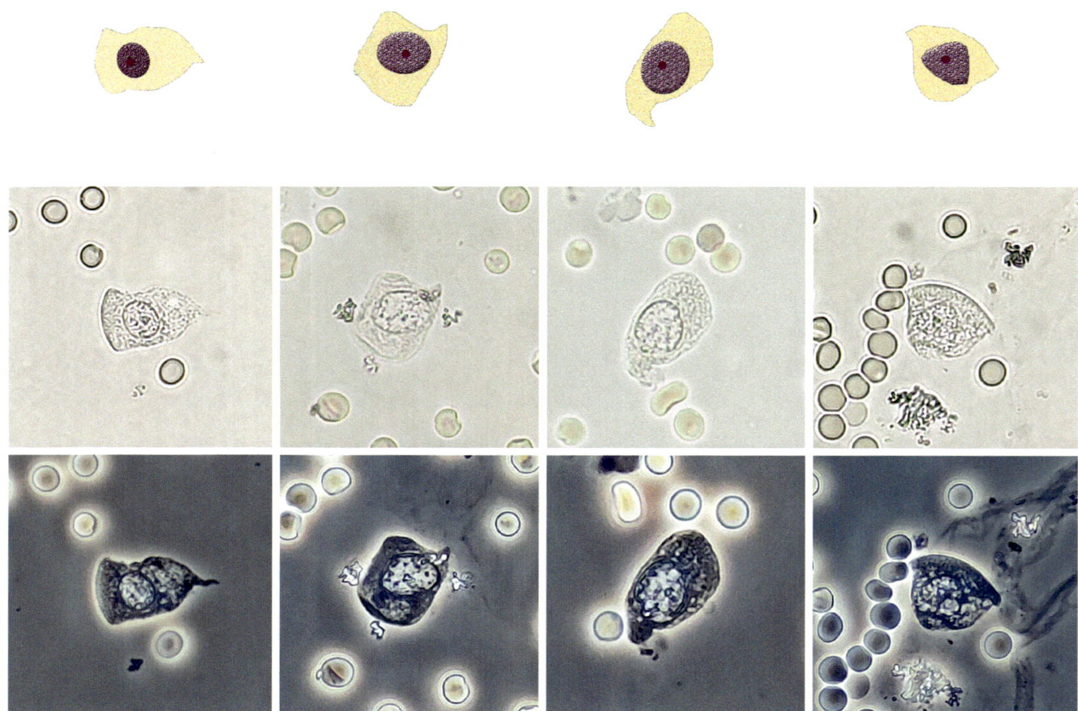

Fig. 2.39 RTE cells. Unstained, bright field, and phase contrast, ×1000

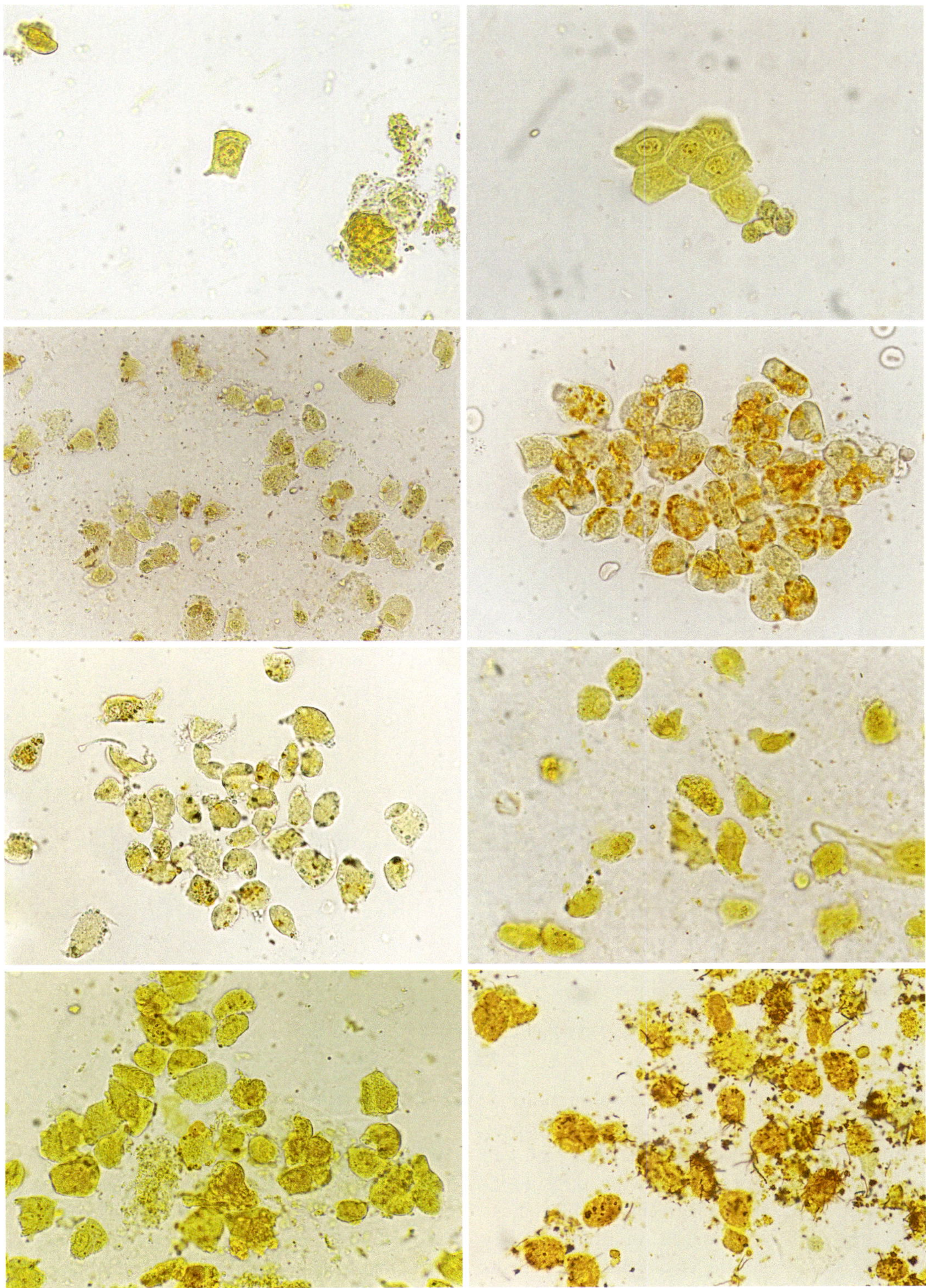

Fig. 2.40 RTE cells. Bilirubinuria, bright field, ×1000

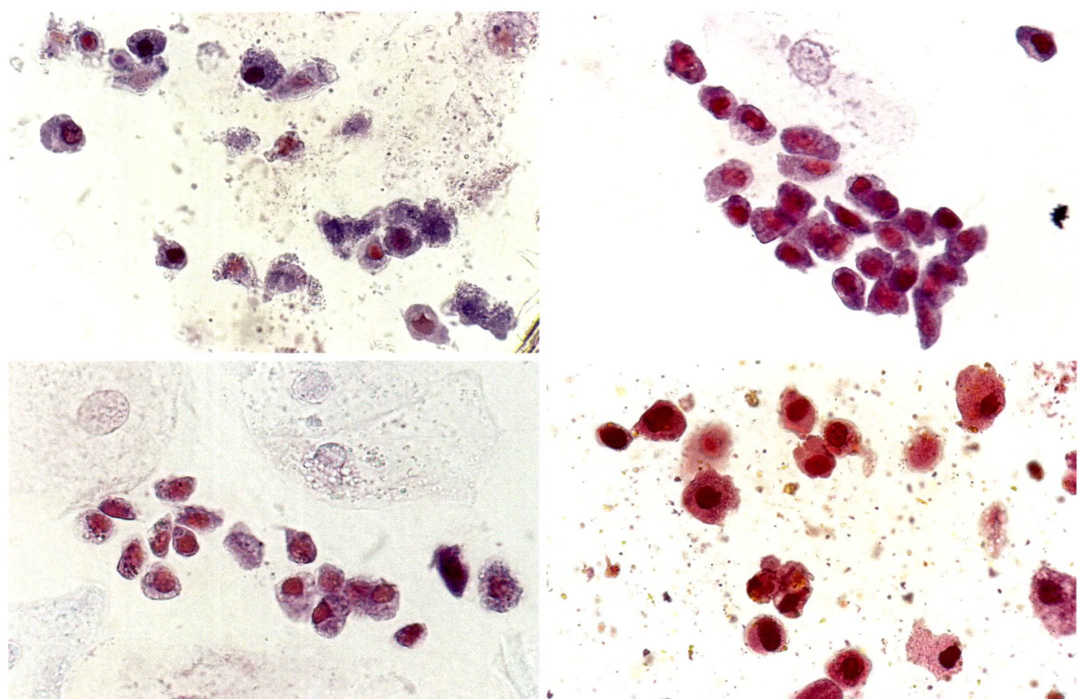

Fig. 2.41 RTE cells. The cytoplasm appears purplish-red, and the nucleus is stained darker. SM stain, ×1000

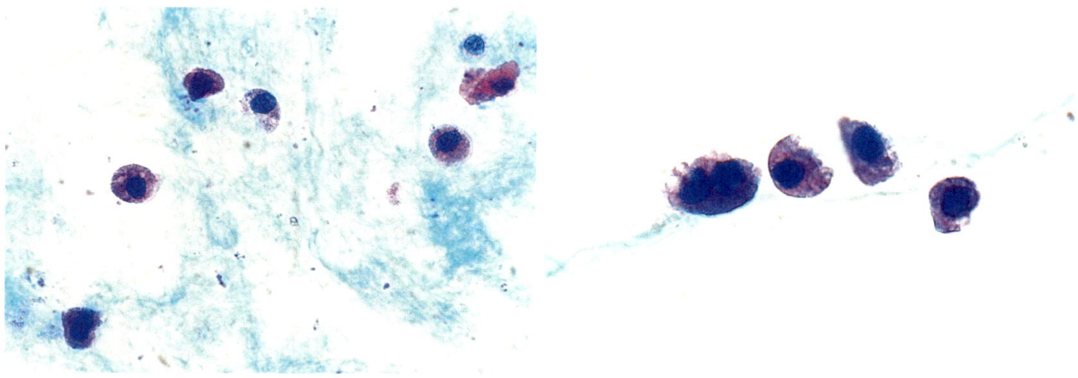

Fig. 2.42 RTE cells. The cytoplasm appears purplish-red, and the nucleus appears blue. S stain, ×1000

and coarsened granules, and variable morphological changes. Some cells may appear as long columnar shapes [18]. After staining, the cell nuclei can be observed, allowing differentiation from other substances (Fig. 2.43). These cells are mainly observed in acute kidney injury (AKI) resulting from various causes (Fig. 2.44).

2.5.4 Wright's Stain

RTE cells exhibit varying sizes and shapes after Wright's staining. They commonly appear polygonal in shape. The cytoplasm shows a purplish-red or bluish-gray color, while the nucleus is round and displays condensed chromatin, resulting in a deeper staining (Fig. 2.45).

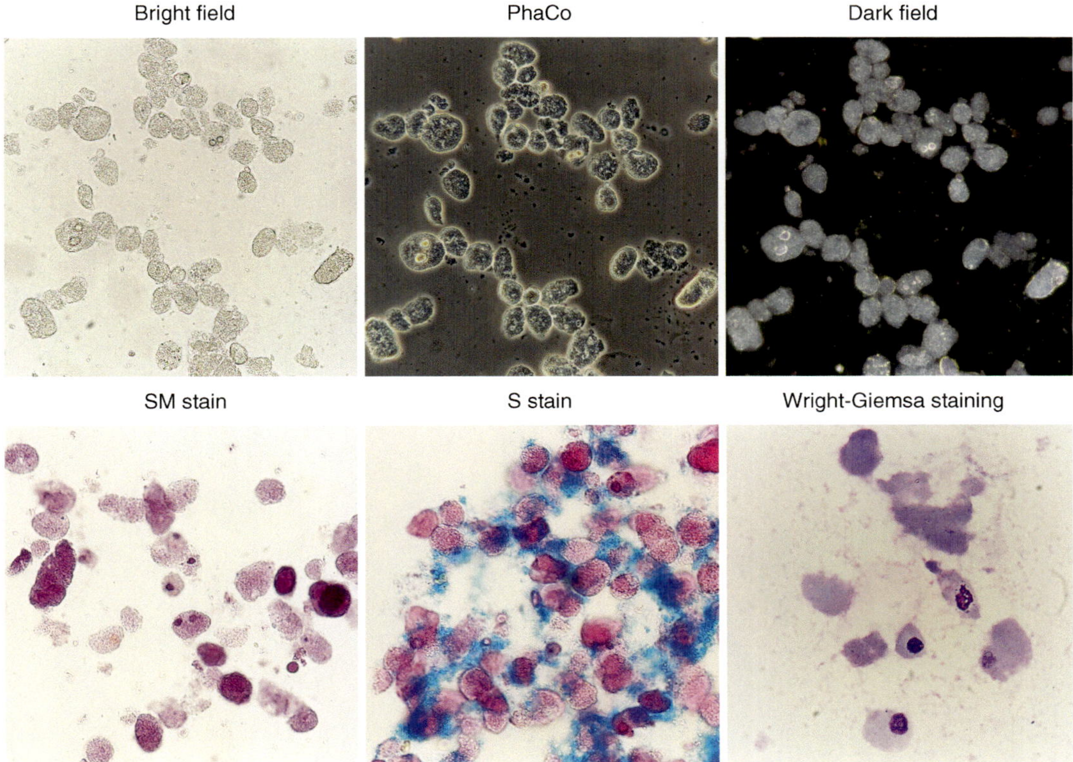

Fig. 2.43 Acute tubular necrosis. The exfoliation of cells is significantly increased, enlargement of cell bodies, increased and coarsened intracytoplasmic granules. The nuclei of most cells are not clearly visible, ×400

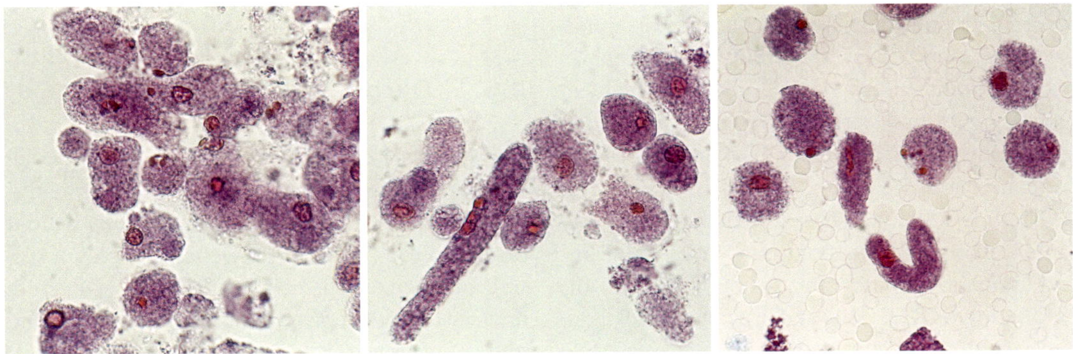

Fig. 2.44 Acute kidney injury caused by trauma, with a significant exfoliation of RTE cells. SM stain, ×1000

2.5.5 Clinical Significance

In normal individuals, RTE cells are rarely or occasionally observed in urine. An increased exfoliation of RTE cells indicates tubular injury, while their presence in clusters often suggests tubular necrosis. Neonatal urine may contain renal tubular epithelial cells [19].

Acute tubular necrosis [20] can be caused by factors such as renal ischemia (due to conditions

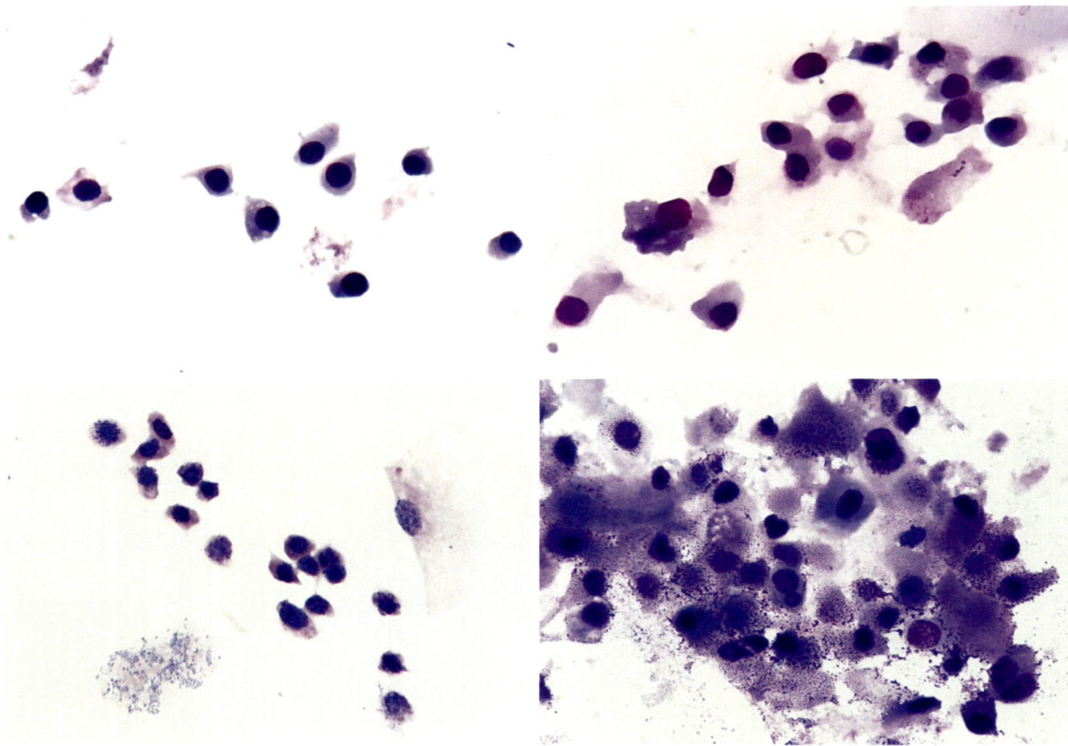

Fig. 2.45 RTE cells. Wright's stain, ×1000

like traumatic shock, surgical or obstetric bleeding, congestive heart failure, cardiac surgery, severe dehydration caused by diarrhea or vomiting, severe burns, severe hemolysis) or nephrotoxicity induced by heavy metals (such as mercury, arsenic), organophosphate pesticides, and nephrotoxic substances like antibiotics and anticancer drugs.

Chronic kidney diseases, including glomerulonephritis, nephrotic syndrome, pyelonephritis, and diabetic nephropathy, often result in the exfoliation of RTE cells and are commonly associated with positive urine protein [21].

In other conditions such as jaundice, amino acid metabolism disorders, rhabdomyolysis, hemolytic uremic syndrome, post-renal transplant and post-transplant rejection reactions, the renal tubular epithelium may also be exfoliated.

2.6 Decoy Cells

Decoy cells are RTE cells or urothelial cells that have been infected by the papillomavirus (polyomavirus, PV). The nuclei of these cells exhibit characteristic changes. These cells display a significant increase in cell and nuclear size, with nuclear changes resembling a balloon or ground glass appearance (Fig. 2.46). Due to the morphological similarity between decoy cells and urothelial cancer cells, staining methods can be used for differentiation.

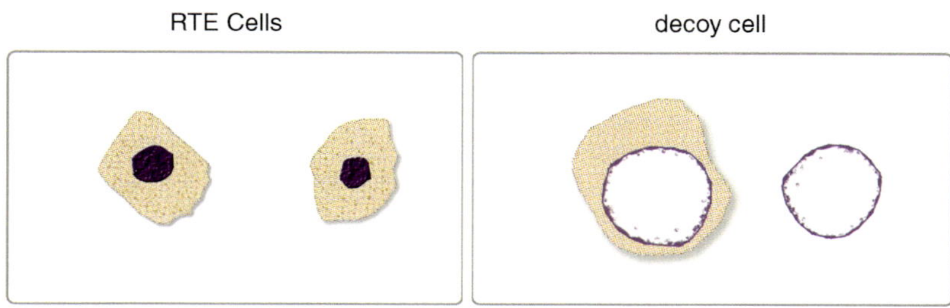

Fig. 2.46 Diagram of RTE cells and decoy cells

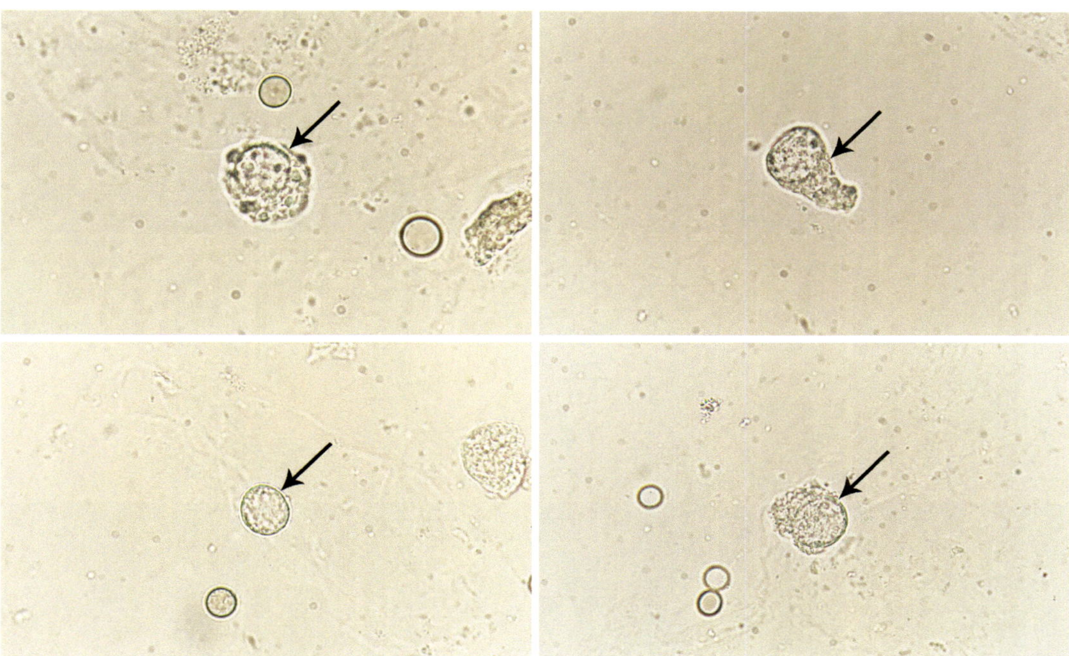

Fig. 2.47 Decoy cells (↑). The nuclei appear vacuolated. Unstained, bright field, ×1000

2.6.1 Unstained

Decoy cells are observed under a bright field microscope. These cells show an increase in cell size and enlarged nuclei with a vacuolated appearance, and some cells may have indistinct structures. Inclusion bodies within the cell nuclei are not easily visible, which can result in potential missed detection (Fig. 2.47). The structures of decoy cells are more discernible during phase contrast microscopy. Observations can reveal vacuole-like cell nuclei and nucleolar inclusions of various sizes (Fig. 2.48).

2.6.2 SM Stain and S Stain

The greatest advantage of SM stain method is the preservation of the cellular morphology. It is simple to perform and can provide quick staining and minimize the risk of missing cells. Decoy cells exhibit varying cell sizes and irregular shapes after SM stain. The cytoplasm appears bluish-purple, while the nuclei exhibit vacuolated changes with a reddish-purple color. The cytoplasmic granularity varies, with coarse granules and enlarged nuclei that are noticeably eccentric, thickened nuclear membranes, and a relatively

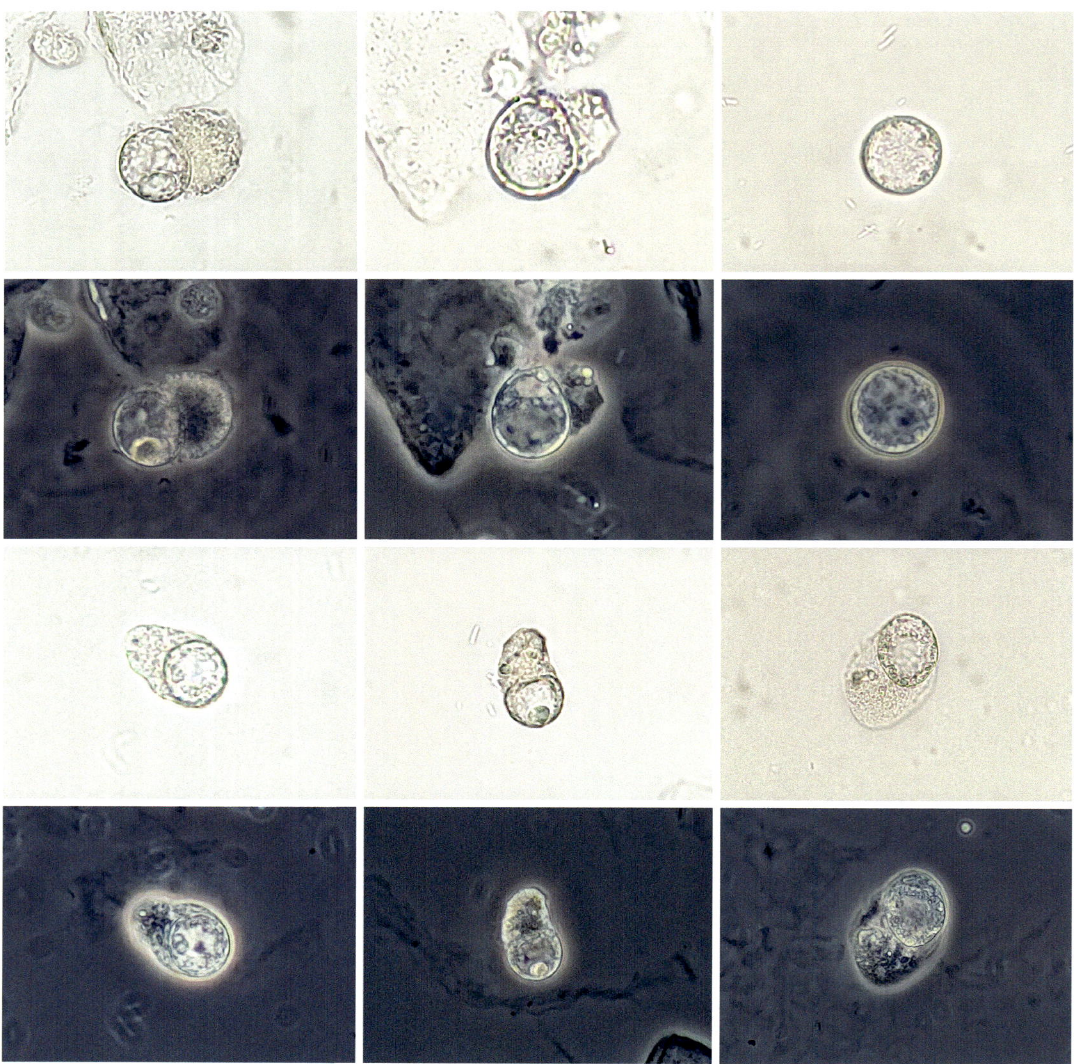

Fig. 2.48 Decoy cells. Unstained, bright field, and phase contrast microscopy, ×1000

higher nuclear-to-cytoplasmic ratio. The nuclear chromatin structure appears disrupted, with coarse granules or clumps. Some cells may contain intranuclear viral inclusions, while a small number of cells may show nuclear extrusion, revealing naked nuclei (Fig. 2.49). Decoy cells show a distinct contrast in color between the cytoplasm and nucleus after S staining. The cytoplasm appears purplish-red, while the nuclei appear deep blue. Intranuclear viral inclusions of varying sizes are observed, exhibiting a deep blue color (Fig. 2.50) [22].

2.6.3 Clinical Significance

Some patients who receive kidney or bone marrow transplants and those who are undergoing prolonged immunosuppressive treatment, as well as individuals with compromised immune function, are at an increased risk of polyomavirus (PV) infection. In the case of such an infection, decoy cells can be detected in the patient's urine. In patients who have undergone kidney transplantation, PV infection can lead to transplant renal dysfunction and polyomavirus-asso-

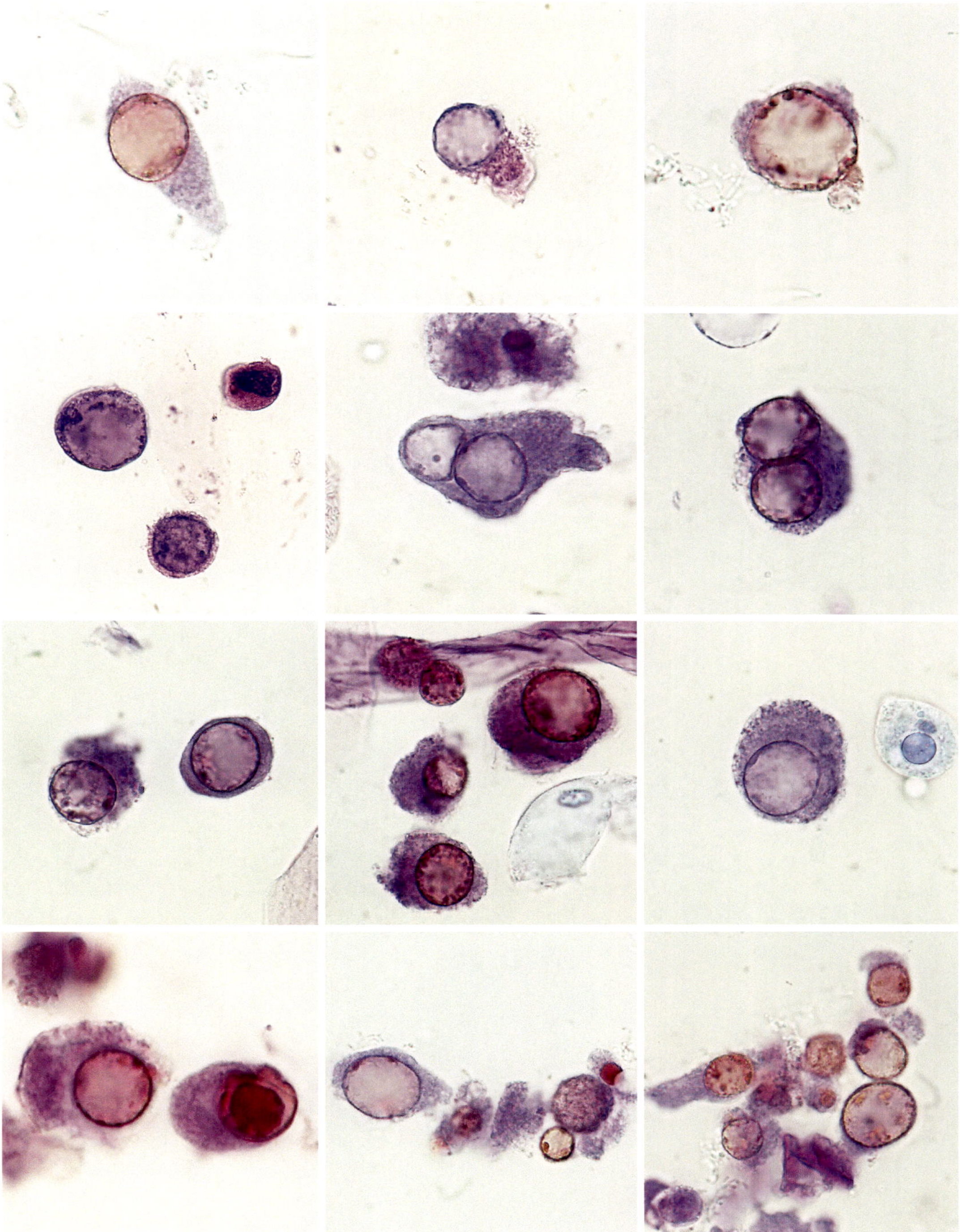

Fig. 2.49 Decoy cells. The cell volume and nucleus size increase, and the nuclei appear vacuolated with thickened nuclear membranes. SM stain, ×1000

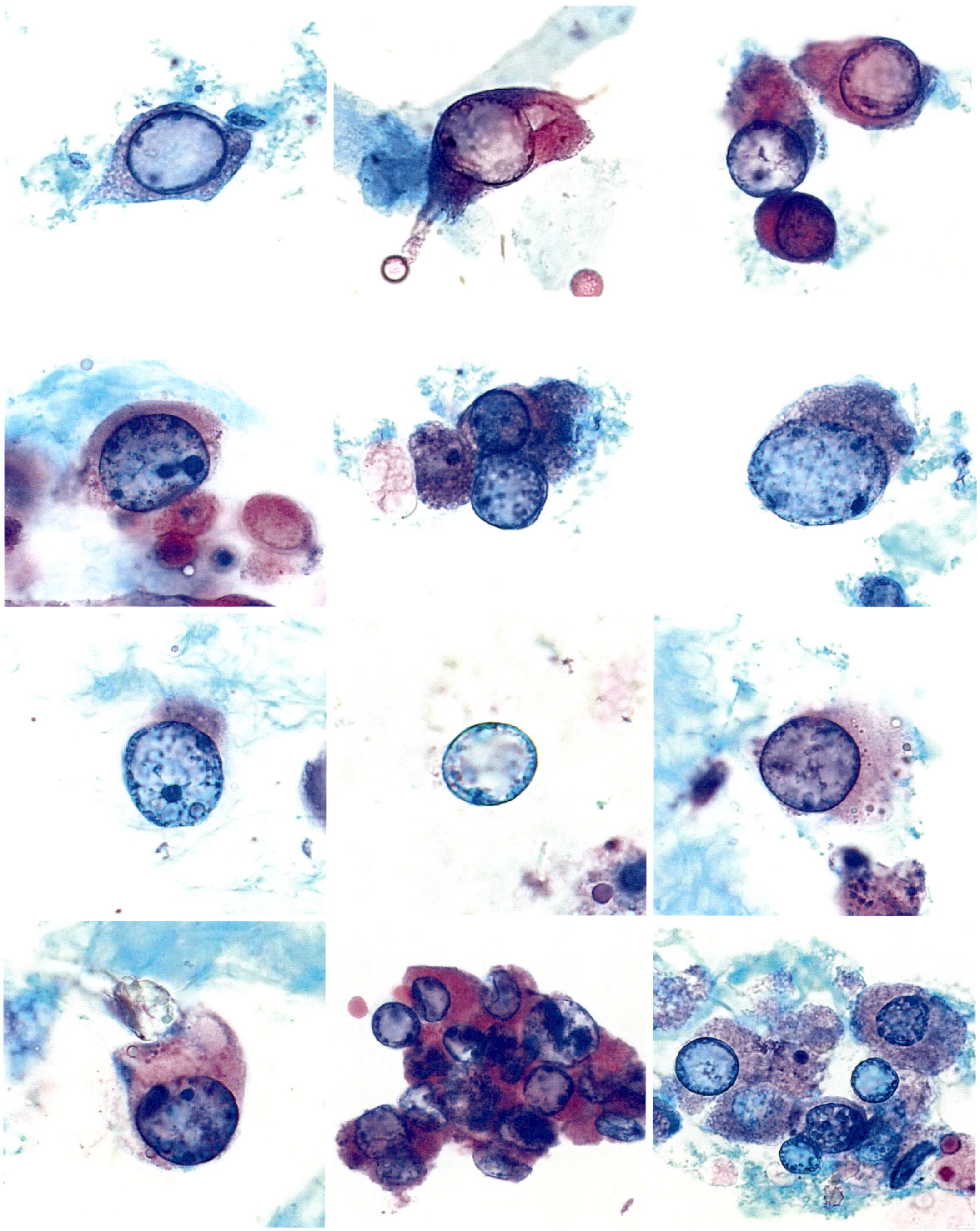

Fig. 2.50 Decoy cells. The cytoplasm appears purplish-red, while the nucleus is blue, and the inclusions are more deeply stained. S stain, ×1000

ciated nephropathy (PVAN). PV can also remain latent in the body and rapidly activate and replicate when the immune system is compromised, resulting in a sudden decline or loss of transplant kidney function. The detection of decoy cells in urine can be followed by specific nucleic acid tests for polyomaviruses such as BK virus and JC virus to confirm the diagnosis.

2.7 Oval Fat Bodies: Intracellular Lipid Droplets

2.7.1 Origin

Oval fat bodies are formed when renal tubular epithelial cells undergo lipid droplet degeneration or accumulate a large amount of fat. They are also known as fatty granular cells.

2.7.2 Unstained

These cells vary in size and are filled with lipid droplets, which are unevenly sized, are highly refractile, and appear pale yellow. They can cover the cell nucleus (Fig. 2.51).

2.7.3 SM Stain or S Stain

The lipid droplets within the cytoplasm are not stained after SM staining or S staining (Figs. 2.52 and 2.53).

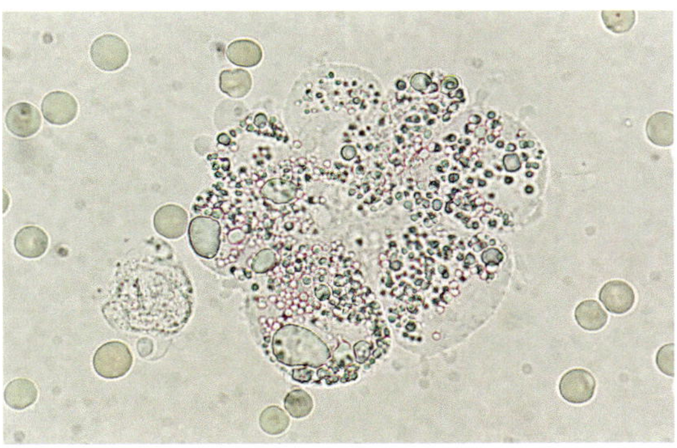

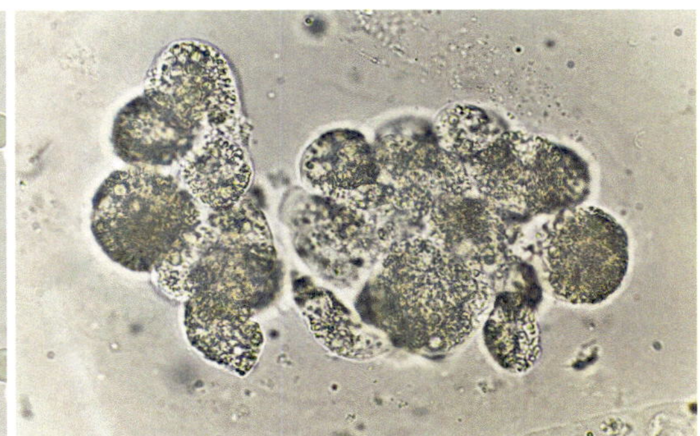

Fig. 2.51 Oval fat bodies. Unstained, bright field, ×1000

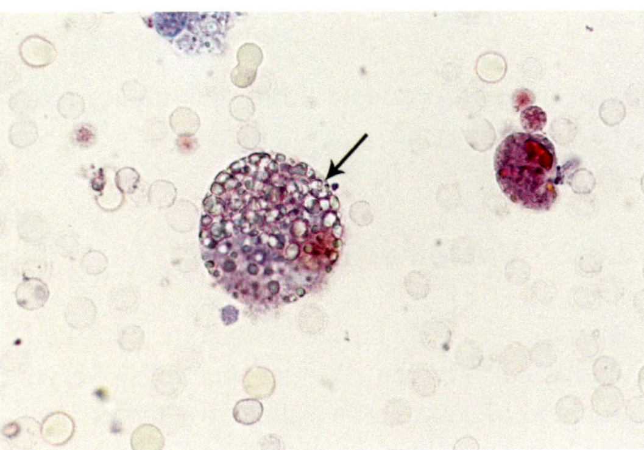

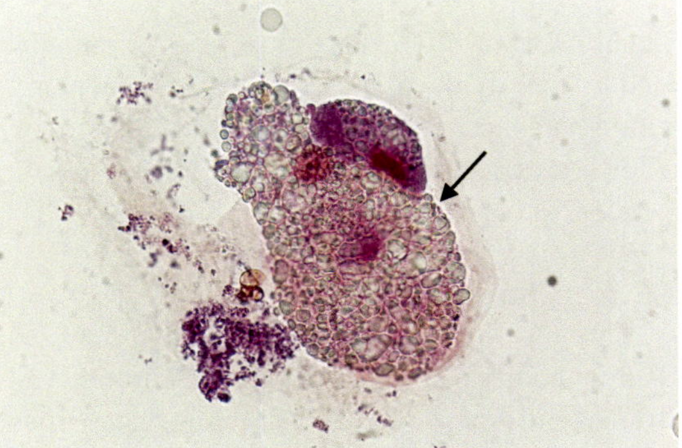

Fig. 2.52 Oval fat bodies (↑). The lipid droplets within the cytoplasm are not stained. SM stain, ×1000

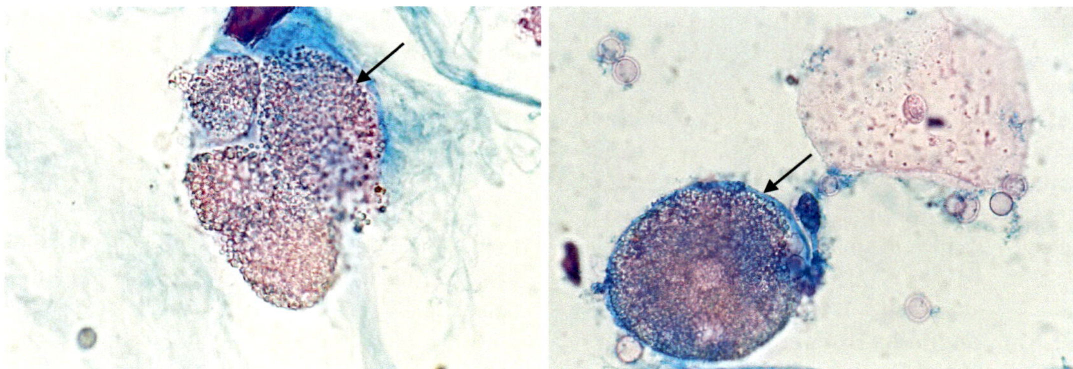

Fig. 2.53 Oval fat bodies (↑). The lipid droplets within the cytoplasm are not stained and appear as small granules. S stain, ×1000

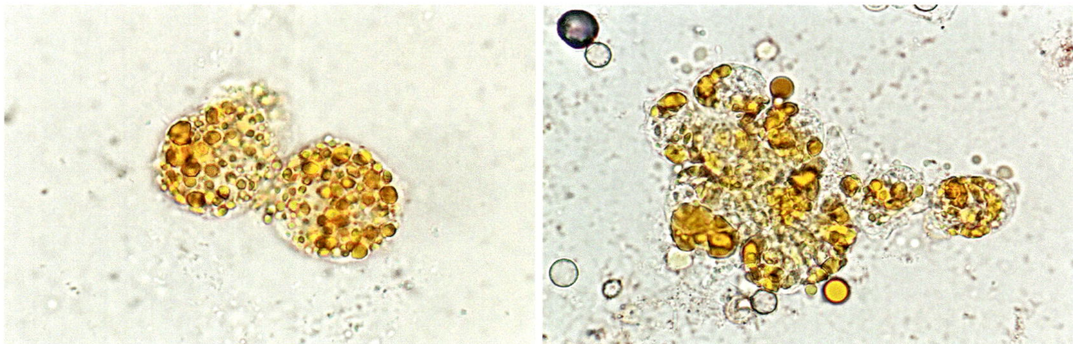

Fig. 2.54 Oval fat bodies. The lipid droplets within the cytoplasm appear orange. Sudan III stain, ×1000

2.7.4 Sudan III Stain or Oil Red O Stain

Sudan III stain or Oil Red O stain is commonly used to identify the presence of lipid components within cells or casts. They appear orange or reddish-orange after staining (Fig. 2.54).

2.7.5 Clinical Significance

Oval fat bodies can be observed in nephrotic syndrome, and some studies have suggested that these cells may also be present in patients with autosomal dominant polycystic kidney disease (ADPKD) [23].

2.8 Macrophages (Histiocytes)

2.8.1 Origin

Macrophages originate from the mononuclear phagocyte system.

2.8.2 Unstained

Macrophages vary in size, with some cells being significantly larger. Within the cells, varying numbers of granules, vacuoles, or larger inclusion bodies may be observed (Fig. 2.55). In some histiocytes, engulfed bacteria, RBCs, or WBCs can be seen. The nuclei of these cells may appear

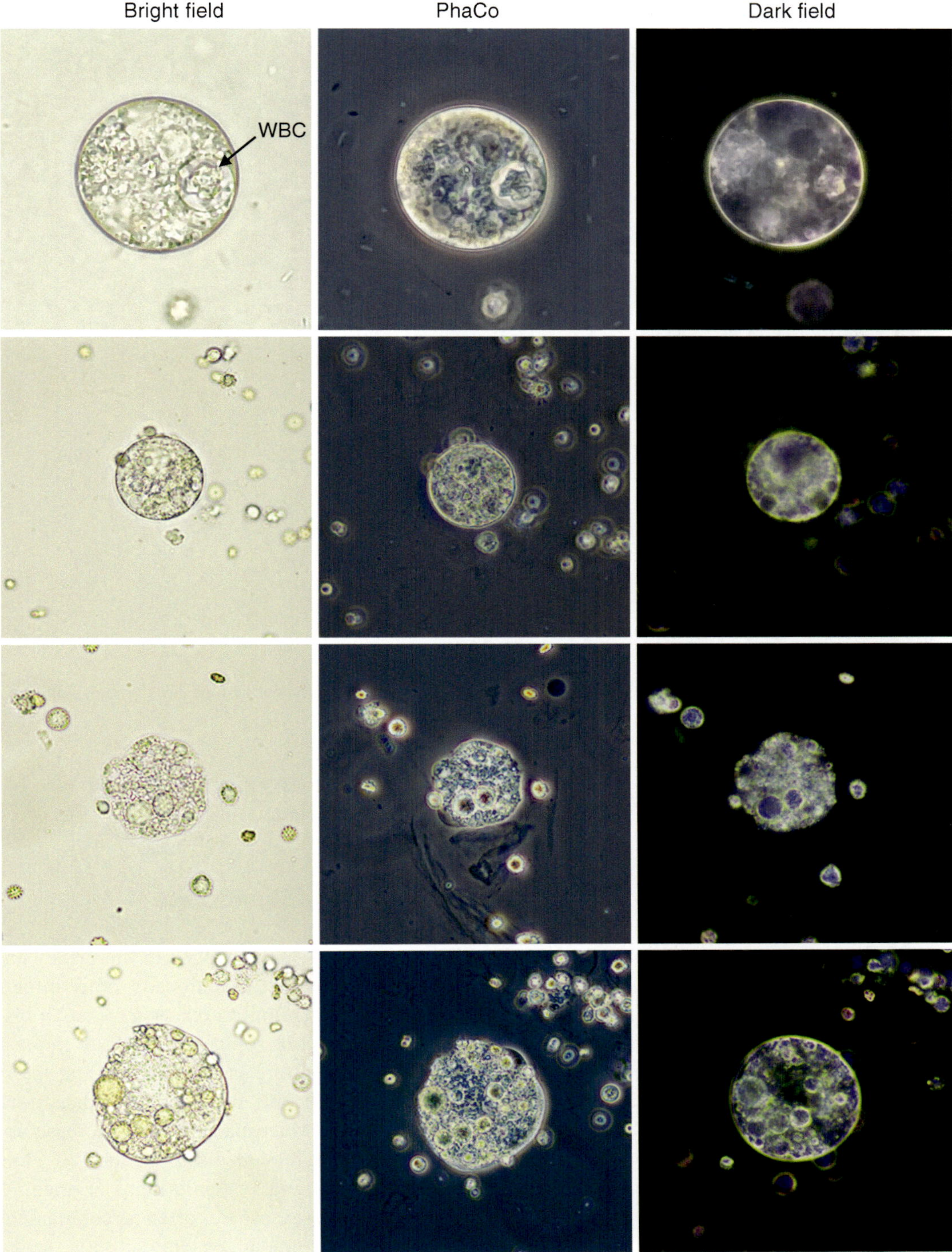

Fig. 2.55 Macrophages. The cell sizes vary, and fat droplets and inclusion bodies can be observed, ×1000

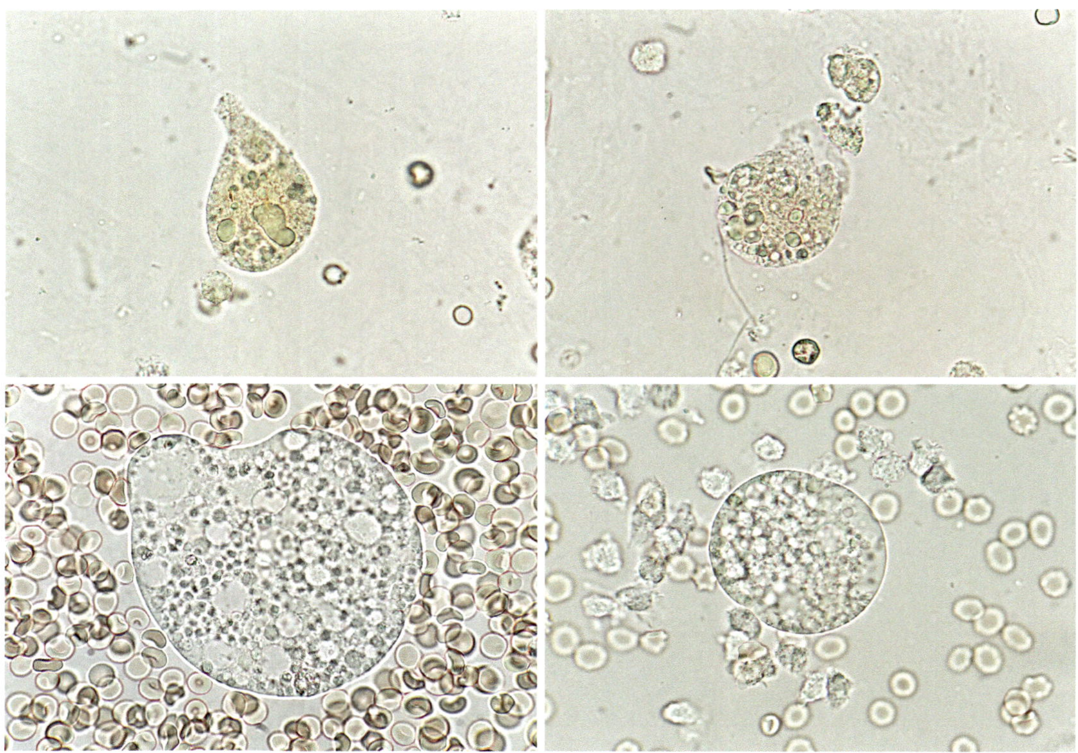

Fig. 2.56 Macrophages, with significant variation in cell size. There are inclusions of various sizes in the cytoplasm, and some cells do not have a visible nucleus. Unstained, bright field, ×1000

indistinct or dissolve. These cells are often mistaken for oval fat bodies (Fig. 2.56).

2.8.3 SM Stain or S Stain

The structure of macrophages is easily recognizable after staining, and the identification of engulfed substances within the cells can be achieved, especially bacteria, RBCs, WBCs, and inclusion bodies. The inclusion bodies within the cytoplasm of macrophages appear in varying sizes and are deeply stained, while lipid substances do not stain after SM staining. The cytoplasm of dead cells appears red or purplish-red (Figs. 2.57 and 2.58), while the cytoplasm of living cells has an overall bluish (Fig. 2.59). After S staining, inclusions within the cells can also be observed (Fig. 2.60).

2.8.4 Clinical Significance

The presence of macrophages in the urine can indicate urinary tract infections or other infections of the genitourinary system, such as pyelonephritis. Macrophages play an important role in engulfing pathogens, making their presence significant for infection detection and diagnosis. Macrophages may increase in certain immune-related diseases, such as glomerulonephritis and systemic lupus erythematosus. These diseases are often accompanied by abnormal immune system activity, lead-

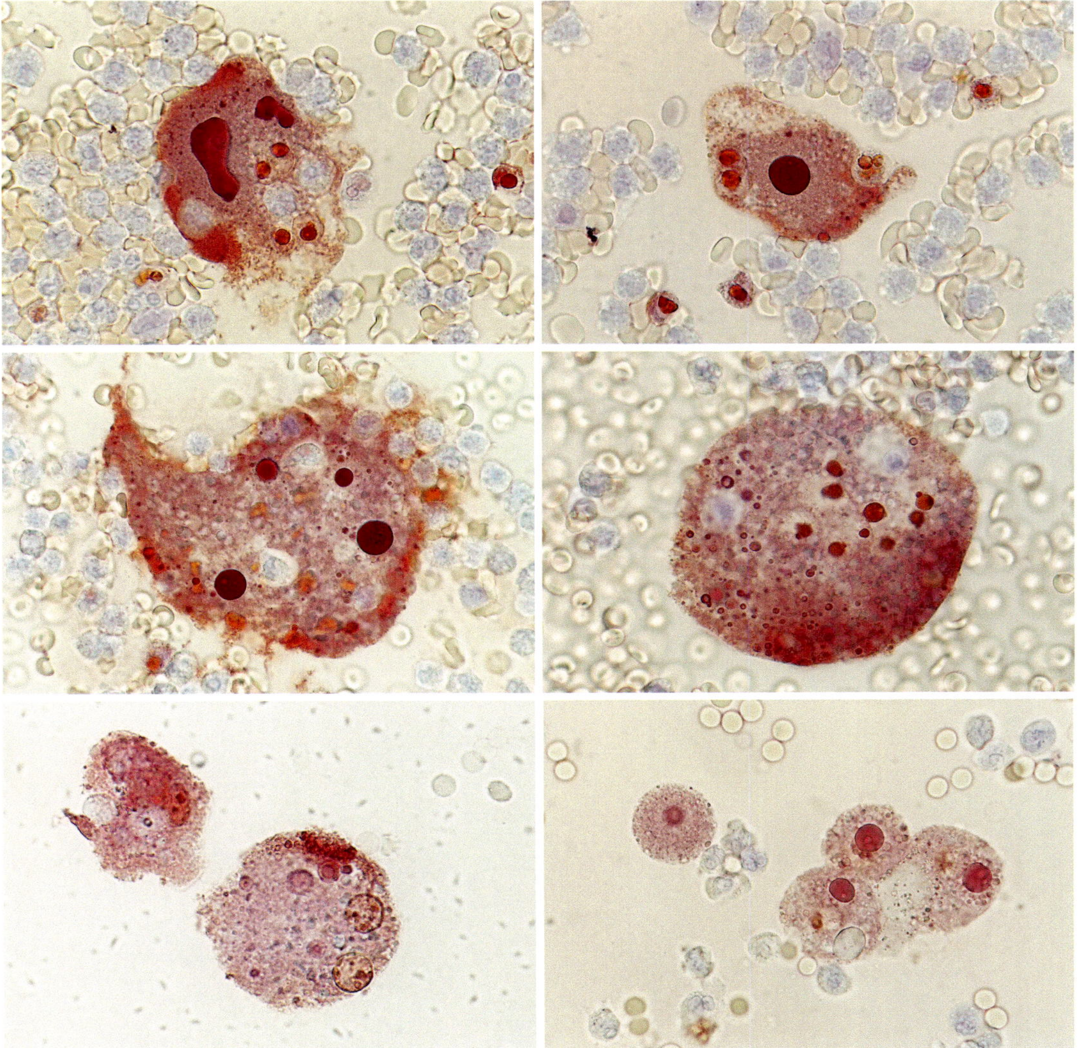

Fig. 2.57 Macrophages exhibit significantly larger cell volumes compared to RBCs in the background, and they can engulf WBCs. SM stain, ×1000

ing to changes in the number and function of macrophages.

Some cases of urinary system tumors can cause an increase in macrophages in the urine. Macrophages are involved in the clearance and regulation of tumors, so their presence may be associated with tumor activity. Macrophages may appear in certain genitourinary system disorders, such as renal tubular dysfunction and glomerular diseases. Their presence may reflect inflammatory responses or tissue damage associated with these diseases.

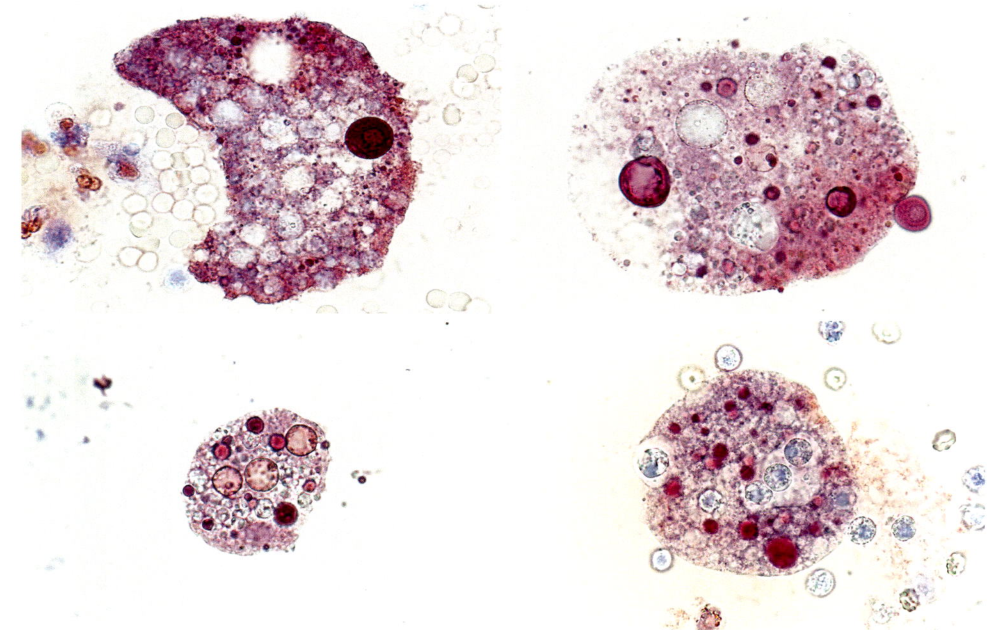

Fig. 2.58 Macrophages vary in size and can engulf WBCs. SM stain, ×1000

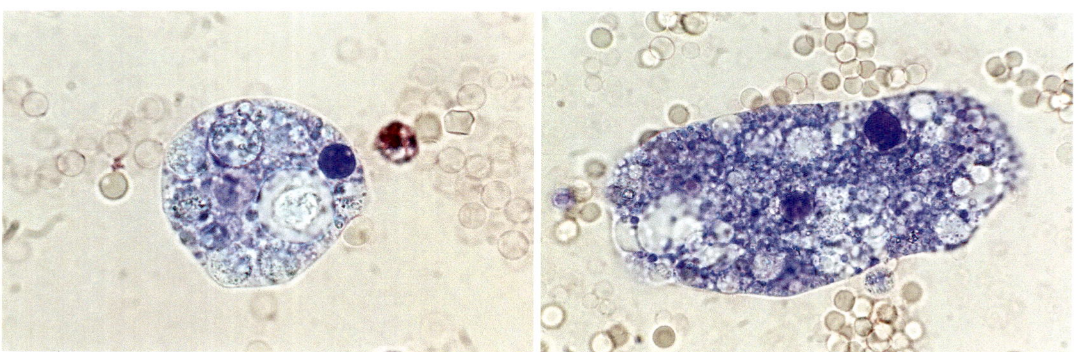

Fig. 2.59 Macrophages. The overall color of viable cells is light blue after staining. SM stain, ×1000

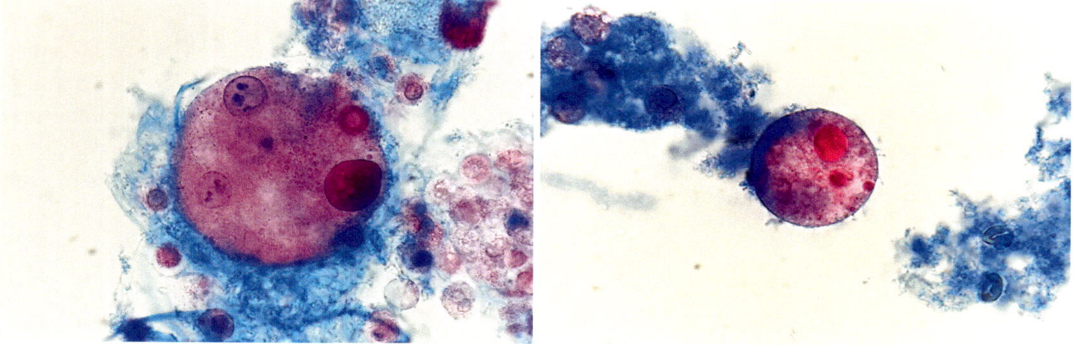

Fig. 2.60 Macrophages. The cell sizes vary, and there may be purple-red inclusion bodies. S stain, ×1000

2.9 Urothelial Cells/Transitional Epithelial Cells

2.9.1 Origin

Urothelial cells, also known as transitional epithelial cells, derive from the sloughing off of epithelial cells in the renal pelvis, ureters, bladder, and the proximal urethra near the bladder segment [24]. Urothelial cells can be divided into superficial, intermediate, and basal urothelial cells, which differ in volume, cytoplasmic content, and nucleus-to-cytoplasm ratio (Fig. 2.61).

2.9.2 Unstained

Urothelial cells in the urine vary in size and can have a round or irregular shape. Based on the cell size, nuclear size and nuclear-cytoplasmic ratio, urothelial cells can be classified into superficial, intermediate, and basal urothelial cells [25]. The deeper the layer of cells, the smaller their size and the higher their nuclear-cytoplasmic ratio. However, compared to squamous epithelial cells, the cytoplasm of these cells has a thicker and more pronounced granular appearance (Fig. 2.62).

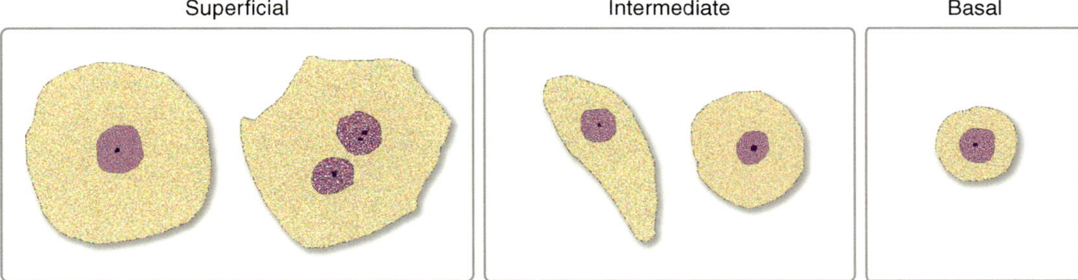

Fig. 2.61 Illustration of urothelial cells

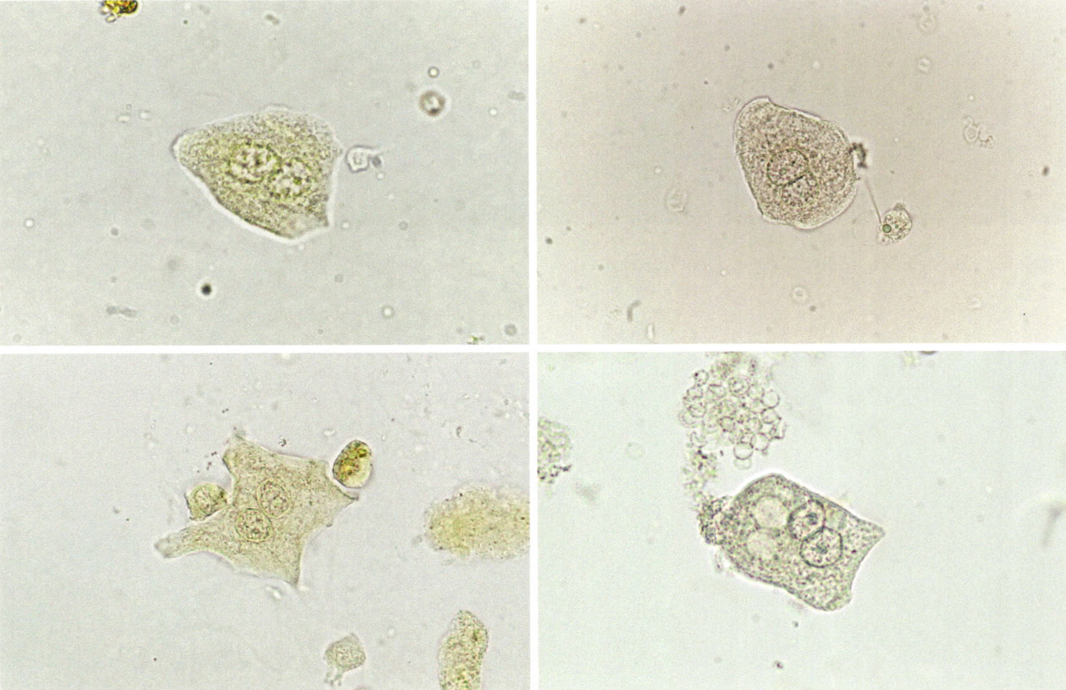

Fig. 2.62 Superficial urothelial cells. Unstained, ×1000

2.9.2.1 Superficial Urothelial Cells

These cells have a size of 15–40 μm. Under the microscope, their cell bodies appear round or irregular in shape. The cell volume varies, and the cytoplasm is thick and granular. The nuclei are round with one or multiple chromatin granules, and small nucleoli can be observed. Using a phase contrast microscope, the cell structure becomes clearer, and it can be distinguished from SECs (Fig. 2.63).

2.9.2.2 Intermediate Urothelial Cells

These cells have a size of 20–30 μm and can appear round, spindle-shaped, tail-like, or irregular. The cytoplasm of these cells are granular, and the nuclei are slightly larger, round, or oval in shape (Fig. 2.64).

2.9.2.3 Basal Urothelial Cells

These cells have a size of 15–30 μm and have a cell body of approximately 2–4 times larger than

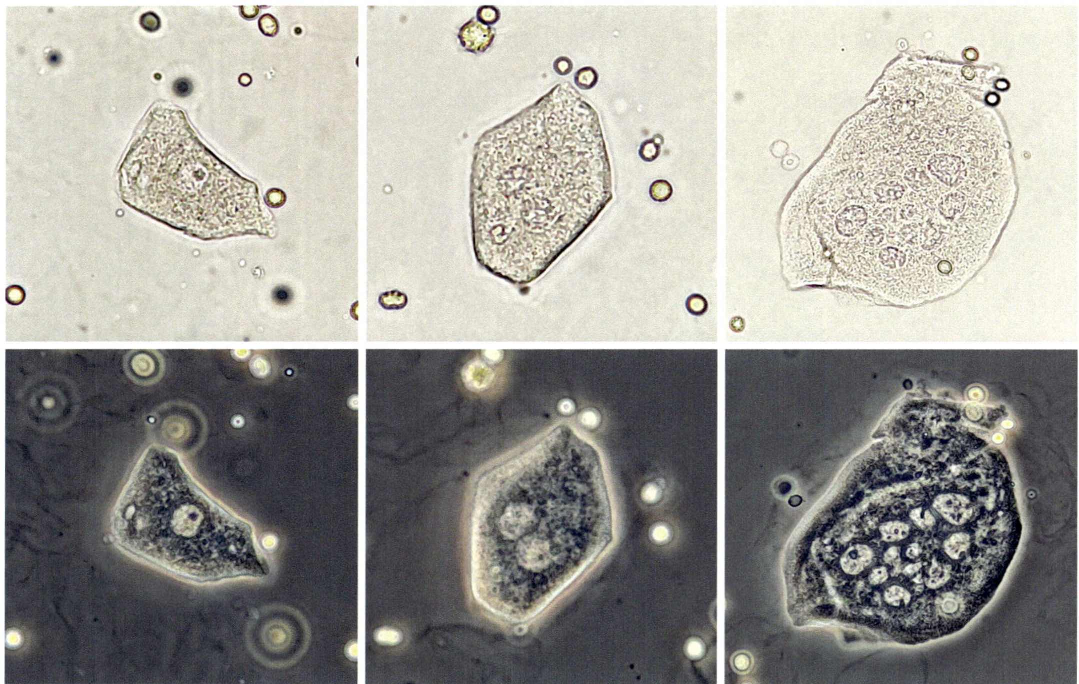

Fig. 2.63 Superficial urothelial cells. Unstained, ×1000

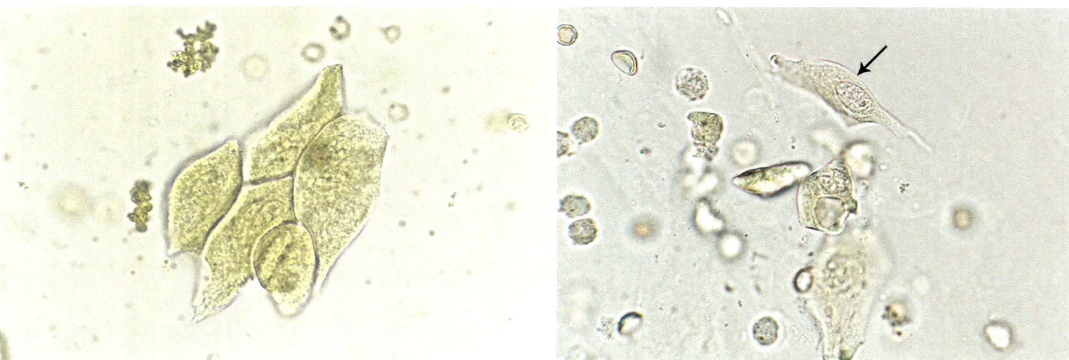

Fig. 2.64 Intermediate urothelial cells. Unstained, ×1000

that of WBCs. Some cells have a similar size to that of renal tubular epithelial cells and are mostly round in shape. The nuclei are slightly larger and round, located centrally or eccentrically. Unstained basal urothelial cells are not easily distinguishable from renal tubular epithelial cells and require staining techniques for differentiation (Fig. 2.65).

In aged urine specimens, old epithelial cells can be observed. These cells have enlarged cell bodies with larger vacuoles or lipid droplets in the cytoplasm. Some cells may exhibit a foamy appearance in the cytoplasm (Fig. 2.66). The cellular structures become more distinct after staining (Fig. 2.67).

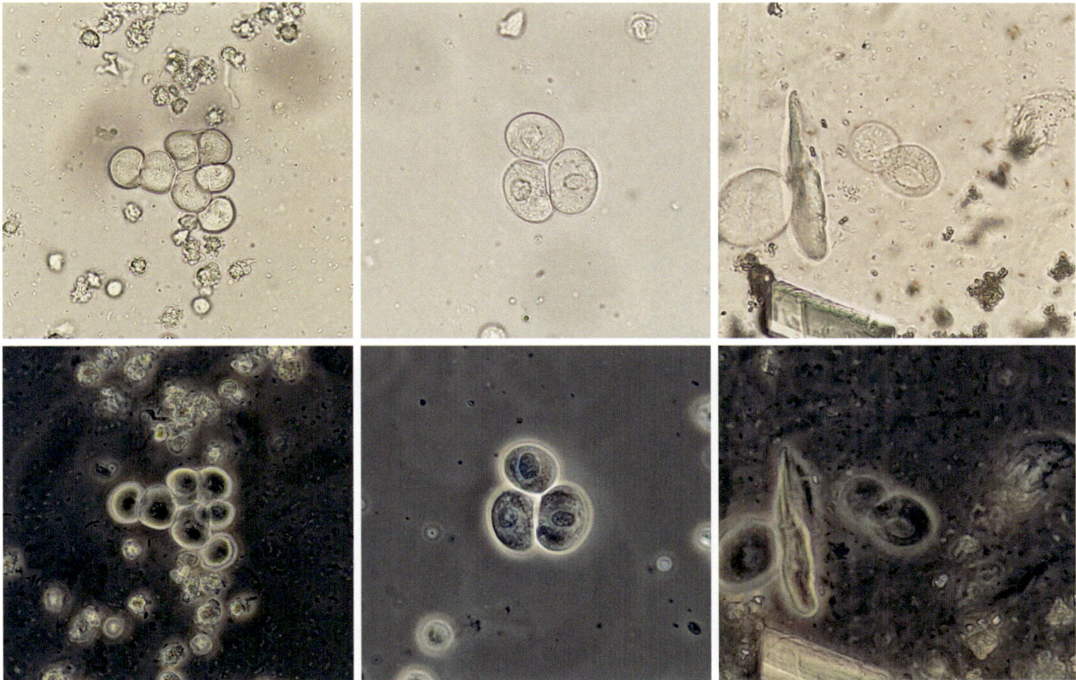

Fig. 2.65 Basal urothelial cells. Unstained, ×1000

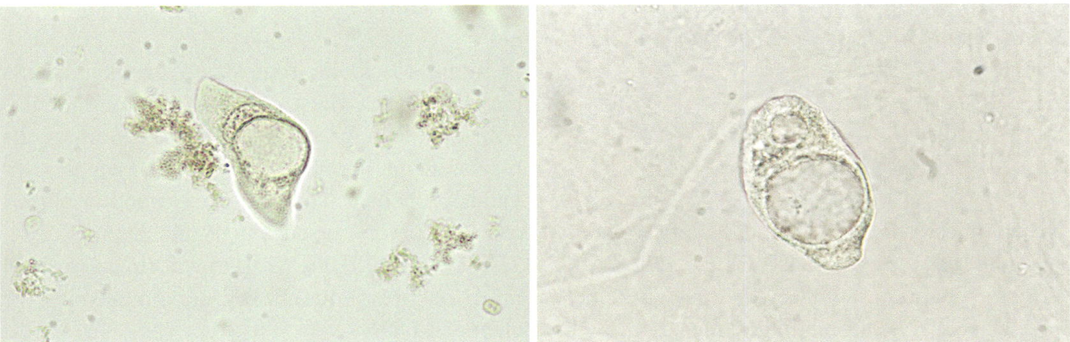

Fig. 2.66 Old urothelial cells. Unstained, ×1000

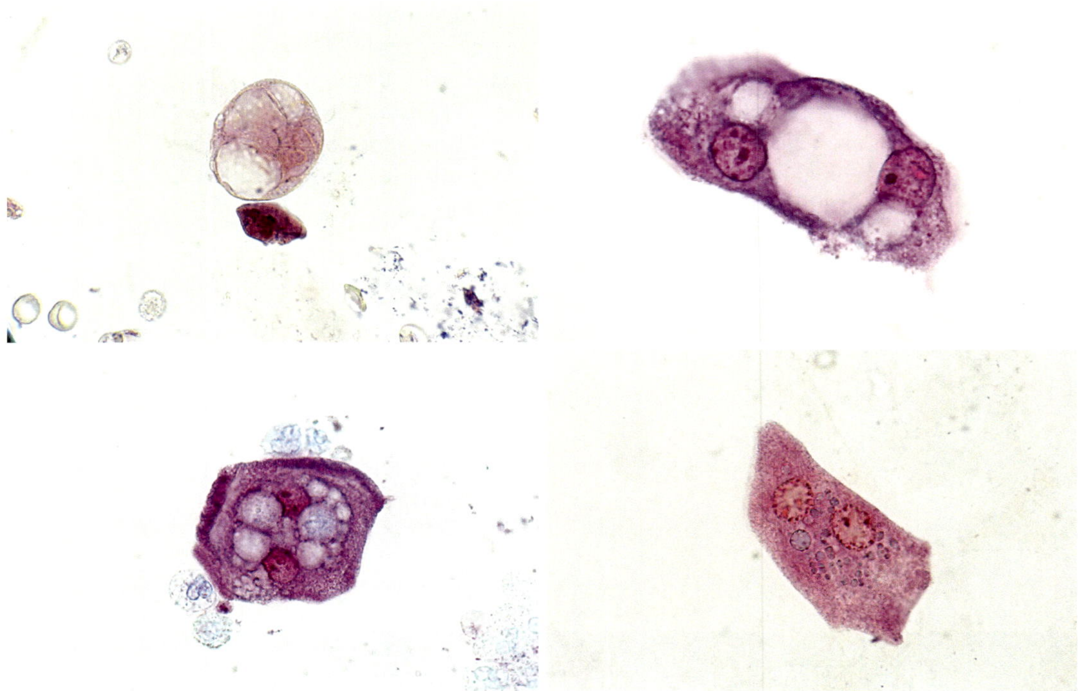

Fig. 2.67 Old urothelial cells. SM stain, ×1000

2.9.3 SM Stain and S Stain

The cytoplasm of urothelial cells appears pink or purplish-red, while the nuclei are stained deeper and exhibit a dark purplish-red after SM staining. It is important to note that some living cells may not be stained well, and their cytoplasm and nuclei appear pale blue (Figs. 2.68 and 2.69). The cytoplasm appears purplish-red, and the nuclei appear blue, with deeply stained nucleoli after S staining (Fig. 2.70).

2.9.4 Wright's Stain

The cytoplasm of urothelial cells appears abundant and has a gray-blue or blue color after Wright's staining, while the nuclei appear purplish-red with chromatin granules. Some cells may exhibit blue-colored nucleoli. These cells can be arranged in clusters (Fig. 2.71) or scattered distribution (Fig. 2.72). Basal urothelial cells have a smaller cell volume and higher nucleus-to-cytoplasm ratio (NCR) (Fig. 2.73).

2.9.5 Multinucleated Urothelial Cells

In some cases, multinucleated urothelial cells may be present. These cells have large cell bodies with abundant granular cytoplasm. Some cells may contain lipid droplets, small vacuoles, or inclusion bodies. The nuclei are round or elliptical, with several or dozens of nuclei (Figs. 2.74, 2.75, and 2.76). These cells may form due to viral infection or stimulation by certain physical or chemical factors.

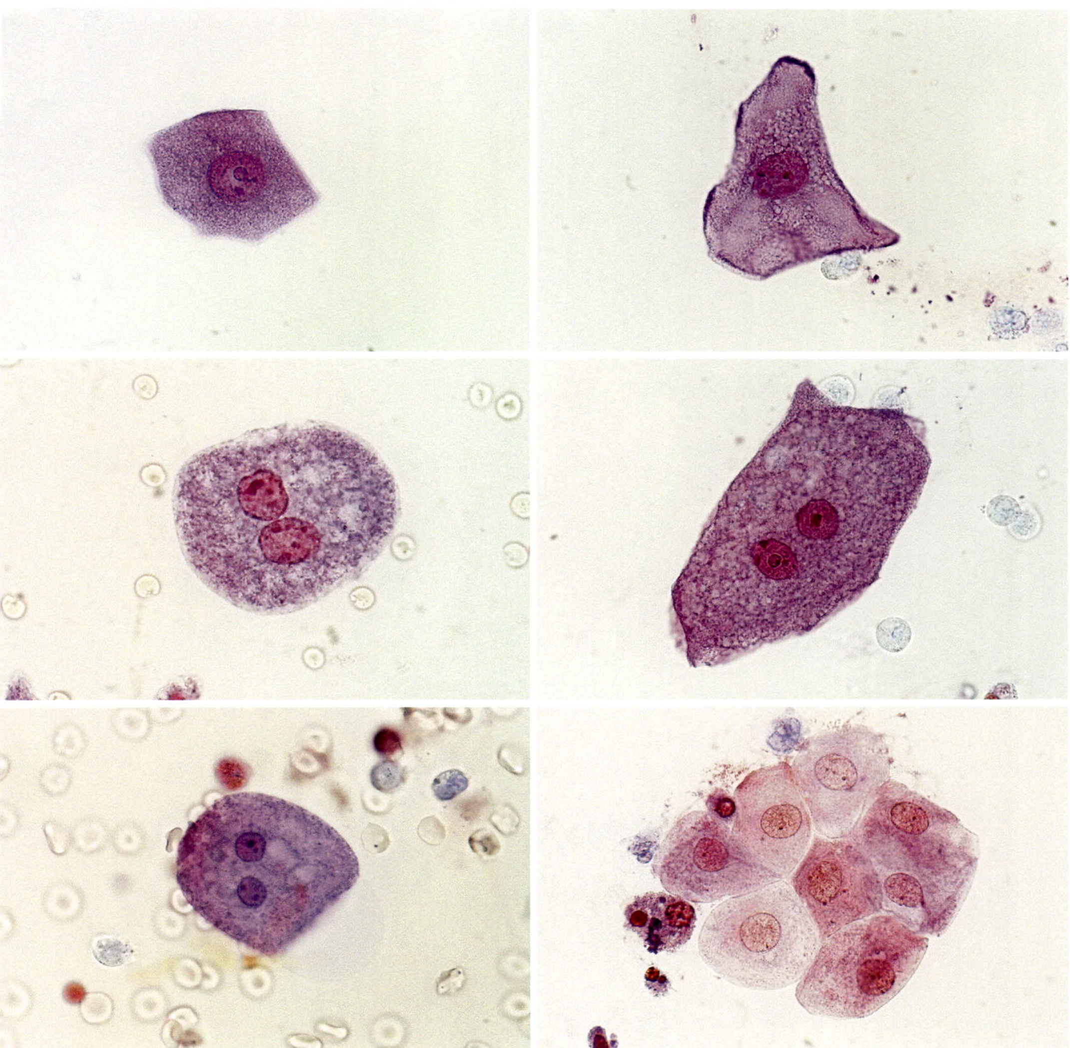

Fig. 2.68 Superficial urothelial cells. SM stain, ×1000

2.9.6 Clinical Significance

In healthy individuals, a small number of urothelial cells can be observed in the urine. However, the presence of a large number of urothelial cells or clusters is frequently associated with conditions such as pyelonephritis, cystitis and urethritis, and can also be observed in cases of urinary tract stones, urinary tract tumors and others. Additionally, the mechanical damage caused by the insertion of a urinary catheter can also result in the presence of a large number of urothelial cells.

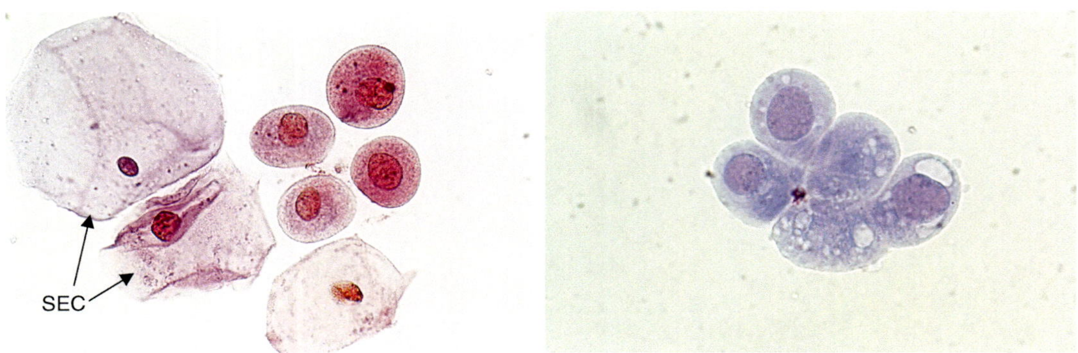

Fig. 2.69 Basal urothelial cells. SM stain, ×1000

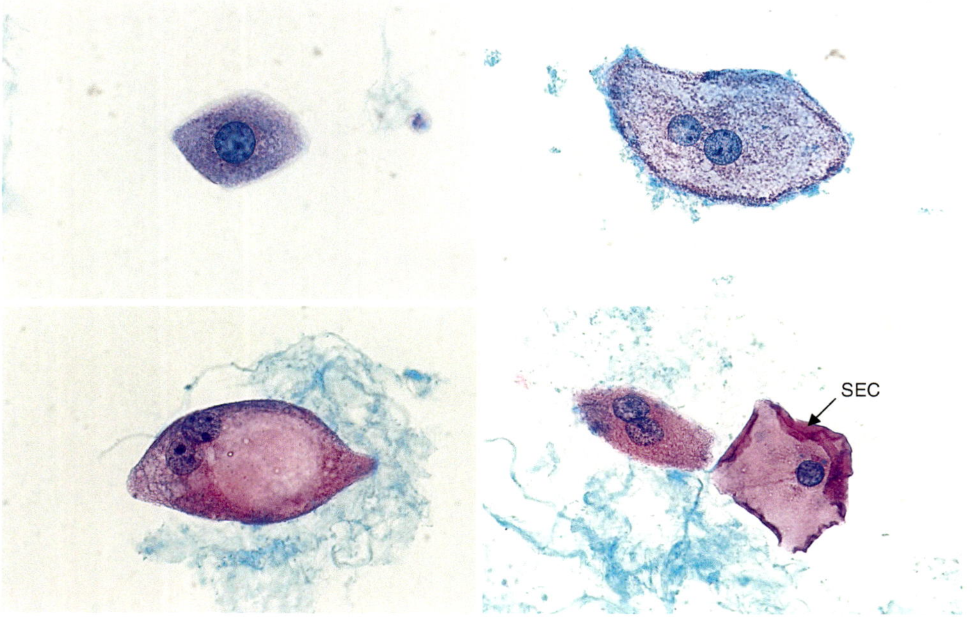

Fig. 2.70 Urothelial cells. The cytoplasm appears purplish-red, while the nucleus appears blue. S stain, ×1000

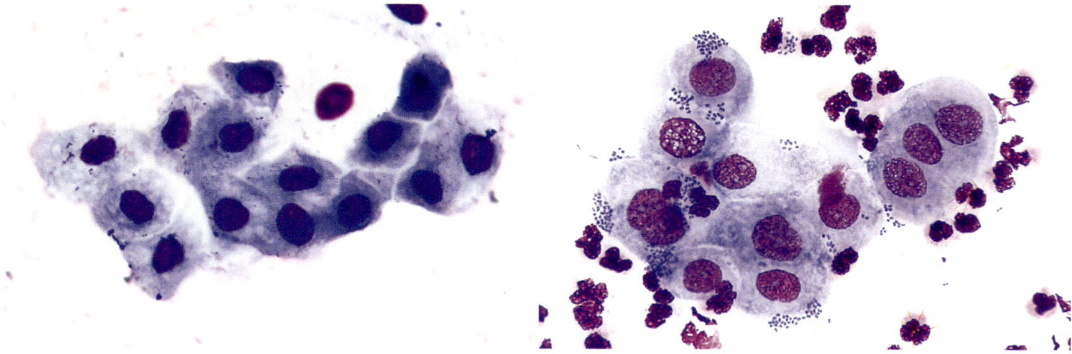

Fig. 2.71 Superficial urothelial cells are arranged in clusters. Wright's stain, ×1000

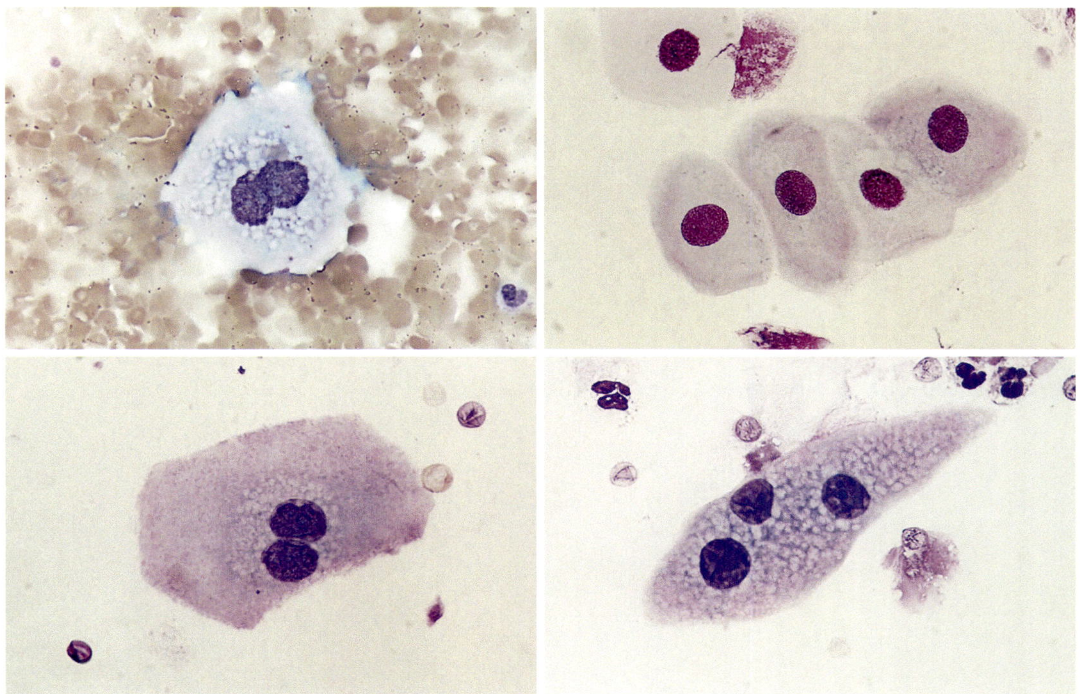

Fig. 2.72 Superficial urothelial cells are scattered individually. Wright's stain, ×1000

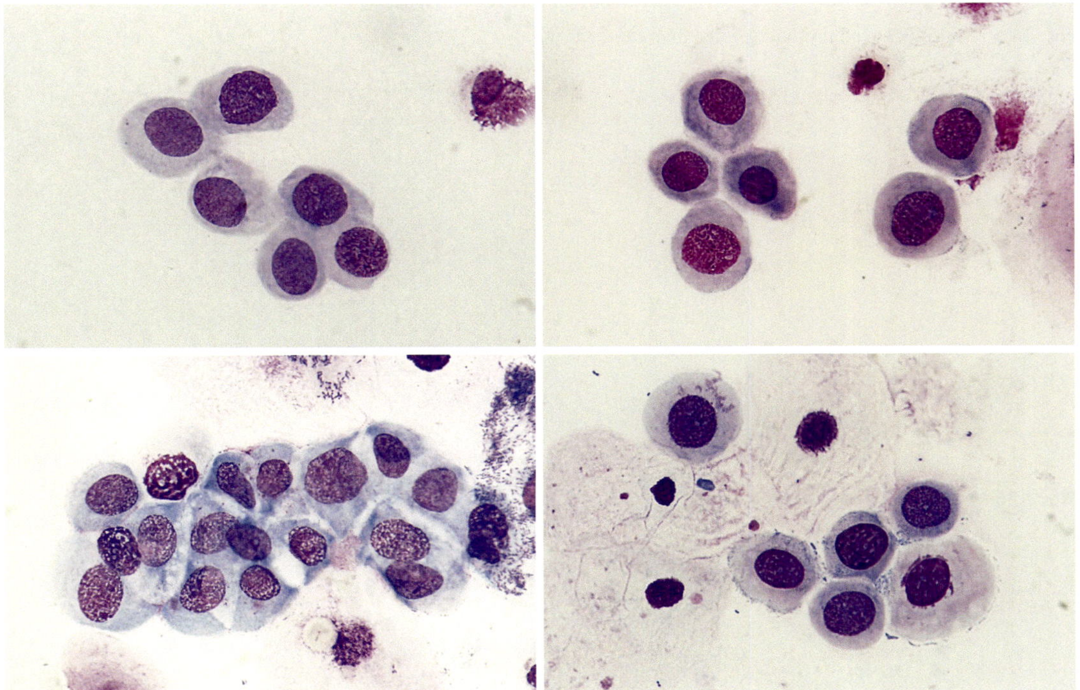

Fig. 2.73 Basal urothelial cells. Wright's stain, ×1000

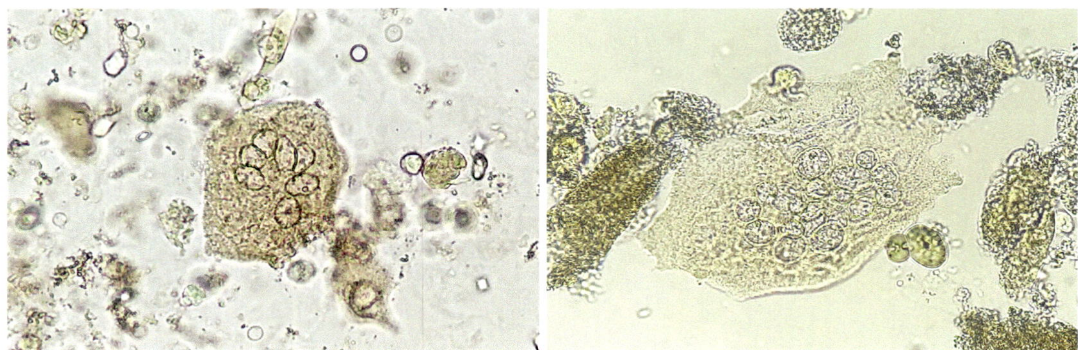

Fig. 2.74 Multinucleated urothelial cells. Unstained, ×1000

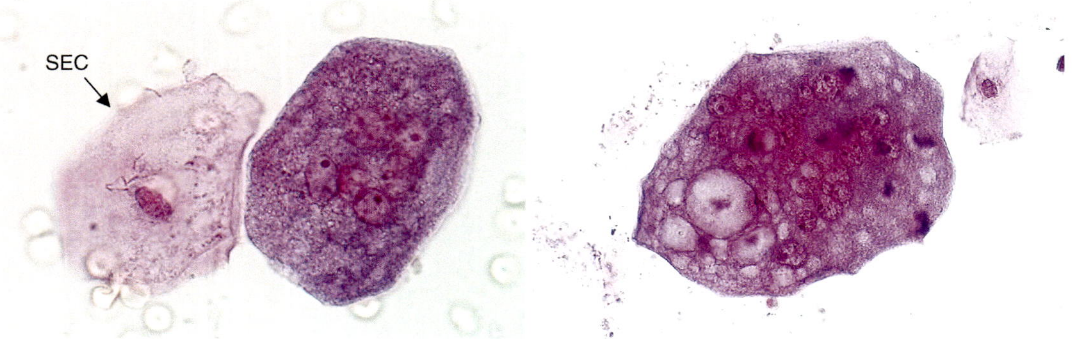

Fig. 2.75 Multinucleated urothelial cells. SM stain, ×1000

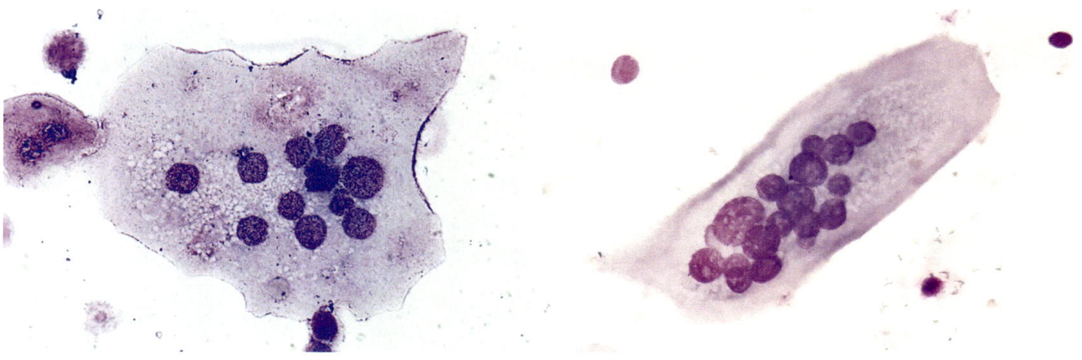

Fig. 2.76 Multinucleated urothelial cells. Wright's stain, ×1000

2.10 Atypical Urothelial Cells

2.10.1 Origin

Atypical urothelial cells refer to morphologically abnormal urothelial cells observed in urine cytology. Although they exhibit features of abnormal proliferation, they do not meet the criteria for diagnosing a tumor. The presence of atypical urothelial cells suggests the possibility of certain pathological processes or potential risks in patients, which require further evaluation and follow-up.

2.10.2 Morphological Features

Atypical urothelial cells show increased heterogeneity in size, shape, and nuclear-cytoplasmic ratio. They may be larger and irregular in shape compared to normal epithelial cells and can occur in clusters or sheets. The nuclear-cytoplasmic ratio may be increased, and there may be an overall increase in nuclear size with regular nuclear contours (Fig. 2.77). Enlarged nucleoli may also be present. Cellular mitosis can be active but without pathological features.

2.10.3 Clinical Significance

Atypical urothelial cells are commonly found in the urine of patients with urinary tract inflammation and urinary tract stones. Additionally, a history of interventions or instillations can reveal the presence of these cells. Severe atypical urothelial cells may indicate pre-cancerous lesions, such as urothelial carcinoma in situ, which serve as an early indication of tumor development and suggest potential malignant tumor risks in patients. If the presence of atypical urothelial cells is identified, further monitoring and follow-up are necessary. This can help physicians detect potential malignant transformation or disease progression in a timely manner and take appropriate treatment measures.

Some atypical urothelial cells cannot be characterized solely based on morphology, requiring further examination and assessment, such as tissue biopsy, immunocytochemistry, or additional

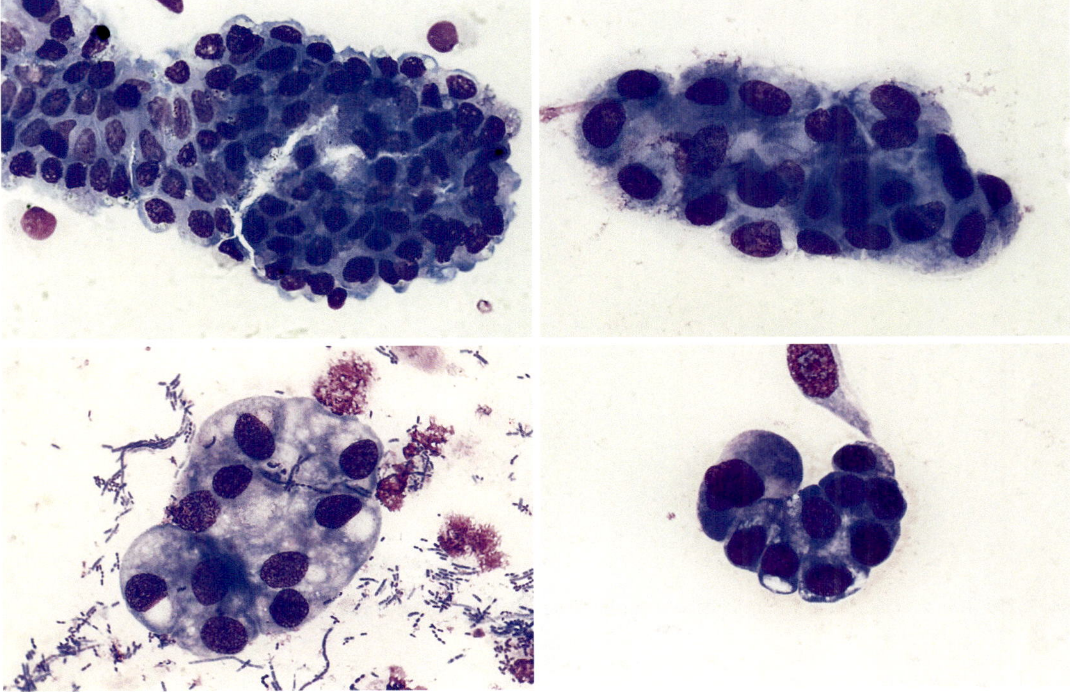

Fig. 2.77 Atypical urothelial cells. Wright's stain, ×1000

imaging studies, to help establish a definitive diagnosis. The final diagnosis should be based on comprehensive clinical history and other diagnostic tests.

2.11 Tumor Cells

2.11.1 Origin

Tumor cells in the urine primarily derive from the sloughing of tumor cells in the renal pelvis, ureter, bladder and urethra. Moreover, tumor cells from other sites infiltrating the bladder may also be identified in the urine.

The majority of tumor cells in the urine are associated with urothelial carcinoma, which predominantly affects individuals over the age of 50. It is more prevalent in males than females, with bladder cancer being the most common type. Bladder cancer ranks ninth worldwide among malignant tumors in terms of incidence. As tumor cells from the renal pelvis, ureter, bladder, and other areas are shed, they can be expelled in the urine, thereby allowing for the detection of tumor cells in urinary samples (Fig. 2.78).

2.11.2 Unstained

The tumor cells exhibit notable cellular pleomorphism. They are found in clusters, sheets, or scattered distribution. These cells have a large size, prominent nuclei, dense chromatin and conspicuous nucleoli. Unstained cells appear unclear in structure and are difficult to identify (Fig. 2.79). Clear identification requires the use of staining techniques.

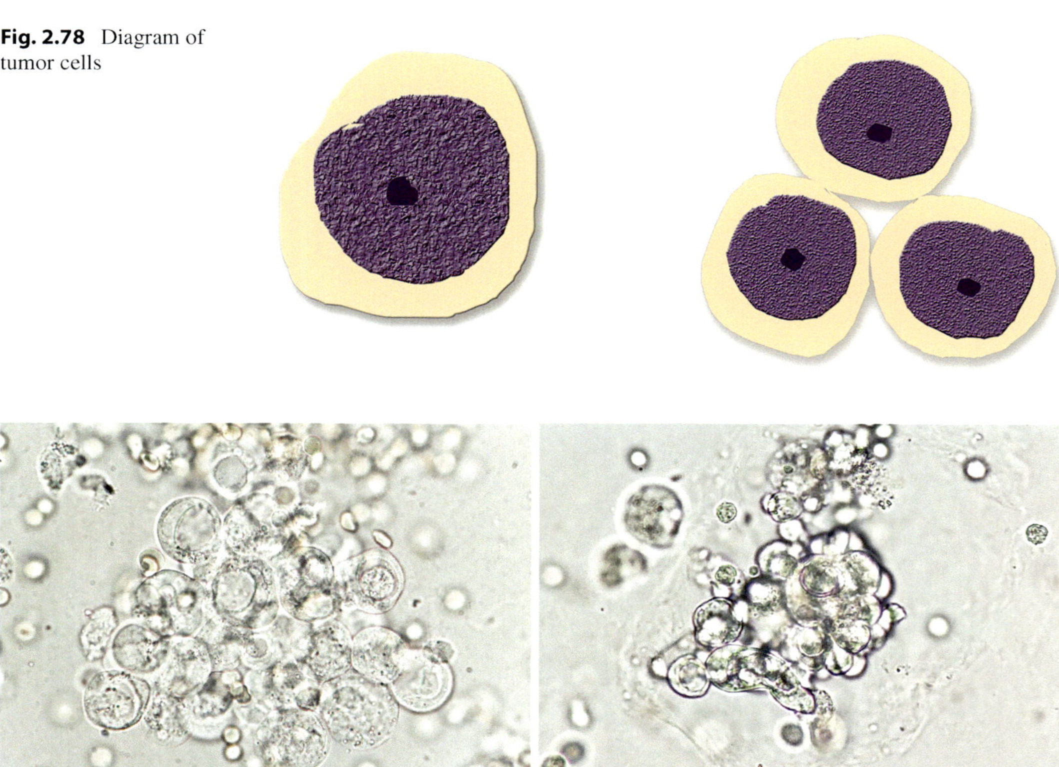

Fig. 2.78 Diagram of tumor cells

Fig. 2.79 Tumor cells. The cells are clustered and show an unclear border. Unstained, ×1000

2.11.3 SM Stain or S Stain

The cytoplasm of tumor cells appears pink, while the nuclei are stained with a dark purplish-red color, and the nucleoli are deeply stained after SM staining (Fig. 2.80). The cytoplasm of tumor cells appears purplish-red, and the nuclei appear blue after S staining (Fig. 2.81).

2.11.4 Wright's Stain

Tumor cells are easily recognizable after Wright's staining. The cytoplasm appears blue, the nucleus is stained purple-red, and the nucleoli are blue (Fig. 2.82). Tumor cells are found in clusters or scattered distribution (Fig. 2.83), varying in size, with some cells exhibiting giant volumes. The nuclei are large, and the chromatin is densely stained, with prominent nucleoli.

2.11.5 Clinical Significance

The examination of tumor cells in urine has significant clinical significance. Here are several aspects of its clinical importance:

Early tumor diagnosis: Urine tumor cell examination helps in the early detection of malignant tumors in the urinary system, such as bladder cancer and renal pelvis cancer. Timely screening and detection can increase the detection rate of early-stage tumors, thus facilitating early treatment and improving patient survival rates.

Assessment of tumor progression and recurrence: Urine tumor cell examination can be used to assess tumor progression and recurrence. Monitoring the presence and quantity of tumor cells in urine helps physicians understand the effectiveness of tumor treatment, determine if the tumor is under control, and predict the risk of tumor recurrence.

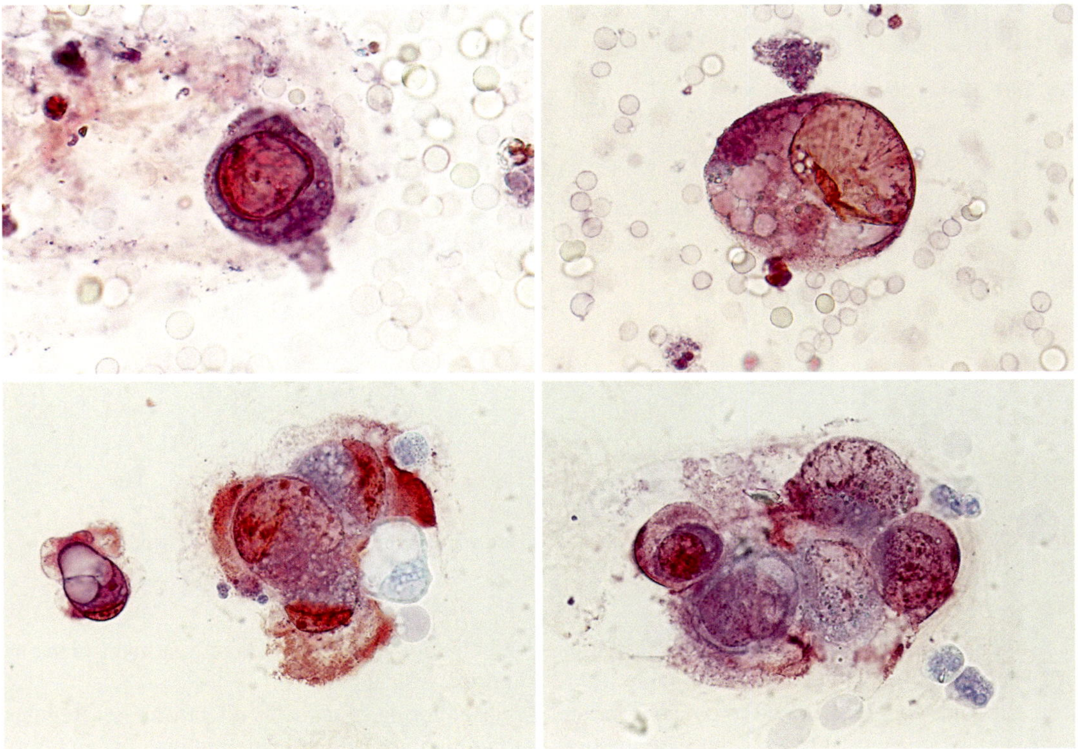

Fig. 2.80 Tumor cells. The cellular volume exhibits significant variation in size, with some cells appearing markedly enlarged. They are scattered or clustered in distribution, and the nuclei exhibit a deep staining intensity. The nucleoli are prominently visible. SM stain, ×1000

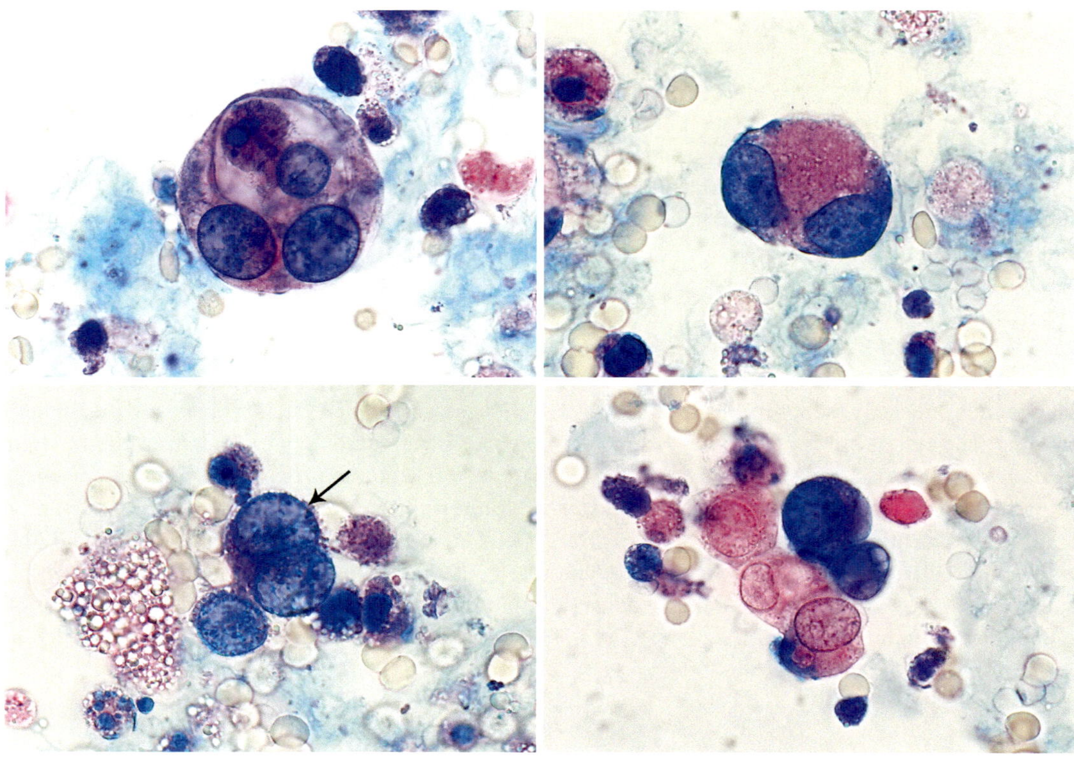

Fig. 2.81 Tumor cells. S stain, ×1000

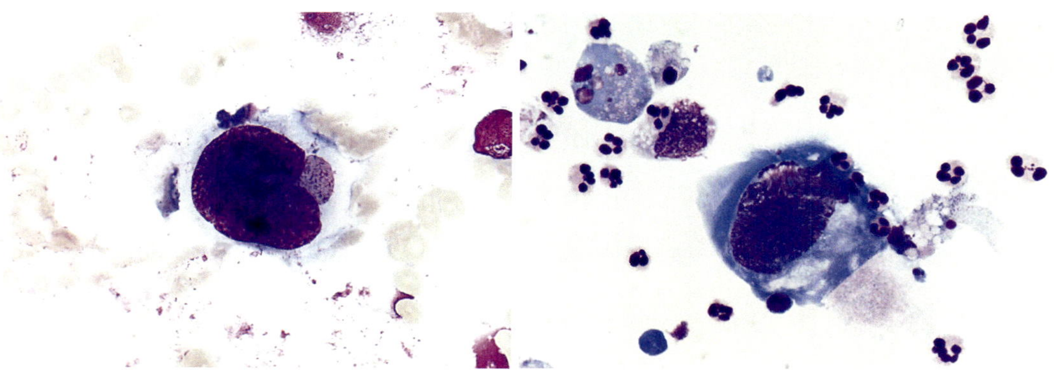

Fig. 2.82 Tumor cells. The cells have large cell volumes and are scattered in distribution. Wright's stain, ×1000

Guidance for treatment strategies: The results of urine tumor cell examination provide valuable guidance for selecting the most appropriate treatment strategies. Based on the examination results, physicians can determine the extent of surgical resection and the use of radiotherapy and chemotherapy and adjust treatment plans to improve efficacy.

Monitoring treatment effectiveness: Regular urine tumor cell examination allows for monitoring the effectiveness of treatment. If the number of tumor cells in urine significantly decreases or

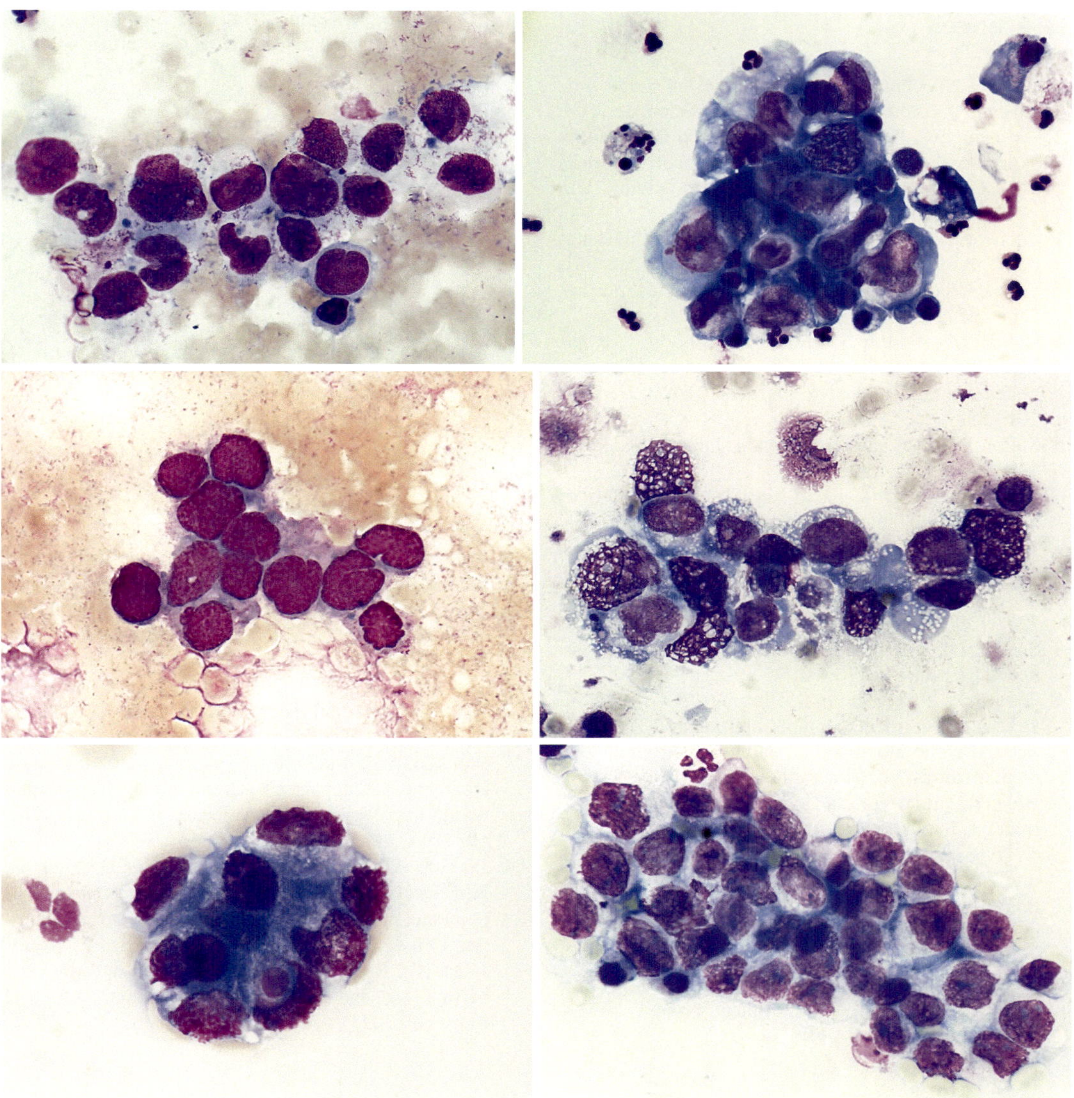

Fig. 2.83 Tumor cells. The cells are arranged in sheets or clusters, with large nuclei and dense chromatin. Wright's stain, ×1000

disappears, it indicates a good treatment response. Conversely, if the number of tumor cells increases or persists, it may be necessary to adjust the treatment plan or consider alternative treatment options.

In summary, urine tumor cell examination is clinically significant in terms of early diagnosis, assessing tumor progression and recurrence, guiding treatment strategies, and monitoring treatment effectiveness. This examination is convenient, cost-effective, and minimally invasive, and it can detect tumor cells or early microscopic lesions shed from sites that are difficult to reach with conventional methods. Combined with cystoscopy, urine cytology serves as an important diagnostic tool for bladder malignancies and recurrence.

References

1. Brunzel NA. Fundamentals of urine and body fluid analysis. Amsterdam: Elsevier Health Sciences; 2021.
2. Cavanaugh C, Perazella MA. Urine sediment examination in the diagnosis and management of kidney disease: core curriculum 2019. Am J Kidney Dis. 2019;73(2):258–72.
3. Pillsworth TJ Jr, Haver VM, Abrass CK, Delaney CJ. Differentiation of renal from non-renal hematuria by microscopic examination of erythrocytes in urine. Clin Chem. 1987;33(10):1791–5.
4. Hebert LA, Parikh S, Prosek J, Nadasdy T, Rovin BH. Differential diagnosis of glomerular disease: a systematic and inclusive approach. Am J Nephrol. 2013;38(3):253–66.
5. Sutton JM. Evaluation of hematuria in adults. JAMA. 1990;263(18):2475–80.
6. Strasinger SK, Di Lorenzo MS. Urinalysis and body fluids. Philadelphia: FA Davis; 2014.
7. Tesser Poloni JA, Bosan IB, Garigali G, Fogazzi GB. Urinary red blood cells: not only glomerular or nonglomerular. Nephron Clin Pract. 2011;120(1):c36–41.
8. Stenzel DJ, Boreham PF. Blastocystis hominis revisited. Clin Microbiol Rev. 1996;9(4):563–84.
9. Chase J, Hammond J, Bilbrough G, DeNicola DB. Urine sediment examination: potential impact of red and white blood cell counts using different sediment methods. Vet Clin Pathol. 2018;47(4):608–16.
10. Hida Y, Yamashita M, Ichikawa M, Masunaga S, Imura T, Suzuki S, Gejyo F. The clinical significance of glitter-cells in the urine during urinary tract infection. Rinsho Byori. 1996;44(10):977–82.
11. Poirier KP, Jackson GG. Characteristics of leukocytes in the urine sediment in pyelonephritis; correlation with renal biopsies. Am J Med. 1957;23(4):579–86.
12. Mody L, Juthani-Mehta M. Urinary tract infections in older women: a clinical review. JAMA. 2014;311(8):844–54.
13. Chen A, Lee K, Guan T, He JC, Schlondorff D. Role of CD8+ T cells in crescentic glomerulonephritis. Nephrol Dial Transplant. 2020;35(4):564–72.
14. Singh N, Samant H, Hawxby A, Samaniego MD. Biomarkers of rejection in kidney transplantation. Curr Opin Organ Transplant. 2019;24(1):103–10.
15. Lusica M, Rondon-Berrios H, Feldman L. Urine eosinophils for acute interstitial nephritis. J Hosp Med. 2017;12(5):343–5.
16. Walter FG, Gibly RL, Knopp RK, Roe DJ. Squamous cells as predictors of bacterial contamination in urine samples. Ann Emerg Med. 1998;31(4):455–8.
17. Amatya R, Bhattarai S, Mandal PK, Tuladhar H, Karki BM. Urinary tract infection in vaginitis: a condition often overlooked. Nepal Med Coll J. 2013;15(1):65–7.
18. Schumann GB, Johnston JL, Weiss MA. Renal epithelial fragments in urine sediment. Acta Cytol. 1981;25(2):147–52.
19. Ridley JW. Fundamentals of the study of urine and body fluids. Berlin: Springer; 2018.
20. Perazella MA. The urine sediment as a biomarker of kidney disease. Am J Kidney Dis. 2015;66(5):748–55.
21. Yokoyama T, Nitta K. Recent advances in urinalysis as a diagnostic indicator of renal diseases. Rinsho Byori. 2015;63(2):252–8.
22. Yan L, Guo H, Han L, Huang H, Shen Y, He J, Liu J. Sternheimer-Malbin staining to detect decoy cells in urine of 213 kidney transplant patients. Transplant Proc. 2020;52(3):823–8.
23. Duncan KA, Cuppage FE, Grantham JJ. Urinary lipid bodies in polycystic kidney disease. Am J Kidney Dis. 1985;5(1):49–53.
24. Jackson AR, Hoff ML, Li B, Ching CB, McHugh KM, Becknell B. Krt5(+) urothelial cells are developmental and tissue repair progenitors in the kidney. Am J Physiol Renal Physiol. 2019;317(3):F757–66.
25. Jafari NV, Rohn JL. The urothelium: a multi-faceted barrier against a harsh environment. Mucosal Immunol. 2022;15(6):1127–42.

3 Casts

Shimin Zhang, Yinfeng Wang, Yue An, Liang Fu, Qiangwu Zeng, Jingfang Li, Lixia Zhang, Xiaoqing Liu, and Wei Yang

3.1 Urinary Casts: Overview

3.1.1 Definition of Casts

Casts are protein aggregates formed by the coagulation of organic or inorganic substances, such as proteins, crystals, fat, cells, or cell fragments, within the renal tubules and collecting ducts.

3.1.2 Conditions for Cast Formation

Several factors contribute to the formation of casts: an abnormal increase in protein content in the glomerular filtrate serves as the matrix for cast formation; the concentrating function of the renal tubules further enhances the protein concentration within the casts; the acidification function of the tubules promotes protein denaturation and coagulation; slow urine flow or local stasis facilitates the components to aggregate; and renal units in the resting state are more prone to cast formation, which is subsequently expelled with urine when the units become active again.

The basic process of cast formation involves the gradual formation of primary fibers within the renal tubules, derived from the glycoprotein Tamm-Horsfall protein (THP), also known as uromodulin, with a monomeric molecular weight of 70 kDa and a polymeric molecular weight of

S. Zhang (✉)
Department of Clinical Laboratory, Peking Union Medical College Hospital, Peking Union Medical College, Beijing, China

Y. Wang
Department of Clinical Laboratory, Ningxia Medical University General Hospital, Yinchuan, Ningxia, China

Y. An
Clinical Laboratory, The Second Affiliated Hospital of Dalian Medical University, Dalian, China

L. Fu
Department of Laboratory Medicine, The Fifth Affiliated Hospital, Southern Medical University, Guangzhou, Guangdong, China

Q. Zeng
Department of Clinical Laboratory, The Second People's Hospital of Guiyang, Guiyang, Guizhou, China

J. Li
Department of Clinical Laboratory, The Third Affiliated Hospital of Kunming Medical University, Kunming, China

L. Zhang
Department of Laboratory Medicine, The First Affiliated Hospital of Nanjing Medical University, Nanjing, China
e-mail: zhanglixia7602@jsph.org.cn

X. Liu
Department of Laboratory Medicine, The Eighth Affiliated Hospital of Sun Yat-sen University, Shenzhen, China
e-mail: LXQFT@126.com.cn

W. Yang
Department of Laboratory Diagnostics, The First Affiliated Hospital of Harbin Medical University, Harbin, Heilongjiang, China

L. Zheng et al. (eds.), *Urine Formed Elements*, https://doi.org/10.1007/978-981-99-7739-0_3

70,000 kDa. THP is secreted by the thick ascending limb of the loop of Henle and the distal tubule epithelial cells. These fibers attach to the luminal surface of tubular cells and bind substances from the glomerular filtrate, including plasma-filtered albumin, to form various types of casts [1]. Casts are formed in the distal renal tubules and collecting ducts and are subsequently eliminated from the body. The length and width of casts vary depending on the diameter and length of the renal tubule segment in which they form (Fig. 3.1, Table 3.1).

3.1.3 Clinical Significance

There is a wide variety of urinary casts, each with its clinical significance. They can provide important clues and valuable information for the diagnosis of kidney diseases and urinary tract disorders (see the clinical significance of various types of casts). During microscopic examination, it is important to accurately classify the types of casts and report their quantities. For special casts that are difficult to distinguish using light microscopy or unstained samples, staining methods, phase contrast microscopy, polarized light microscopy, and other techniques can be used for identification. Certain specific casts, such as muddy brown casts, can serve as sensitive indicators of acute kidney injury and acute tubular necrosis, and should be promptly reported.

3.2 Hyaline Casts

3.2.1 Composition of Hyaline Casts

Hyaline casts mainly consist of THP and a small amount of albumin. When urine acidity increases, urine flow decreases or slows down, and urine

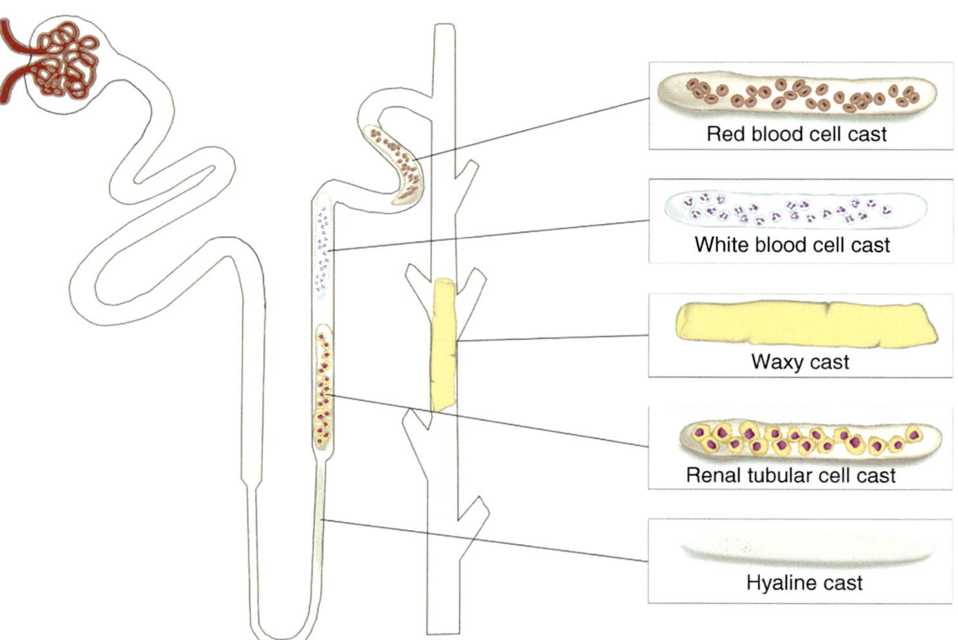

Fig. 3.1 Diagram illustrating the formation of casts

Table 3.1 Morphological characteristics of common casts

Types	Characteristics	Diagram
Hyaline casts	• Colorless and transparent • Thin texture • Lack of refractivity • Cylindrical shape with varying lengths and thicknesses • Parallel sides with blunt-rounded ends • May contain few granules, cells, or fat droplets	
Granular casts	• Finely granular casts: Small granules dispersed throughout matrix • Coarsely granular casts: coarse granules within matrix • The granules appear as grayish-white or pale yellow in color (excluding high bilirubinuria)	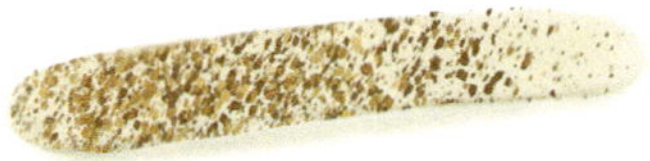
Muddy brown casts	• Brownish-brown granules within matrix	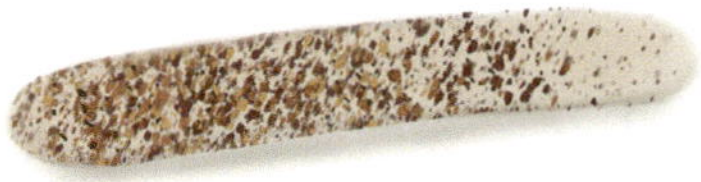
Waxy casts	• The matrix resembles wax-like consistency • Homogeneous matrix • High refractive index • Cracks or fissures often present	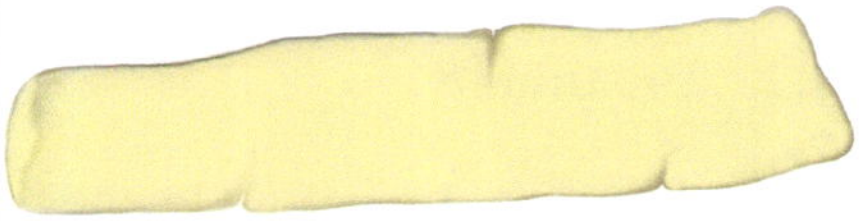
Red blood cell (RBC) casts or erythrocyte casts	• Intact RBCs within matrix	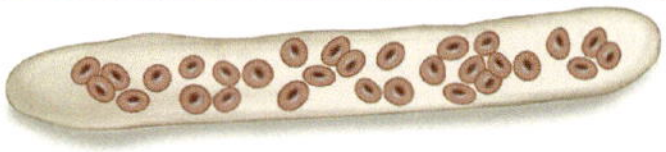
Blood casts	• The granules within the matrix exhibit a reddish-brown or red coloration • The granules vary in size	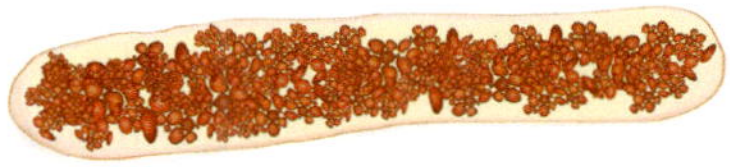
Hemoglobin casts	• Homogeneous matrix • Orange-red or red • The casts are prone to fragmentation or breakage	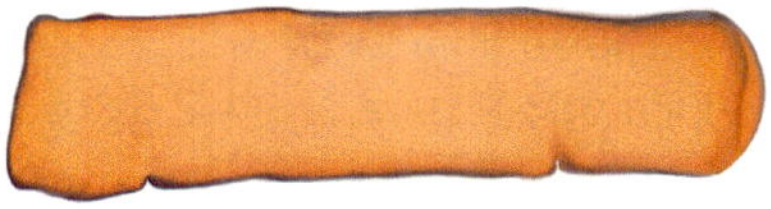
White blood cell casts	• Intact WBCs within the matrix • WBCs arranged either closely or loosely	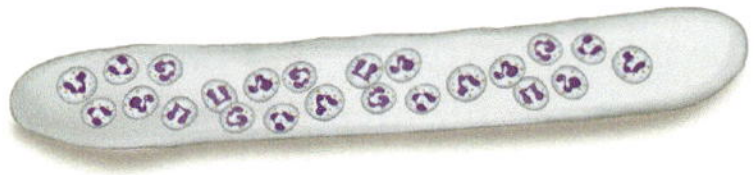
Renal tubular epithelial (RTE) cell casts	• Intact RTE cells within the matrix • RTE cells have a larger cell volume compared to WBC	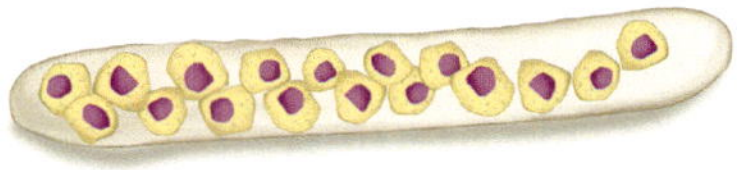
Fatty casts	• Fat droplets within the matrix • Highly refractile • Fat droplets have yellowish (bright field microscopy) • Triglycerides stain orange or red using Sudan III or Oil Red O	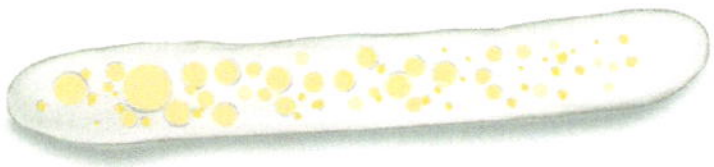

(continued)

Table 3.1 (continued)

Types	Characteristics	Diagram
Crystal casts	• Crystals within the matrix • Crystals exhibit strong birefringence	
Broad casts	• The cast width is relatively wide, exceeding 50 μm • It could be broad waxy casts, broad granular casts, or other types of broad casts	

becomes highly concentrated, hyaline casts may appear [1–3].

3.2.2 Unstained

Hyaline casts are colorless and transparent, with a thin texture and poor refractivity. They are cylindrical, varying in length and thickness, with most being narrow and short, although some can be larger. Hyaline casts have parallel sides and blunt-rounded ends, sometimes with one end slightly pointed or tapered, and can be curved or straight. Some hyaline casts may contain a few granules, a small number of cells, or fat droplets. Due to their thin texture, hyaline casts are easily overlooked or missed under light microscopy. However, they can be clearly observed using phase contrast microscopy. In dark field observation, the matrix of hyaline casts appears thin (Fig. 3.2).

3.2.3 S Stain or SM Stain

The matrix of the casts is relatively thin, resulting in a lighter color compared to waxy casts. They appear blue or light blue with S stain (Fig. 3.3), while with SM stain, they appear pink (Fig. 3.4).

3.2.4 Clinical Significance

Hyaline casts are a relatively common type of casts found in urine, which can be observed in both healthy individuals and during various disease states. Under physiological conditions, such as heavy physical labor or intense exercise, hyaline casts may occasionally be present in the urine. Non-renal conditions, such as fever, dehydration, diuretic use, and severe vomiting, can cause transient increases in hyaline casts [1, 2]. In many kidney diseases, there is a significant increase in the number of hyaline casts, either occurring alone or in conjunction with other types of casts. The presence of a large number of hyaline casts indicates renal damage caused by decreased renal blood flow. This is commonly seen in conditions such as acute and chronic glomerulonephritis, acute pyelonephritis, nephrotic syndrome, chronic renal failure, malignant hypertension and congestive heart failure [4].

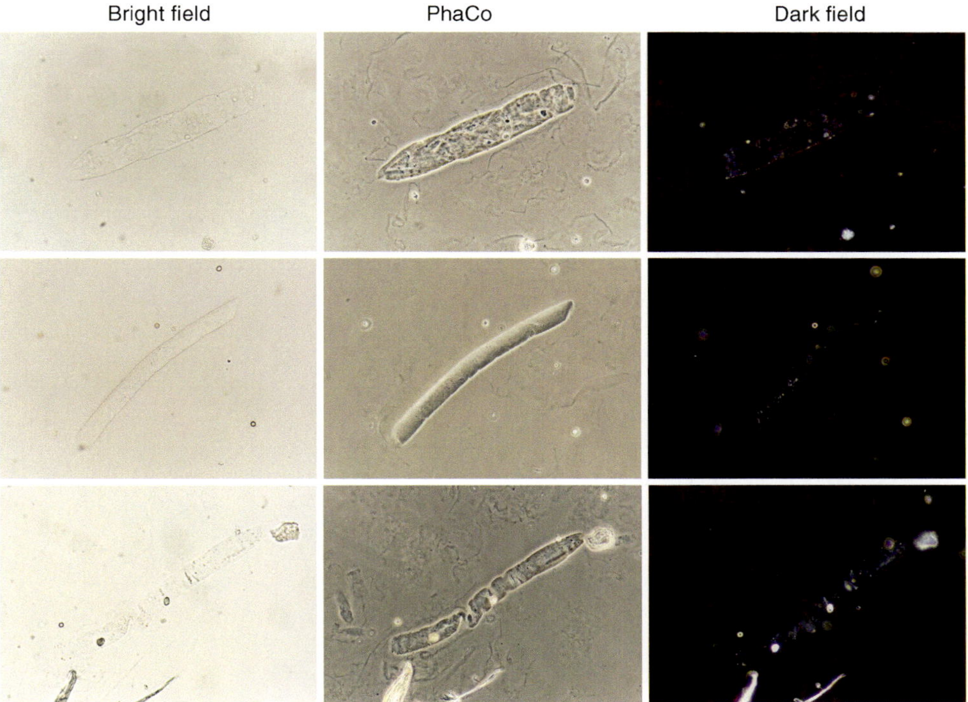

Fig. 3.2 Hyaline casts. They have a thin matrix, their structure is clear under contrast microscopy, and their refractivity is weak under dark field, ×400

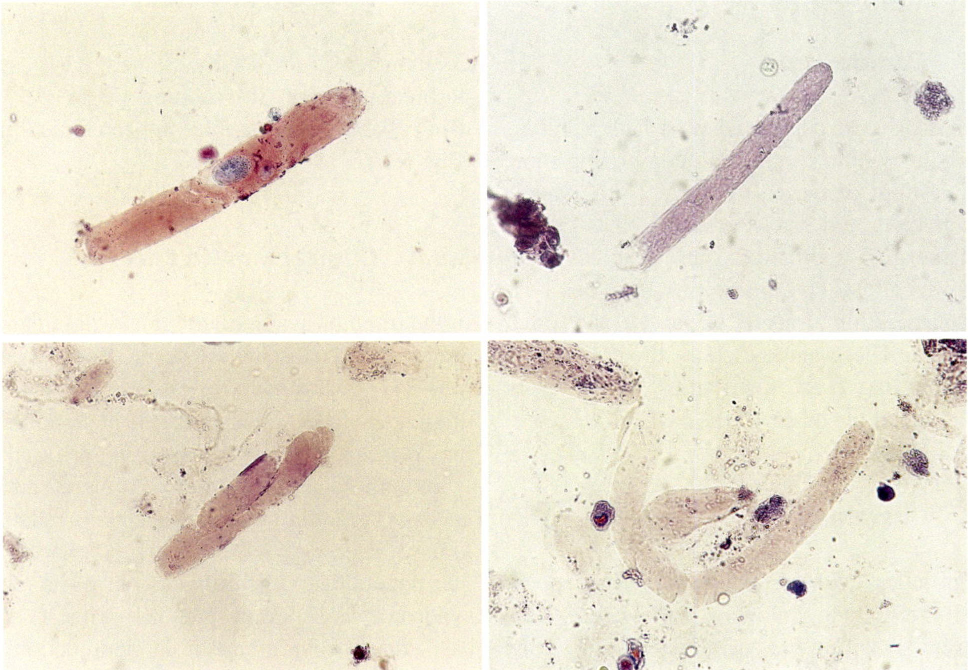

Fig. 3.3 Hyaline casts. Pink or pale red cast matrix. SM stain, ×400

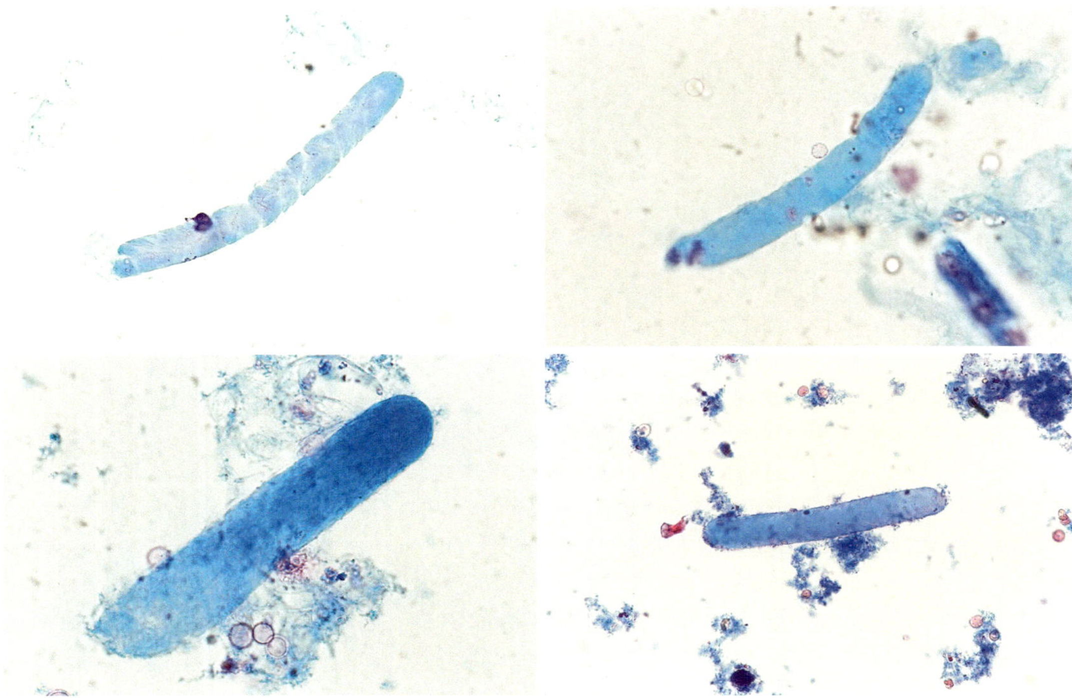

Fig. 3.4 Hyaline casts. The matrix appears light blue. S stain, ×400

3.3 Granular Casts

3.3.1 Composition

Granular casts are composed of variable numbers of granules within the matrix, comprising more than one-third of the cast volume [5]. Coarsely granular casts and finely granular casts can be found in urinary sediments. These granules originate from cellular debris resulting from cell lysis and degeneration, plasma proteins, and other substances. The granules within the cast matrix exhibit varying sizes, distributing uniformly or aggregating at the edges of the cast [6].

3.3.2 Unstained

The granules within the cast matrix appear grayish-white, pale yellow, or yellow (Fig. 3.5). The granules within the cast appear deep yellow in bilirubinuria (Figs. 3.6 and 3.7). Granular casts have a more distinct structure under contrast microscopy and dark field. Compared to hyaline casts, they have stronger refractivity (Fig. 3.8).

3.3.3 SM Stain or S Stain

Granular casts are easily stained. They appear purplish-red after SM staining (Fig. 3.9), while using S stain, the granules appear bluish-purple (Fig. 3.10).

3.3.4 Clinical Significance

In the urine of healthy individuals, granular casts are generally absent. However, finely granular casts may occasionally be observed during dehydration and fever, and an increase in granular casts may be seen after intense physical exercise [5].

In pathological conditions, an increased presence of granular casts suggests parenchymal kidney diseases such as acute or chronic glomerulonephritis, interstitial nephritis, nephrotic syndrome and chronic pyelonephritis. Granular casts may occur alone or in conjunction with other types of casts.

In some urine samples, the granules within the casts may exhibit a darker color, appearing as dark brown, known as muddy brown casts

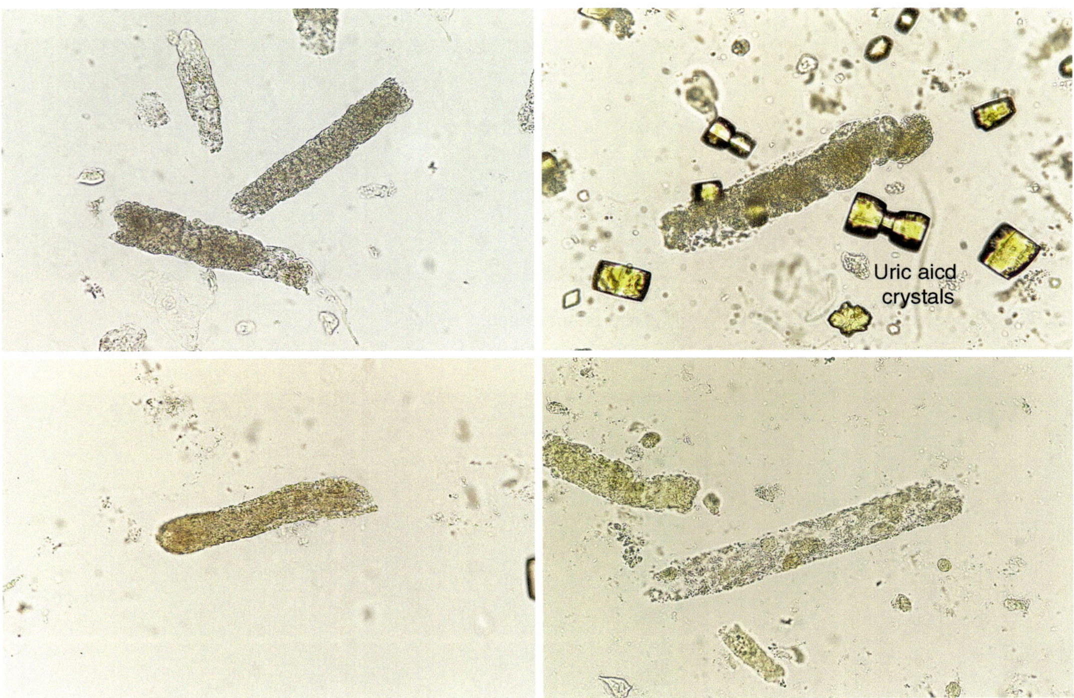

Fig. 3.5 Granular casts, bright field, unstained, ×400

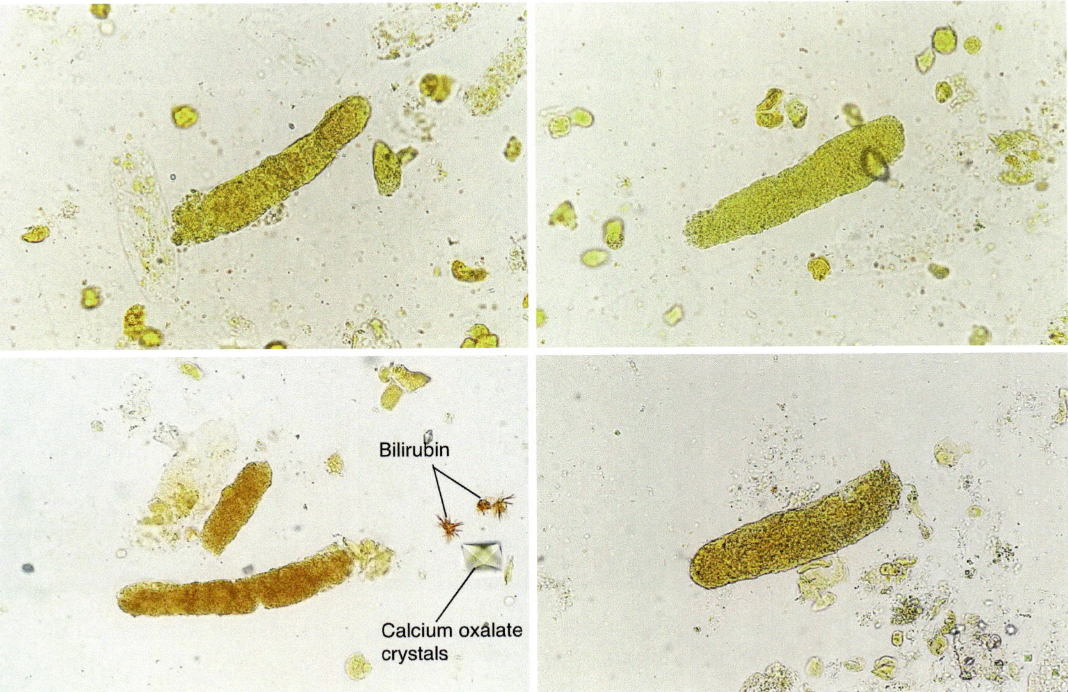

Fig. 3.6 Granular casts. The granules appear deep yellow in bilirubinuria. Unstained, ×400

Bright field
PhaCo
Dark field

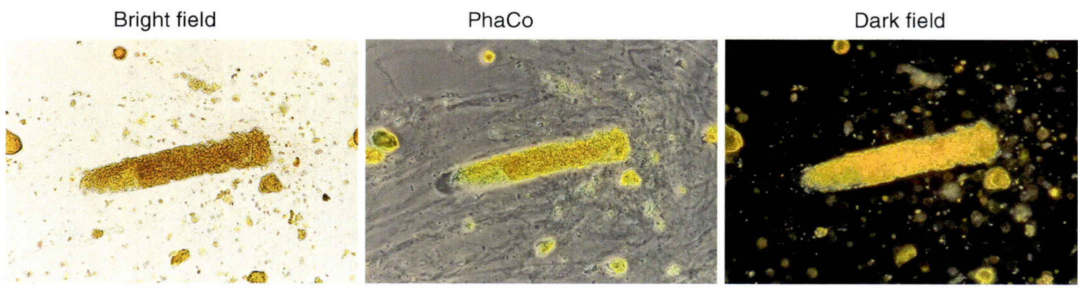

Fig. 3.7 Granular casts appear yellow in bilirubinuria, unstained, ×400

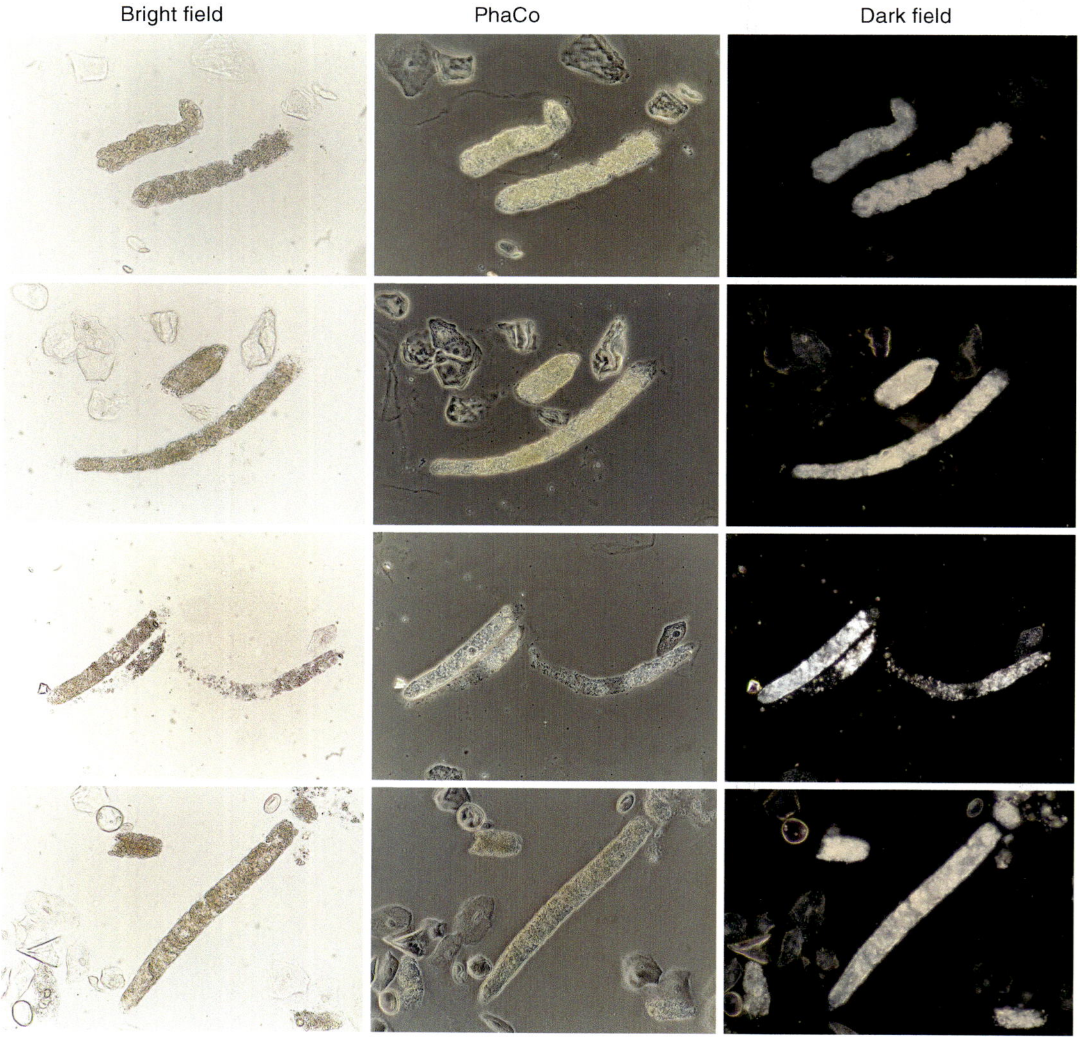

Bright field
PhaCo
Dark field

Fig. 3.8 Granular casts. The number of granules in their matrix varies, and the structure is clear under contrast microscopy. Compared to hyaline casts, their refractivity is stronger under dark field, ×400

(Fig. 3.11). They stain more deeply after supravital staining (Figs. 3.12 and 3.13). The abundance of muddy brown casts is often associated with a dirty background and is commonly seen in acute kidney injury caused by acute tubular necrosis [1].

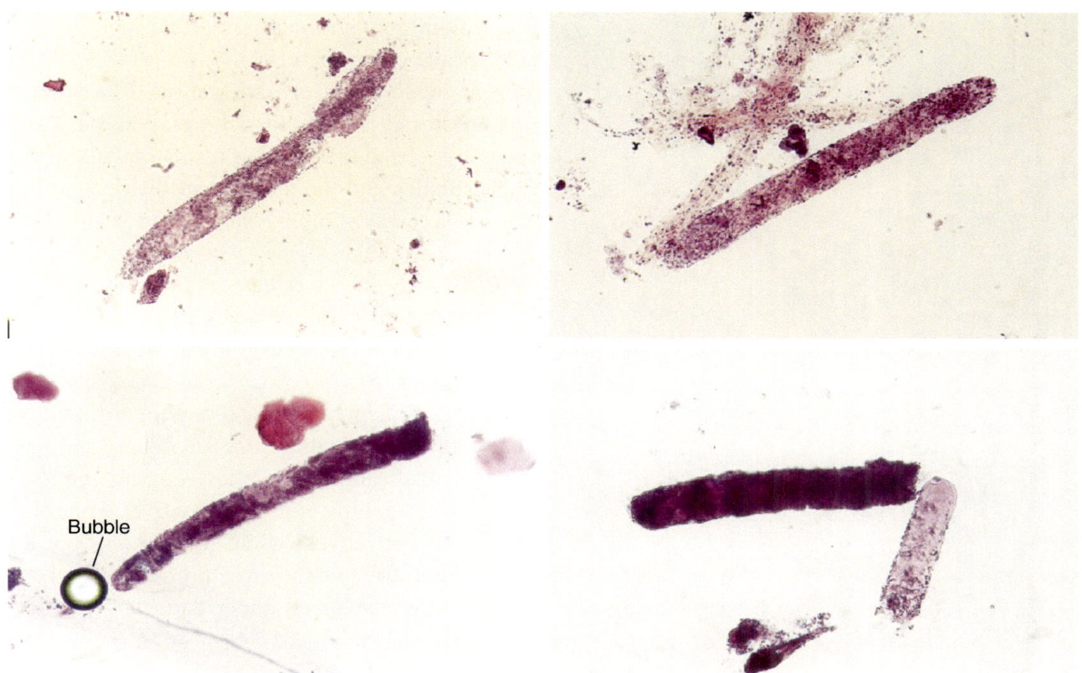

Fig. 3.9 Granular casts. The granules appear purplish-red or bluish-purple. SM stain, ×400

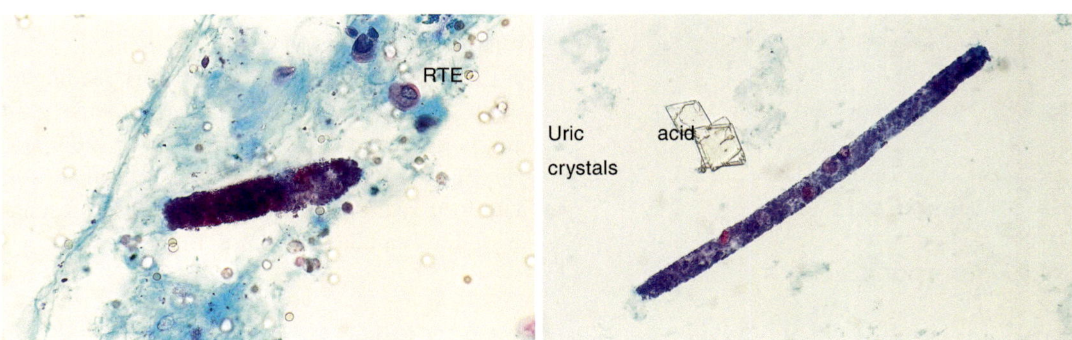

Fig. 3.10 Granular casts. The granules appear bluish-purple. S stain, ×400

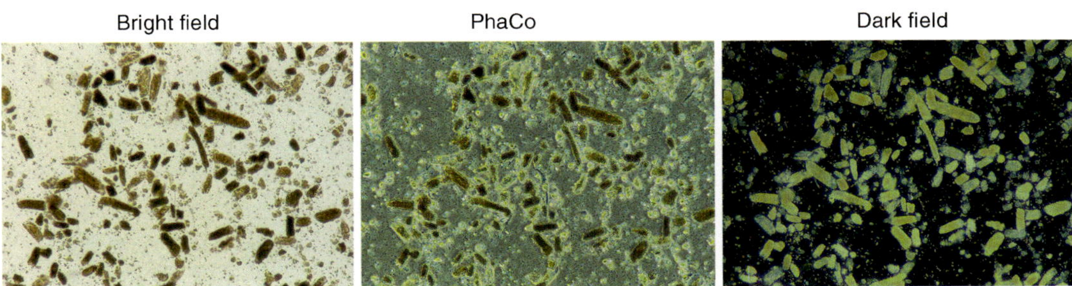

Fig. 3.11 Muddy brown casts. The granules within the cast matrix have a darker color and appear muddy brown. Unstained, ×400

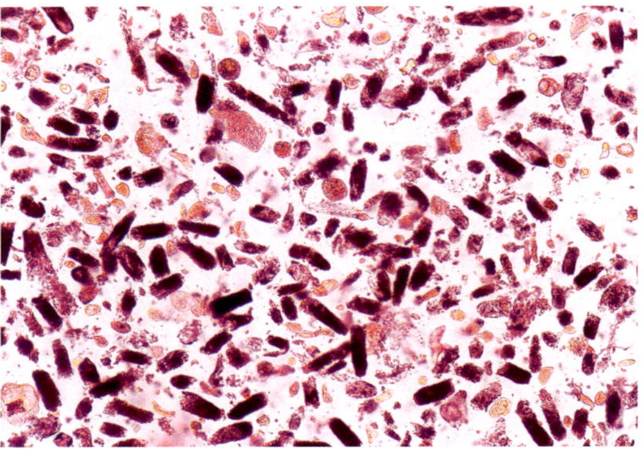

Fig. 3.12 Muddy brown casts. SM stain, ×400

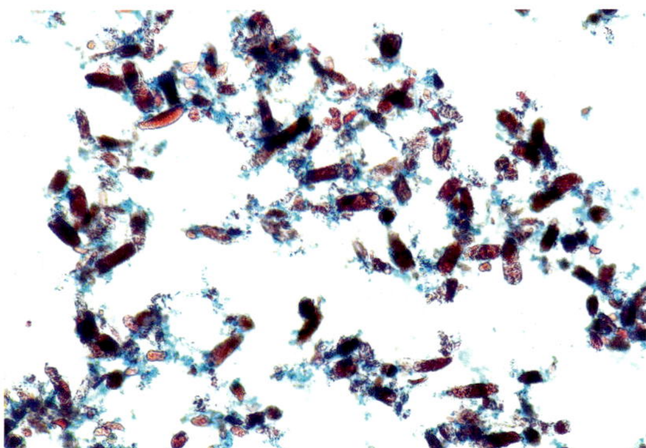

Fig. 3.13 Muddy brown casts. S stain, ×400

3.4 Waxy Casts

3.4.1 Composition

Waxy casts are formed either by the prolonged retention and degeneration of granular or cellular casts within the renal tubules or by the direct dissolution of epithelial cells undergoing amyloid-like degeneration. They can also evolve from the prolonged retention and transformation of transparent casts within the renal tubules [7].

3.4.2 Unstained

Waxy casts exhibit a thick cast matrix with a distinct waxy texture. They may show signs of twisting, folding, notches and are prone to breakage. They have a strong refractive property and can appear pale yellow or dark yellow. The length, thickness and morphological variations of waxy casts are related to the site of formation within the renal tubules and the duration of their retention. Most waxy casts appear parallel on both sides, although irregular shapes can also be observed (Fig. 3.14). Some waxy casts may exhibit a granular texture, representing an intermediate stage in the transformation from granular casts to waxy casts (Fig. 3.15).

The casts display distinct three-dimensionality, well-defined structural characteristics and are readily observable under phase contrast microscopy. They exhibit strong refractive properties along the cast edges, while the matrix appears transparent or contains a minimal number of granules, as visualized under dark field microscopy (Fig. 3.16).

3.4.3 SM Stain or S Stain

When using either SM stain or S stain, the color of casts can be influenced by urine pH, leading to slight variations. After SM staining, the cast matrix appears as either purple-red or blue-purple (Fig. 3.17). After S staining, the cast matrix is a uniform reddish-purple to deep purple, presenting a thick and heavy texture (Fig. 3.18).

3.4.4 Clinical Significance

Waxy casts are not normally found in the urine of healthy individuals. The presence of waxy casts indicates severe renal pathology with a poor prognosis. They are commonly observed in serious kidney diseases such as nephrotic syndrome, renal failure, end-stage chronic kidney disease, renal amyloidosis, and chronic rejection in kidney transplantation [8]. Broad waxy casts may be seen in advanced stages of progressive renal failure, also known as renal failure casts [9].

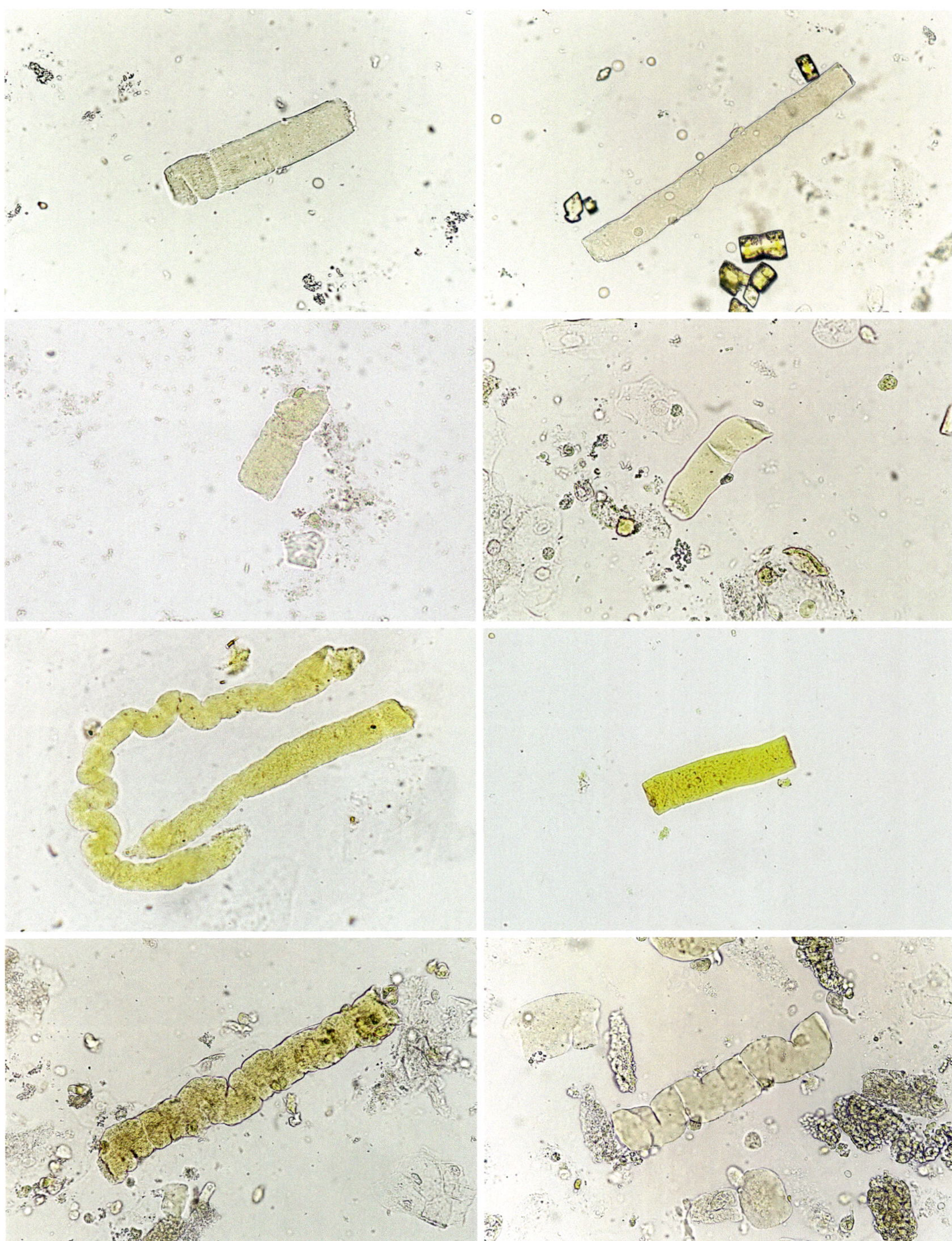

Fig. 3.14 Waxy casts. Unstained, bright field, ×400

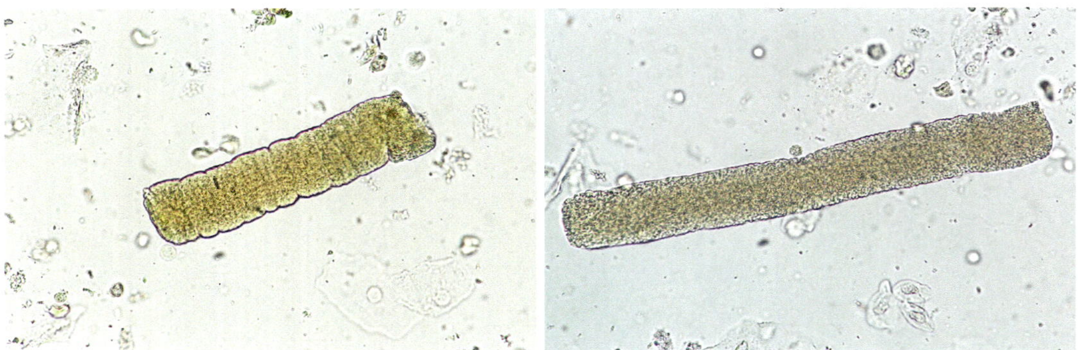

Fig. 3.15 Granular casts becoming waxy casts. Unstained, bright field, ×400

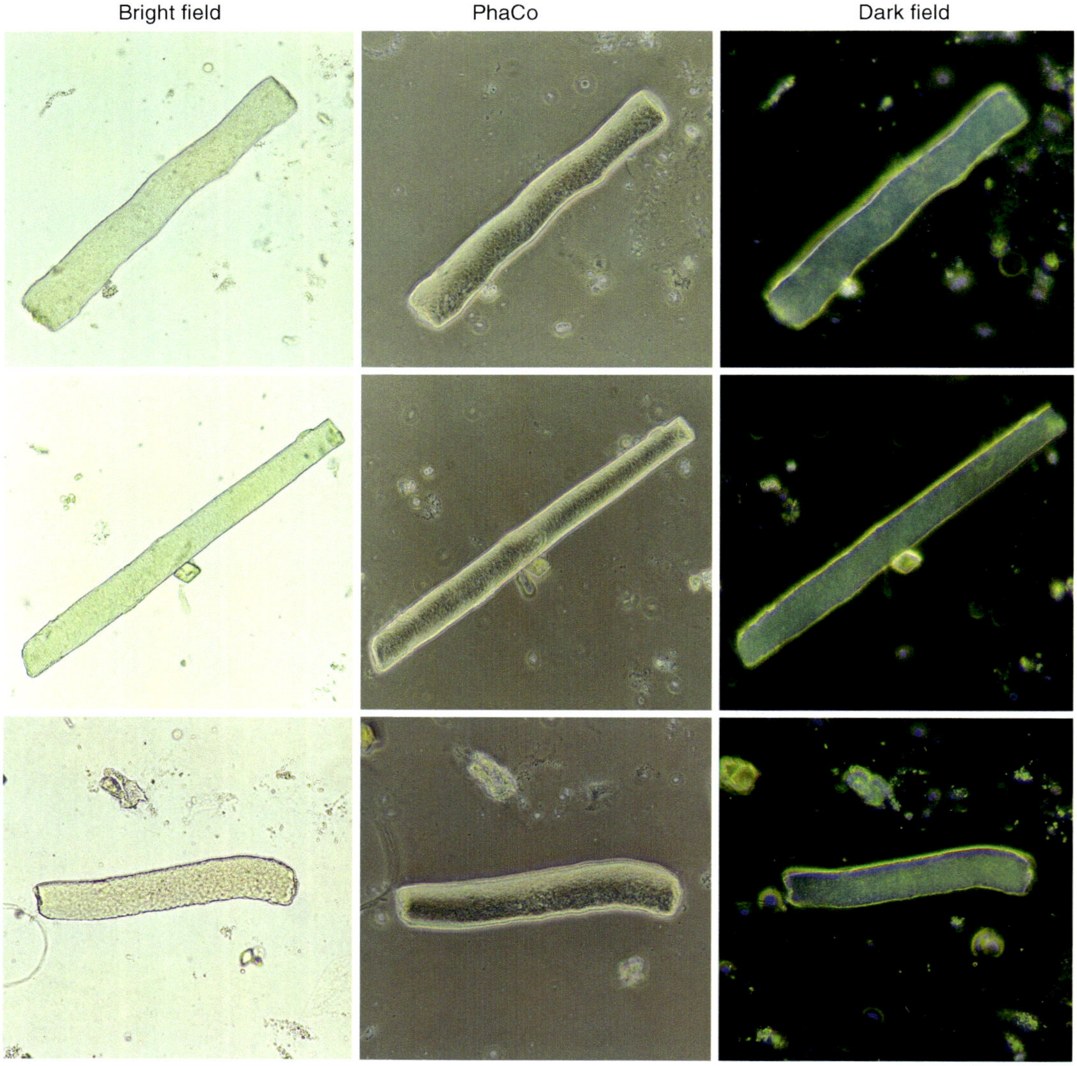

Bright field PhaCo Dark field

Fig. 3.16 Waxy casts. Unstained, ×400

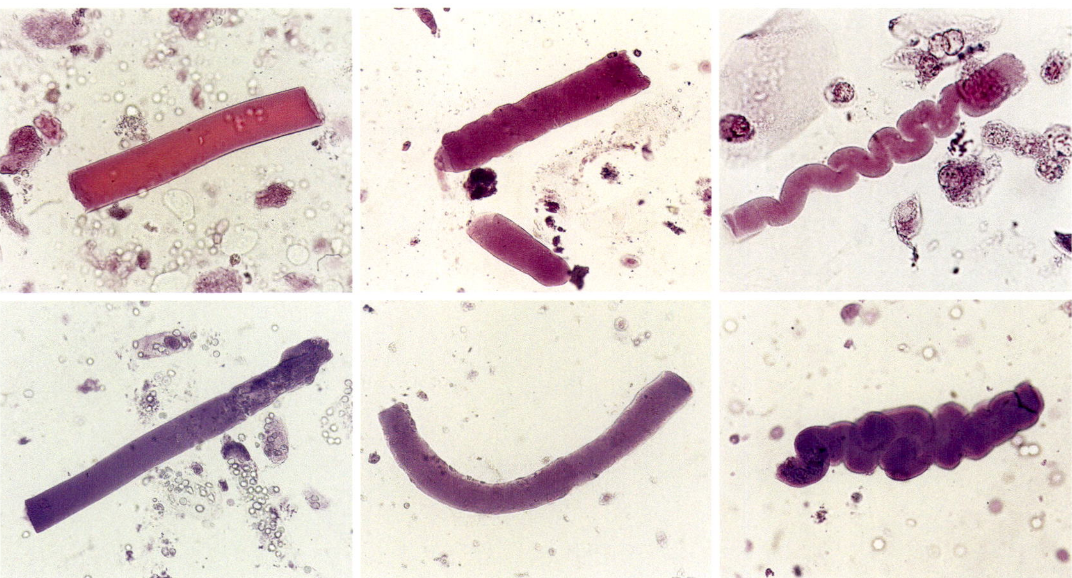

Fig. 3.17 Waxy casts. The color of casts matrix may vary slightly depending on urine pH. They appear purplish-red or bluish-purple. SM stain, ×400

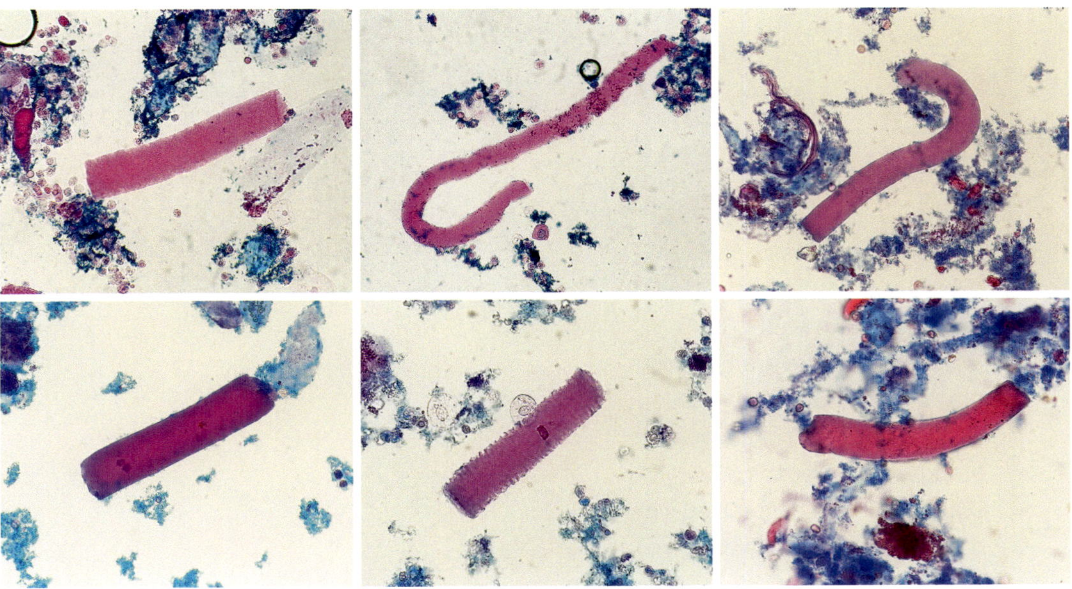

Fig. 3.18 Waxy casts. The matrix appears pinkish-red or purplish-red. S stain, ×400

3.4.5 Identification with Similar Casts

Waxy casts and hemoglobin casts exhibit distinct morphological similarities, but the colors of the cast matrix and the background cells are slightly different, and they each have different clinical significance (Fig. 3.19).

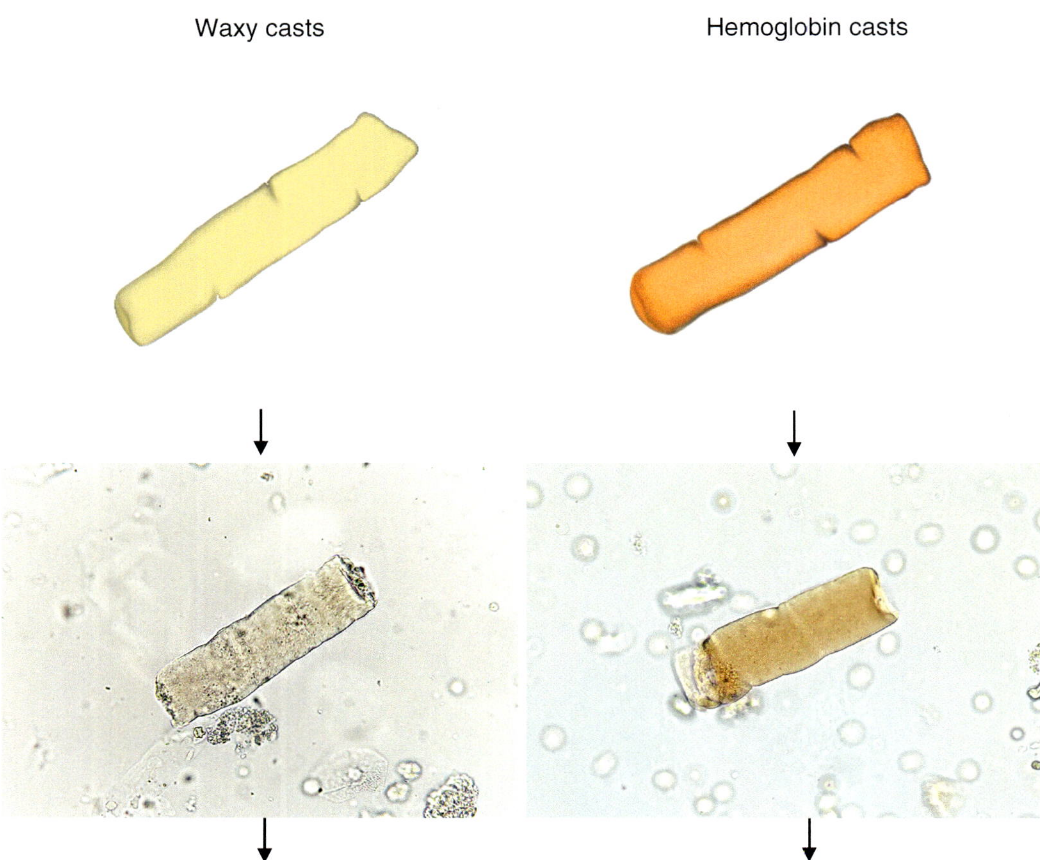

Points of differentiation

- Matrix: Both types of casts exhibit a relatively thick and homogenous matrix.
- Color: Waxy casts are typically grayish-white or pale yellow, while hemoglobin casts appear orange-red or red in color. Waxy casts are associated with dark yellow color in the
- Background: Hemoglobin casts are often accompanied by red blood cells or ghost cells and may coexist with red blood cell casts or blood casts. Waxy casts are commonly observed alongside granular casts or hyaline casts.

Fig. 3.19 Key distinguishing points between waxy casts and hemoglobin casts

3.5 White Blood Cell Casts (WBC Casts)

3.5.1 Composition

These casts contain varying numbers of intact white blood cells [10, 11].

3.5.2 Unstained

The WBC casts can contain different numbers of white blood cells (Fig. 3.20). They may be densely or loosely arranged, with small cell volumes and a three-dimensional structure. The cytoplasm often exhibits granular appearance, and the nuclear structure is usually not well-defined (Fig. 3.21). Under phase contrast microscopy, the WBC casts exhibit prominent three-dimensional characteristics and clear structural details. The WBCs within the casts demonstrate small cell volumes and strong refractivity under dark field (Fig. 3.22).

3.5.3 SM Stain and S Stain

WBC casts matrix appears pink after SM staining, while the WBCs may not stain well or appear purplish-red. The nuclear structure is not clearly visible, and small lipid droplets are often observed within the cytoplasm (Fig. 3.23). WBC casts matrix appears light blue, and the white blood cells may not appear blue or purplish-red with S stain (Fig. 3.24).

3.5.4 Peroxidase Staining

The neutrophils within the casts show a positive reaction (Fig. 3.25), while the renal tubular epithelial cells show a negative reaction.

3.5.5 Clinical Significance

WBC casts are not normally found in the urine of healthy individuals. They may be present in the urine specimens of patients with conditions such as pyelonephritis, glomerulonephritis and interstitial nephritis. The predominant WBCs in these casts are usually neutrophils, but in cases of renal transplant rejection or certain cancer drug treatments, there may be an increase in lymphocytes or monocytes [12].

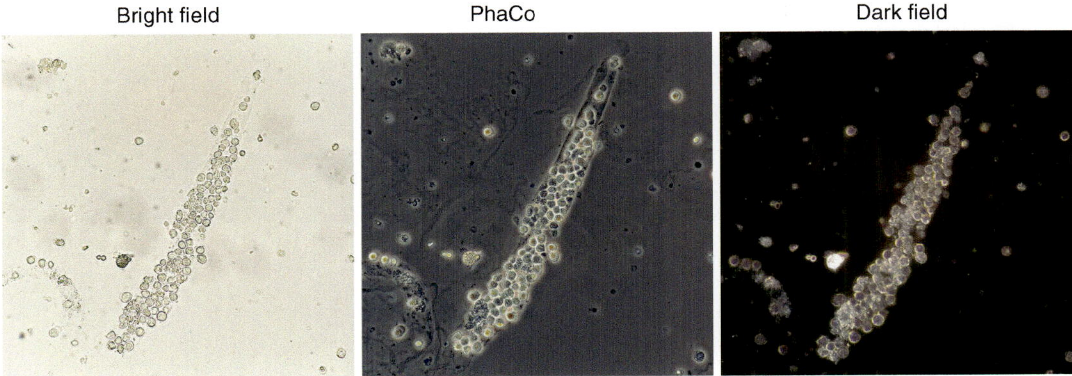

Fig. 3.20 WBC casts. The cast matrix contains a large number of WBCs. Unstained, ×400

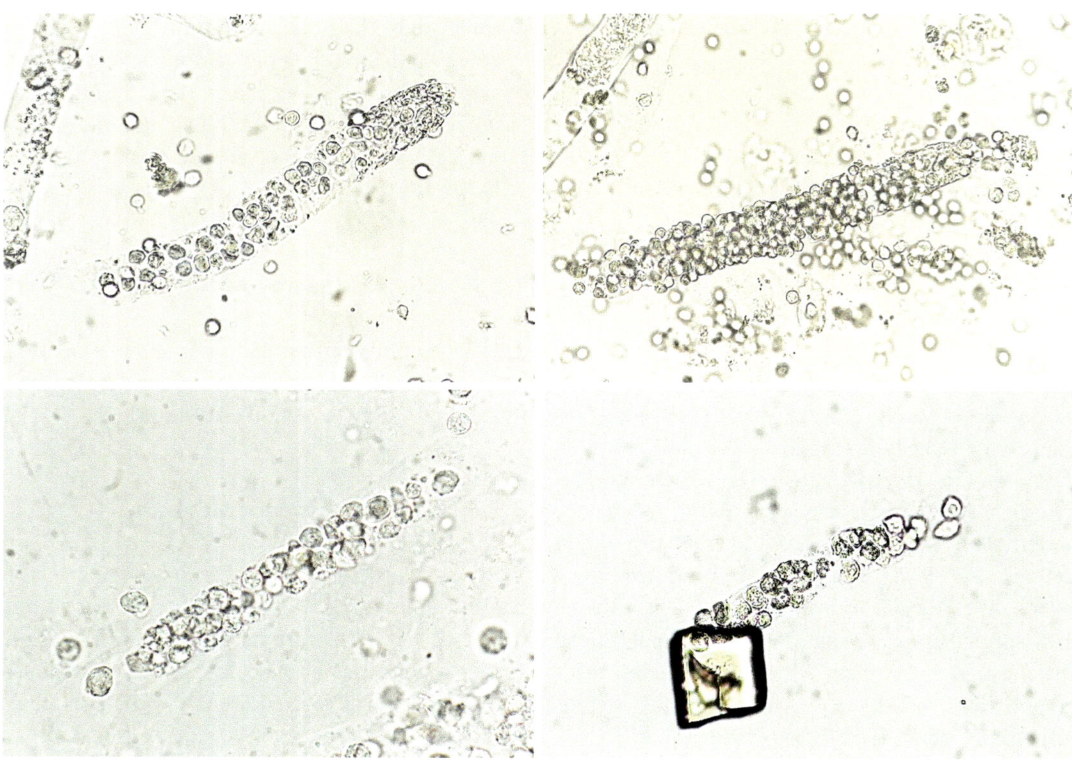

Fig. 3.21 WBC casts. Unstained, bright field, ×400

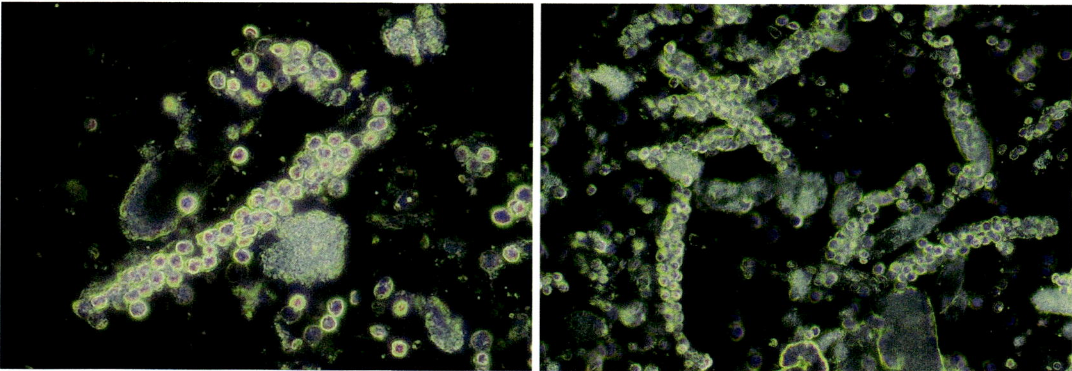

Fig. 3.22 WBC casts. Unstained, dark field, ×400

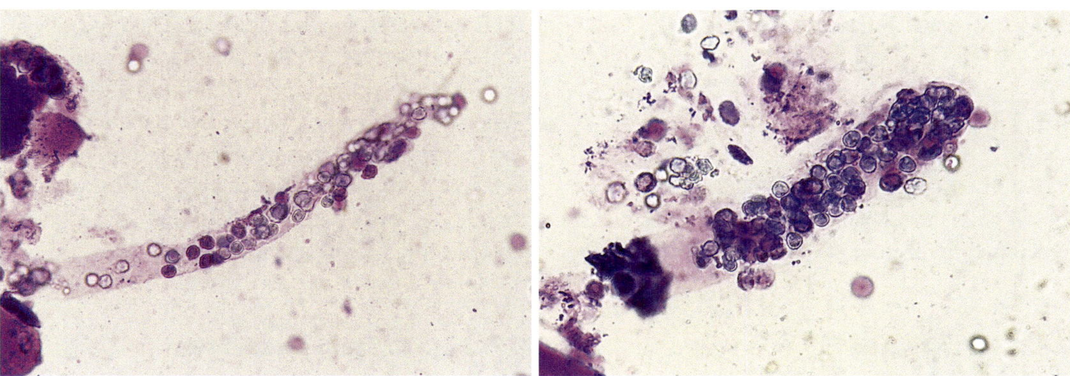

Fig. 3.23 WBC casts. The matrix of the casts appears pink, and the WBCs exhibit purplish-red or bluish-purple. SM stain, ×400

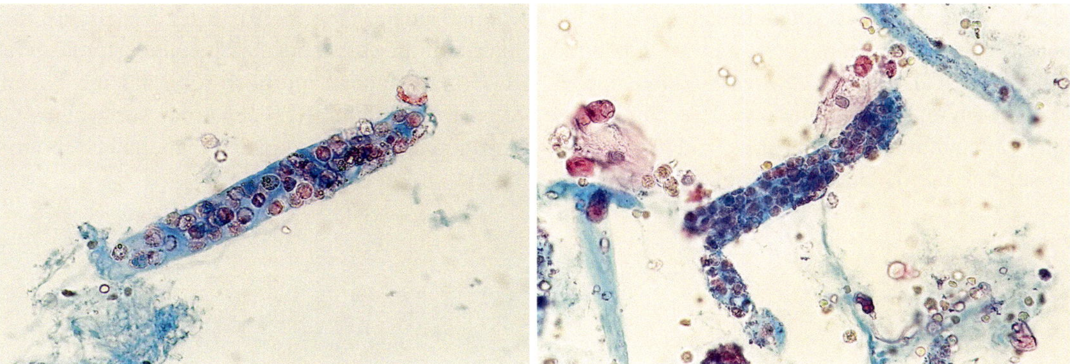

Fig. 3.24 WBC casts. The matrix of the casts appears pale blue, and the WBCs exhibit deep blue or bluish-purple color. S stain, ×400

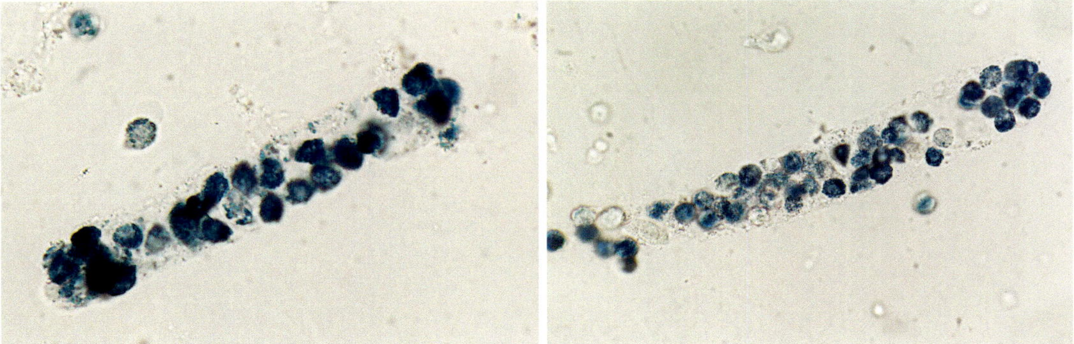

Fig. 3.25 WBC casts. Peroxidase staining, bright field, ×1000

3.6 Renal Tubular Epithelial (RTE) Cell Casts

3.6.1 Composition

RTE cell casts are formed when renal tubular epithelial cells detach due to various causes and are enveloped by proteins to form casts [10].

3.6.2 Unstained

The RTE cells within the casts are slightly larger than WBCs on bright field microscopy, exhibit irregular morphology, and have a granular cytoplasm. They have a single nucleus, and the nuclear structure of some cells may be indistinct. Unstained RTE cells in the casts often appear grayish-white or light yellow. The number of RTE cells within the casts varies, and they can be loosely or tightly arranged (Fig. 3.26). Typical RTE cell casts show a tile-like stacking pattern, with scattered RTE cells in the background. They appear dark yellow in bilirubinuria (Fig. 3.27). When observed under phase contrast microscopy, the matrix of the casts is relatively thin, the RTE cells have enlarged volumes and irregular shapes, and some cells exhibit increased and coarser cytoplasmic granules (Fig. 3.28).

3.6.3 SM Stain and S Stain

The matrix of RTE cell casts appears pink after SM staining, while the RTE cells themselves may exhibit shades of red or purplish-red, with darker-colored nuclei (Fig. 3.29). After S staining, the matrix of the casts appears blue, the cytoplasm of RTE cells appears purplish-red, and the nuclei appear blue. Some RTE cells may show signs of degeneration, with fragmented nuclei and granular cytoplasm (Fig. 3.30).

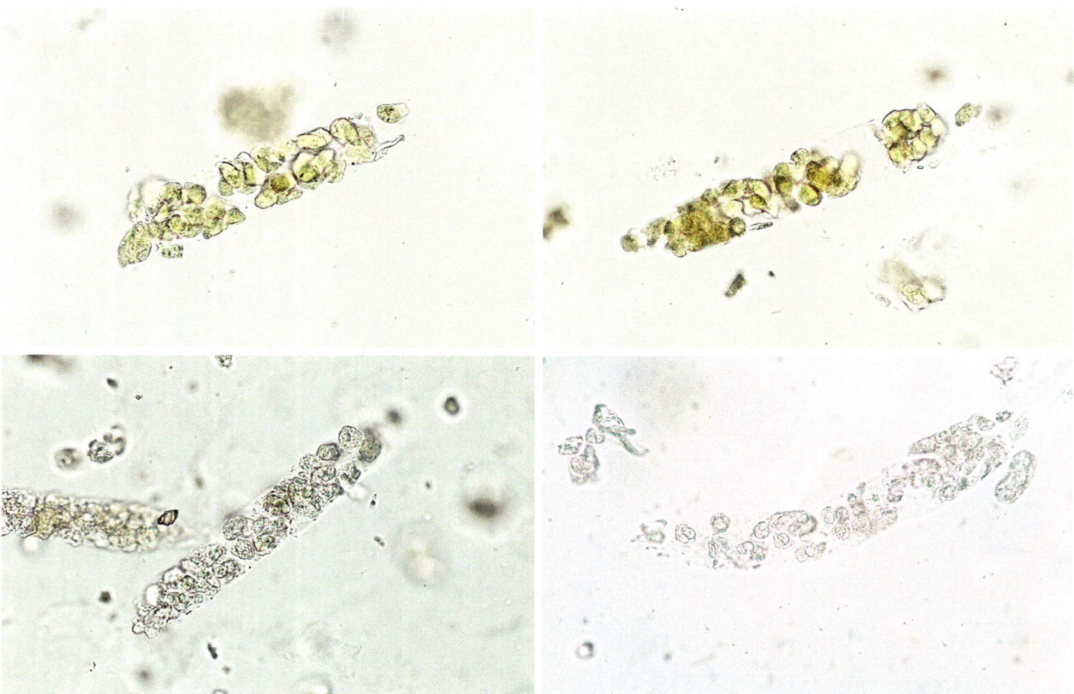

Fig. 3.26 RTE cell casts. The number of cells within the cast matrix varies, and they are arranged either densely or loosely. Unstained, bright field, ×400

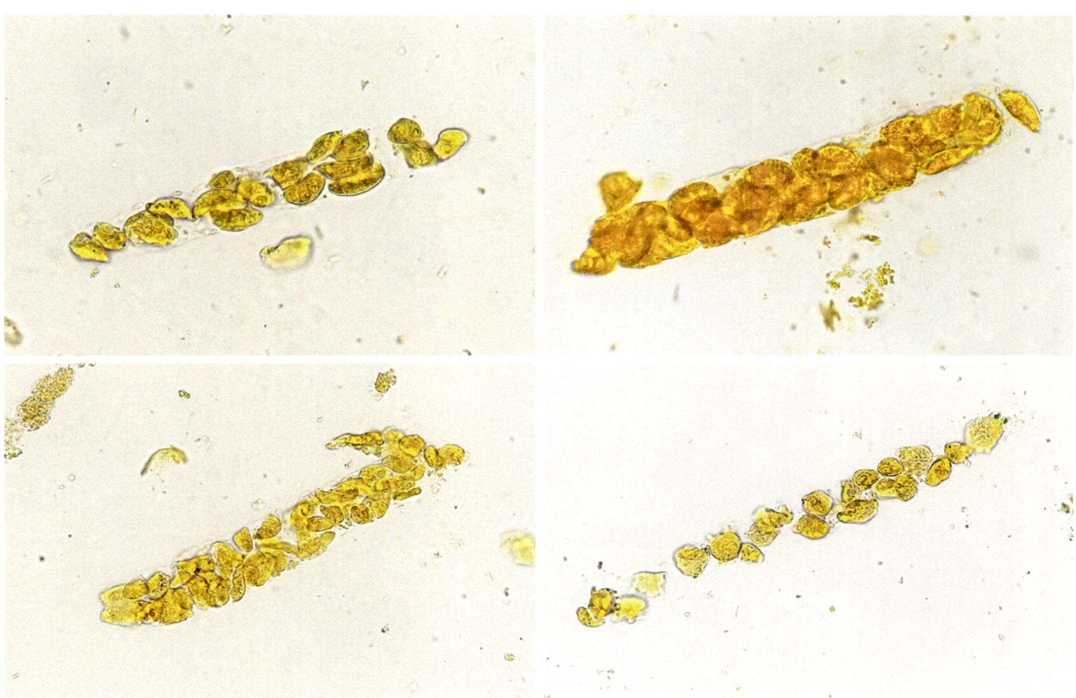

Fig. 3.27 RTE cell casts. RTE cells arranged tightly or loosely within the cast, bilirubinuria, ×1000

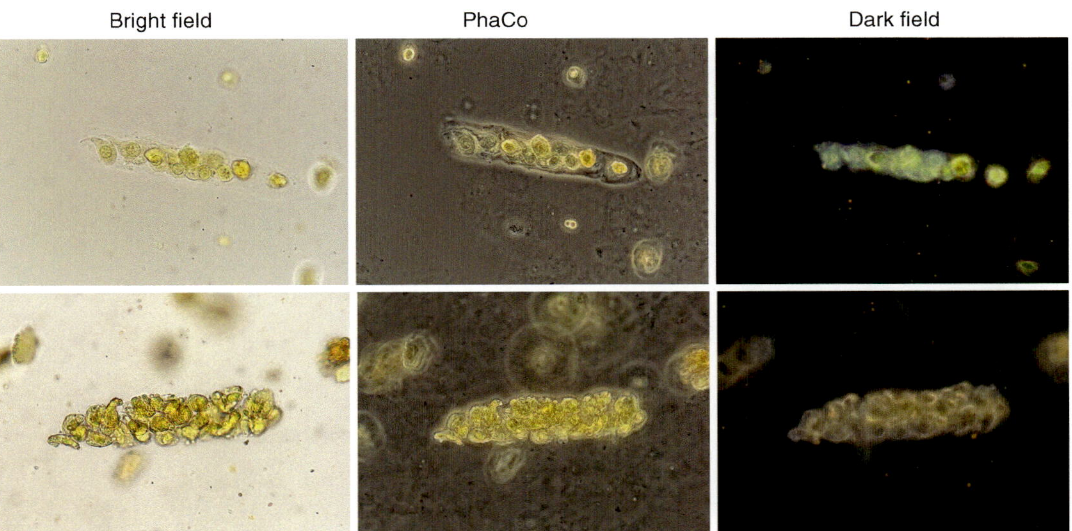

Fig. 3.28 RTE cell casts. Unstained, ×400

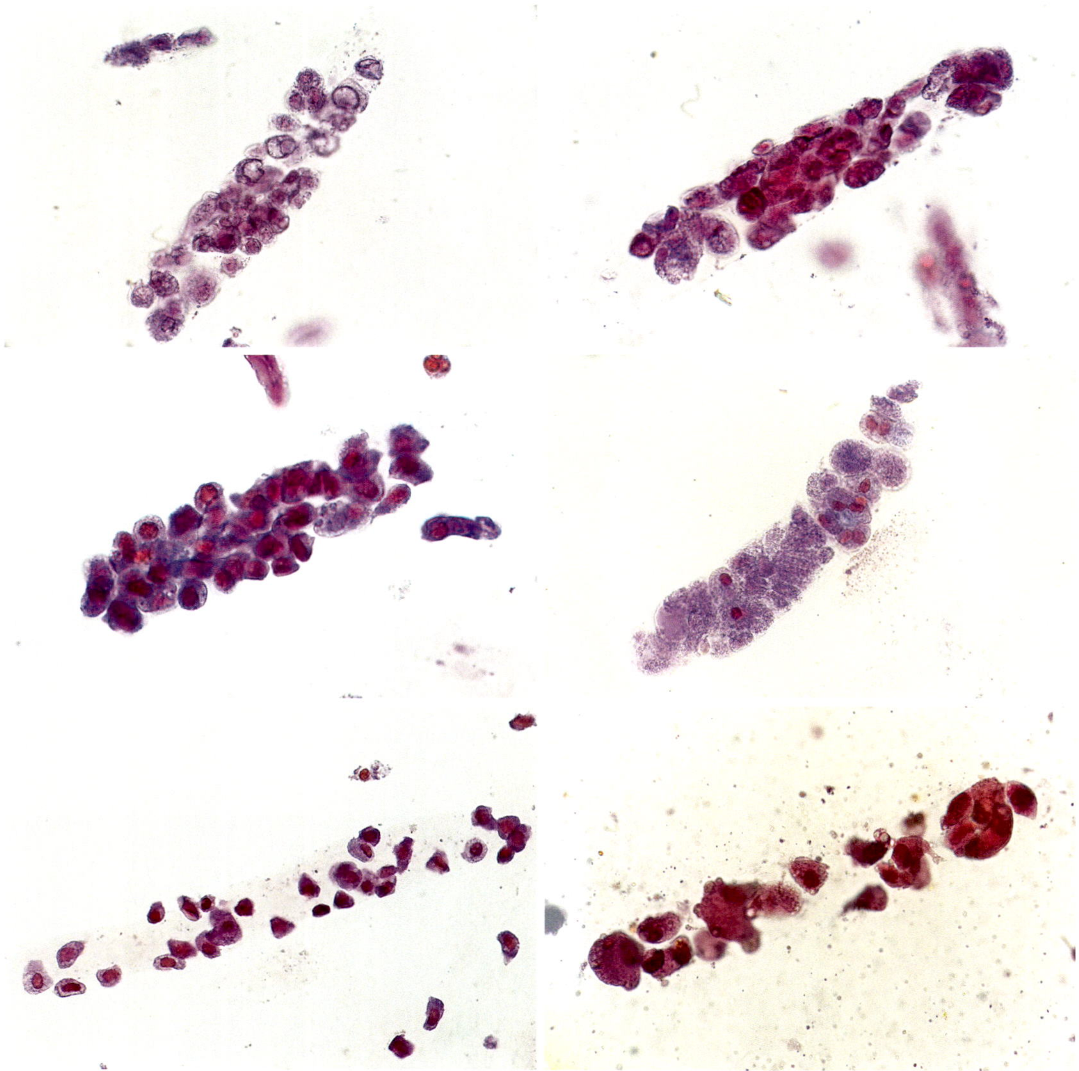

Fig. 3.29 RTE cell casts. SM stain, ×1000

3.6.4 Clinical Significance

RTE cell casts are absent in the urine of healthy individuals. The presence of RTE cell casts suggests renal tubular injury and is commonly observed in conditions such as acute tubular necrosis, heavy metal or chemical poisoning, renal transplant rejection and renal amyloidosis [10, 13, 14].

3.6.5 Differentiation from Similar Casts

When RTE cell casts have a small cell volume, tight arrangement, and unclear cell structure, they may be easily confused with WBC casts (Fig. 3.31).

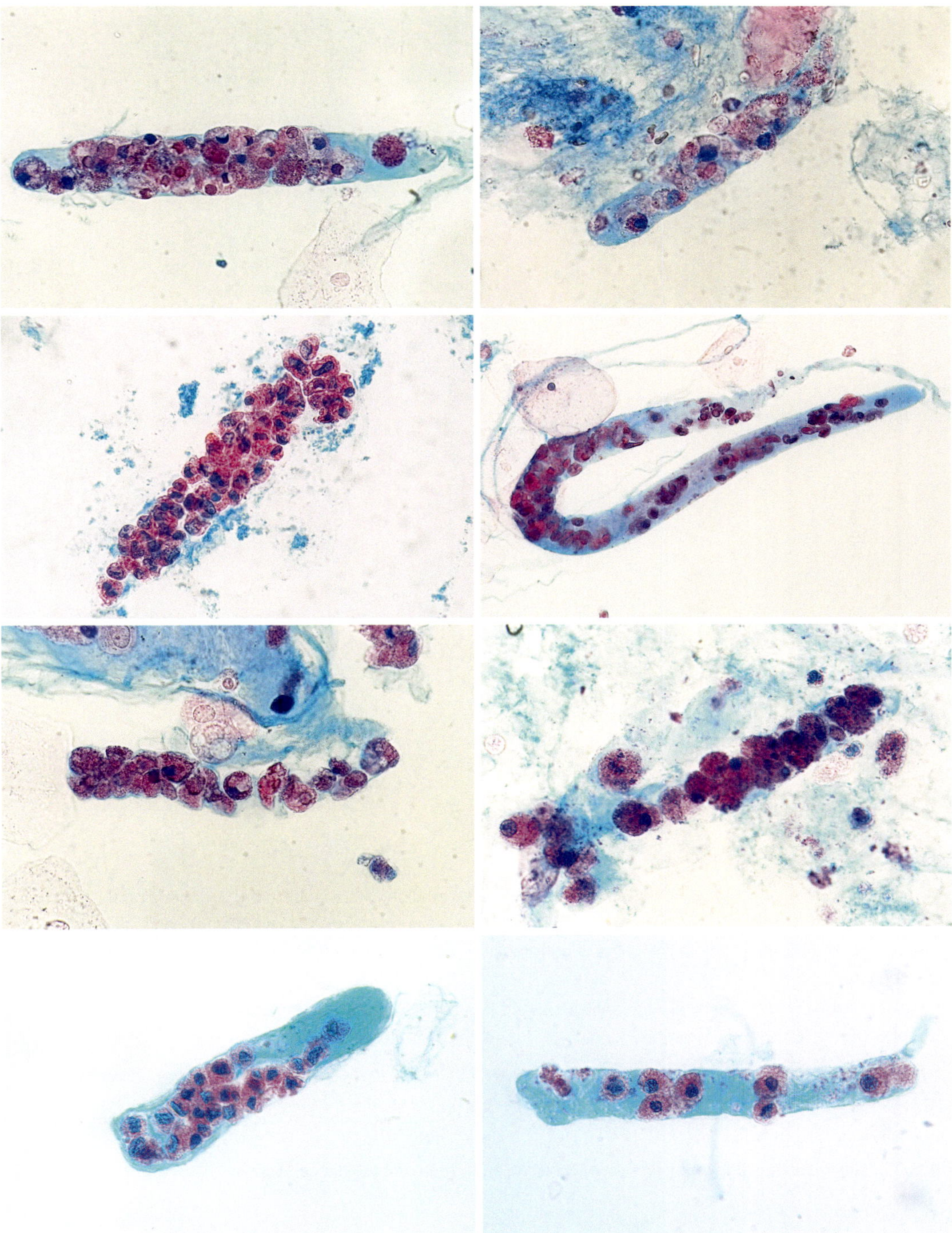

Fig. 3.30 RTE cell casts. The matrix appears blue, and the structure of the renal tubular epithelial cells is clear. S stain, ×1000

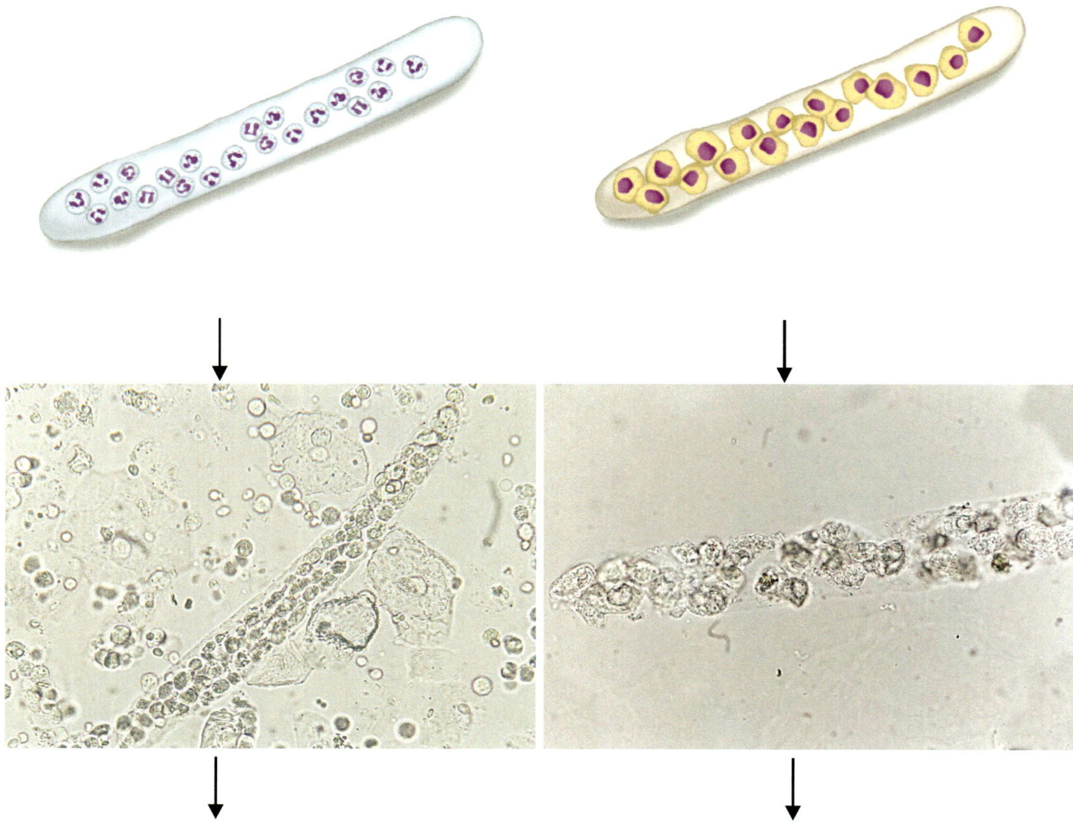

Points of differentiation

Cell volume: The leukocytes within the casts are usually small in size, exhibit a three-dimensional structure, and often show signs of degeneration, typically making the cell nucleus difficult to visualize clearly. The volume of RTE cells within the casts is generally larger, ranging from 2 to 4 times the size of leukocytes or even larger.

Cell arrangement: RTE cells are typically arranged in a tile-like pattern, they may be arranged densely or loosely. The WBCs may be arranged loosely or densely within the WBC casts.

Background cells: WBC casts are primarily composed of WBCs in the background, and the background of RTE cell casts is commonly observed to contain varying numbers of RTC cells.

Fig. 3.31 Key distinguishing points between leukocyte casts and renal tubular cell casts

3.7 Red Blood Cell Casts (RBC Casts or Erythrocyte Casts)

3.7.1 Composition

RBC casts are formed when RBCs pass through the glomerular basement membrane and are enveloped by proteins such as THP, resulting from various causes of glomerular injury [5].

3.7.2 Unstained

RBC casts contain a varying number of intact RBCs or ghost cells. They may be densely packed or scattered within the cast matrix (Fig. 3.32). When RBC casts are present, a large number of RBCs can be seen in the background (Fig. 3.33).

3.7.3 SM Stain and S Stain

The cast matrix appears pale red after SM staining, while the RBCs within the cast may appear purplish-red or unstained (Fig. 3.34). The cast matrix appears blue, and the RBCs within the cast appear pale red color or unstained after S staining (Fig. 3.35).

3.7.4 Clinical Significance

The presence of RBC casts in the urine suggests glomerular disease and hemorrhage within the renal units. They can be observed in conditions such as acute glomerulonephritis, acute exacerbation of chronic nephritis, renal hematuria, acute tubular necrosis, renal transplant rejection,

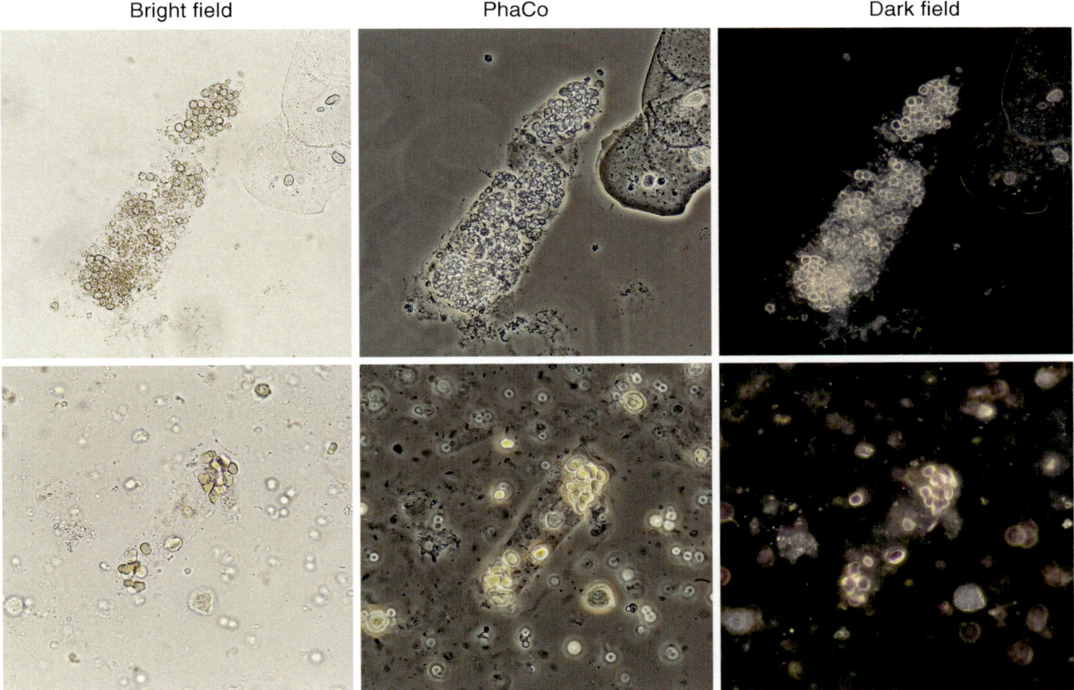

Fig. 3.32 RBC casts. Unstained, ×1000

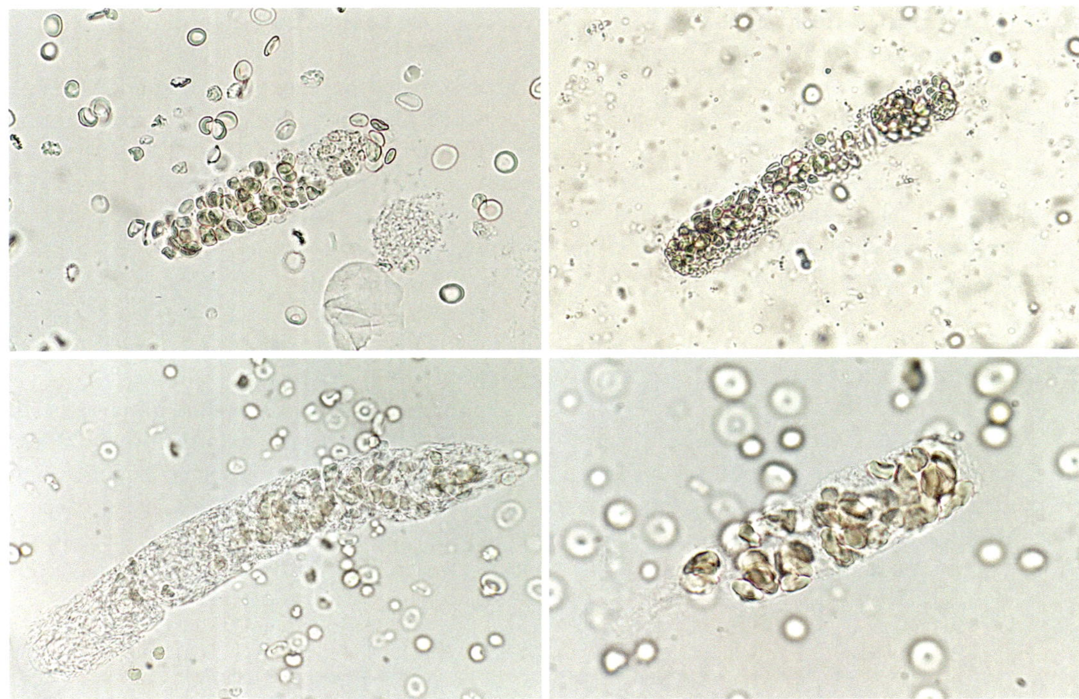

Fig. 3.33 RBC casts. The number of RBCs within the cast varies. Unstained, bright field, ×1000

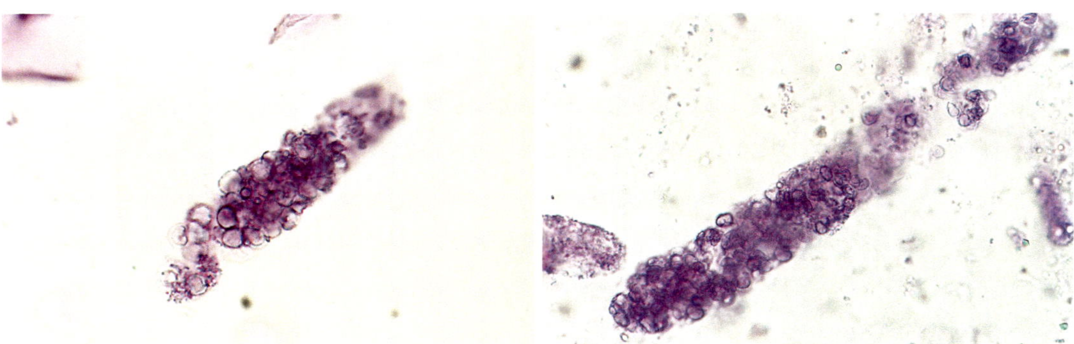

Fig. 3.34 RBC casts. Varying numbers of ghost cells can be seen within the cast. SM stain, ×1000

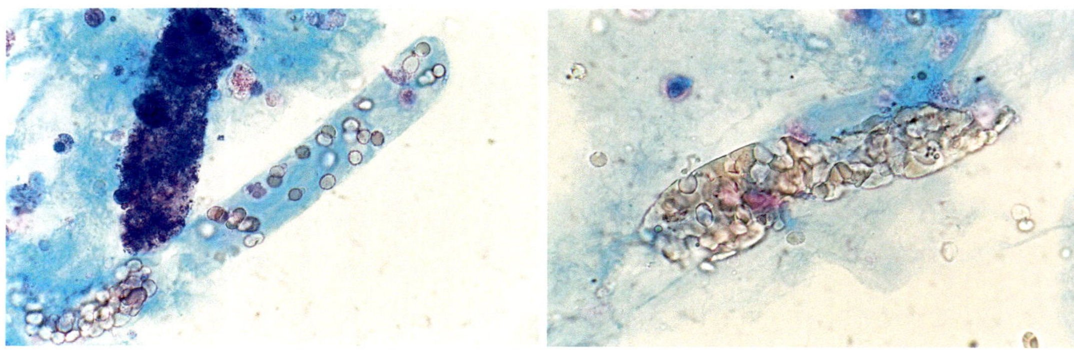

Fig. 3.35 RBC casts. The cast matrix is blue, and the RBCs are not easily stained. S stain, ×1000

interstitial nephritis and renal tumors. RBC casts can also be seen in healthy individuals following vigorous exercise [6, 15].

3.8 Blood Casts

3.8.1 Composition

Blood casts are formed when RBCs become trapped and gradually disintegrate within the renal tubules.

3.8.2 Unstained

Blood casts contain a large amount of hemoglobin and fragments of RBCs. They resemble granular casts and appear red or brownish-red when unstained under dark field or phase contrast microscopy (Fig. 3.36). A large number of RBCs are present in the background (Fig. 3.37). In some cases, the granules within the cast matrix are small (Fig. 3.38).

3.8.3 SM Stain and S Stain

The granules within the casts appear purplish-red after SM staining (Fig. 3.39), and they appear bluish-purple after S staining (Fig. 3.40).

3.8.4 Clinical Significance

Blood casts share the same clinical significance as RBC casts. They indicate renal bleeding, and the presence of blood casts suggests more severe urinary stasis and obstruction [5, 6].

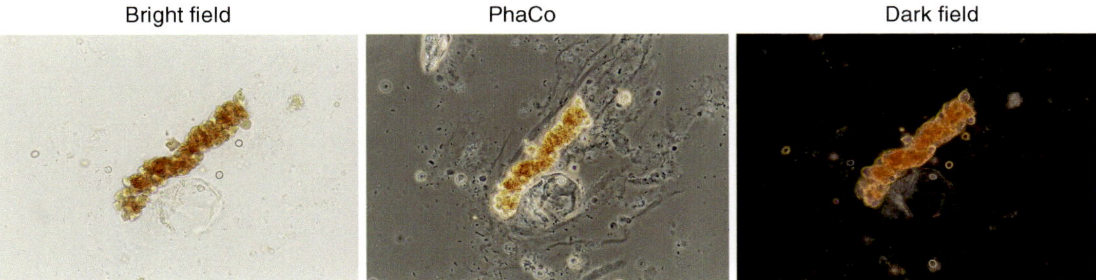

Fig. 3.36 Blood casts. The granules appear orange-red under dark field or phase contrast microscopy. Unstained, ×400

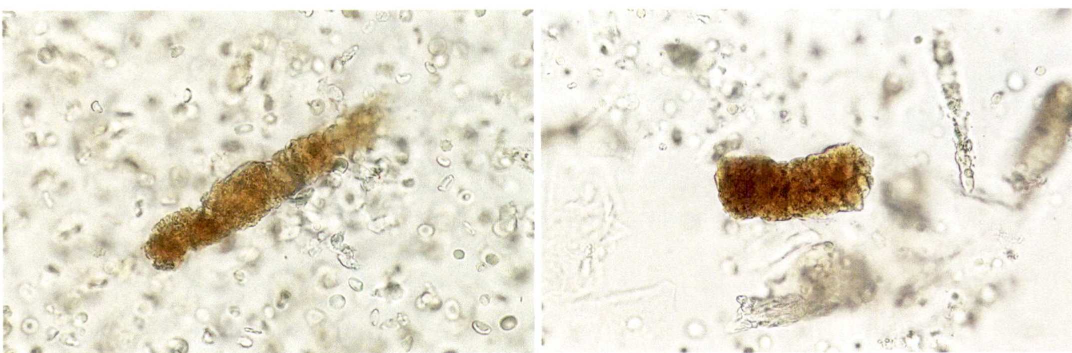

Fig. 3.37 Blood casts. A large number of red blood cells can be observed in the background. Unstained, bright field, ×400

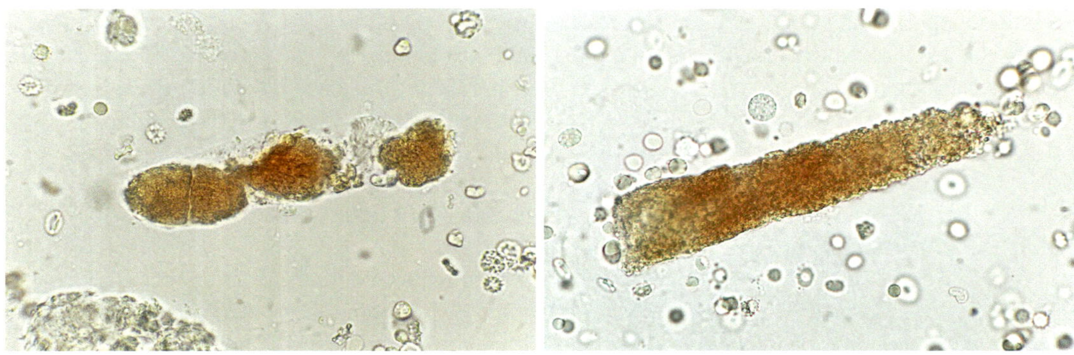

Fig. 3.38 Blood casts. The granules within the matrix are small and appear orange-red. Unstained, bright field, ×1000

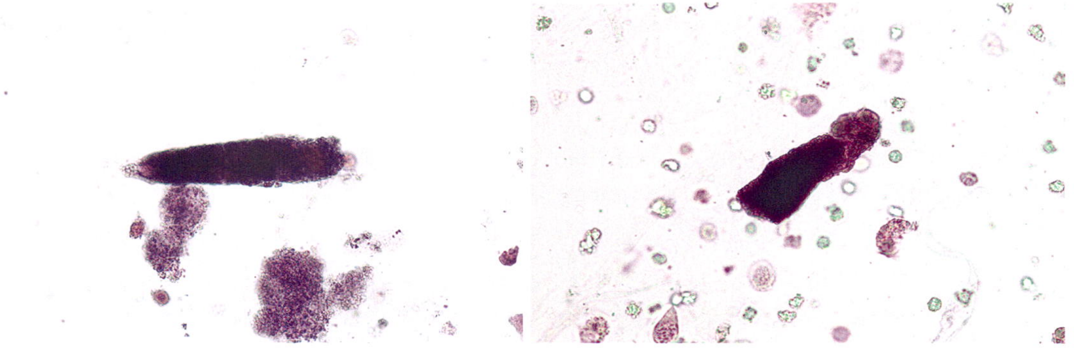

Fig. 3.39 Blood casts. The granules within the casts appear purplish-red in color. SM stain, ×400

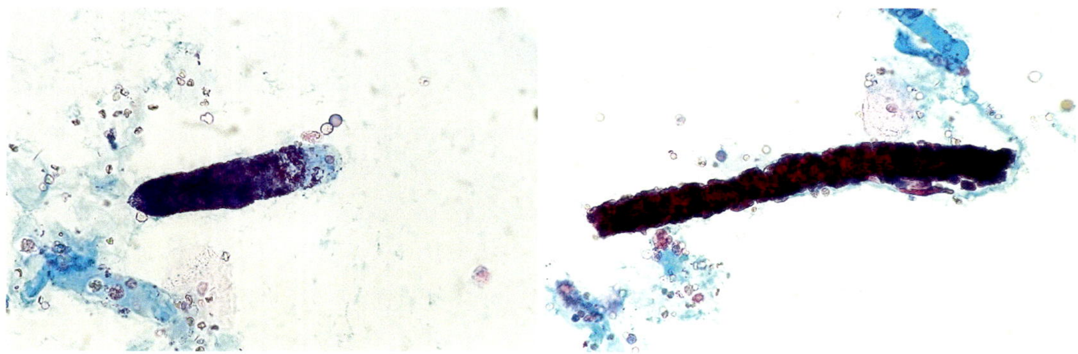

Fig. 3.40 Blood casts. The granules within the casts appear bluish-purple in color. S stain, ×400

3.8.5 Identifying Blood Casts from Similar Casts

Blood casts, granular casts and muddy brown casts are morphologically similar, all of them contain a varying amount of granules within the matrix. But the origin of the granules in the matrix, their colors and clinical implications are all different (Fig. 3.41).

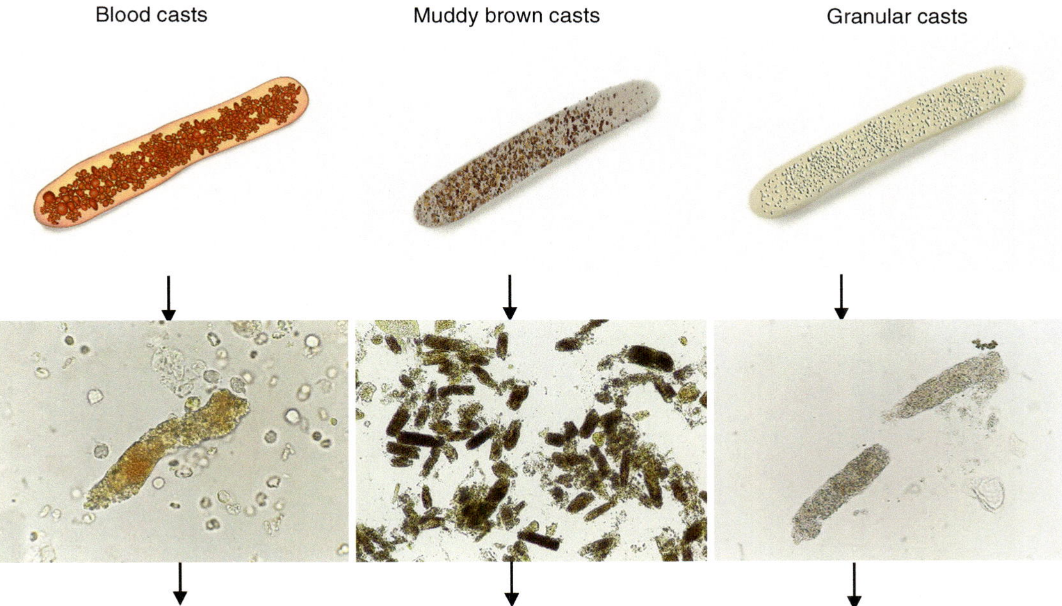

Key points for differentiation

Composition: Blood casts are composed of fragmented RBCs and hemoglobin, while granular casts are composed of cellular debris and precipitated proteins. Muddy brown casts are formed by the presence of dark brown granules.

Color: Blood casts appear red or reddish-brown. Granular casts can vary in color, but they are typically yellowish or brownish. Muddy brown casts have a characteristic brown color.

Clinical significance: The presence of blood casts indicates active bleeding within the renal system, such as glomerular injury or inflammation. Granular casts can be seen in various renal conditions, including acute tubular injury, glomerulonephritis, and pyelonephritis. Muddy brown casts are typically associated with acute tubular necrosis.

Fig. 3.41 Key distinguishing points between blood casts, granular casts and muddy brown casts

3.9 Hemoglobin Casts

3.9.1 Composition

The breakdown of RBCs within the cast results in the formation of hemoglobin casts, where the granular content gradually homogenizes [10].

3.9.2 Unstained Appearance

The cast matrix appears waxy and homogeneous, resembling waxy casts. However, the color of hemoglobin casts differs from waxy casts, displaying a pale red or orange (Fig. 3.42). Some casts exhibit a transitional phase from blood casts to hemoglobin casts, with small granules within their matrix.

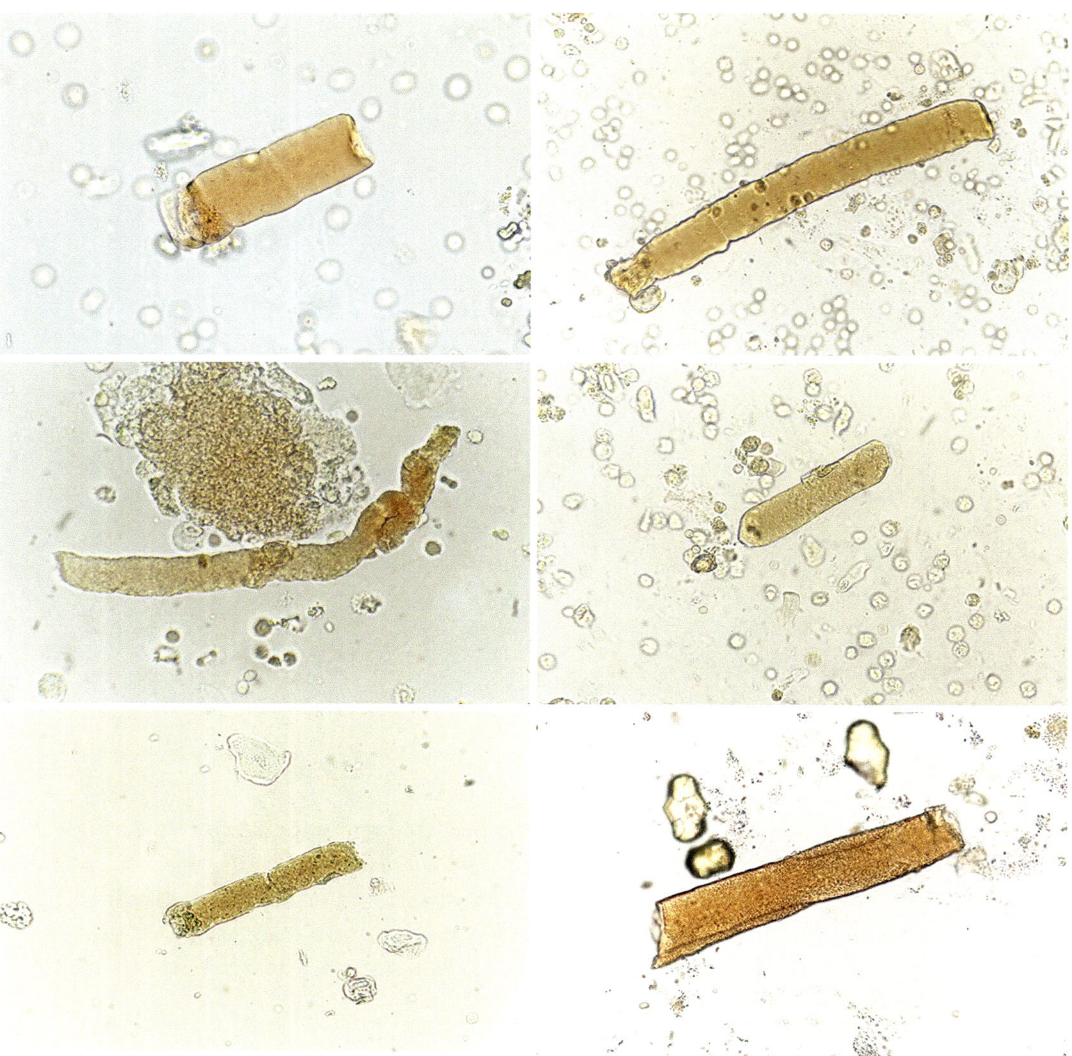

Fig. 3.42 Hemoglobin casts. The matrix of the casts appears orange-red. Unstained, bright field, ×400

Unstained hemoglobin casts exhibit similar color and morphology to myoglobin. A comprehensive analysis considering the patient's medical history is necessary. The presence of myoglobin in the urine can be confirmed using the ammonium sulfate saturation test. ELISA or radioimmunoassay utilizing monoclonal antibodies against myoglobin offer higher sensitivity and specificity. Positive results for myoglobin and negative results for hemoglobin indicate myoglobinuria.

3.9.3 Clinical Significance

Hemoglobin casts merely indicate the presence of hemoglobin within the cast, which may be an indicator of non-renal diseases such as in severe hemolytic anemias (e.g., PNH, autoimmune hemolytic anemia). If urine stasis is sufficient, RBC casts or blood casts degenerate into hemoglobin casts, accompanied by lysis of RBCs and homogenization of hemoglobin. In such cases, the significance of hemoglobin casts is similar to that of RBC casts and blood casts, indicating renal hematuria [5].

3.10 Broad Casts

3.10.1 Composition

Broad casts have a width exceeding 50 μm, which is two to six times wider than other casts. They are predominantly observed as broad granular casts and broad waxy casts, varying in length, appearing either straight or twisted. Some casts are prone to fragmentation.

3.10.2 Unstained

The most prominent characteristic of broad casts is their significantly increased width. Broad casts can contain components such as granules and cells, and they can appear transparent or waxy. Based on the identification of broad casts, further differentiation can be made according to the specific components present, such as broad granular casts, broad waxy casts and broad cellular casts (Fig. 3.43).

3.10.3 SM Stain and S Stain

The staining characteristics are the same as those for casts of the same type (Figs. 3.44 and 3.45).

3.10.4 Clinical Significance

Broad casts are not normally present in urine. They originate from dilated and damaged renal tubules, indicating severe urinary stasis in the local area of the kidney. They are commonly observed in conditions such as early diuresis in acute renal failure, acute kidney injury following hemolytic transfusion reaction, crush syndrome, acute kidney injury after extensive burns, end-stage kidney disease caused by various reasons, and other related conditions.

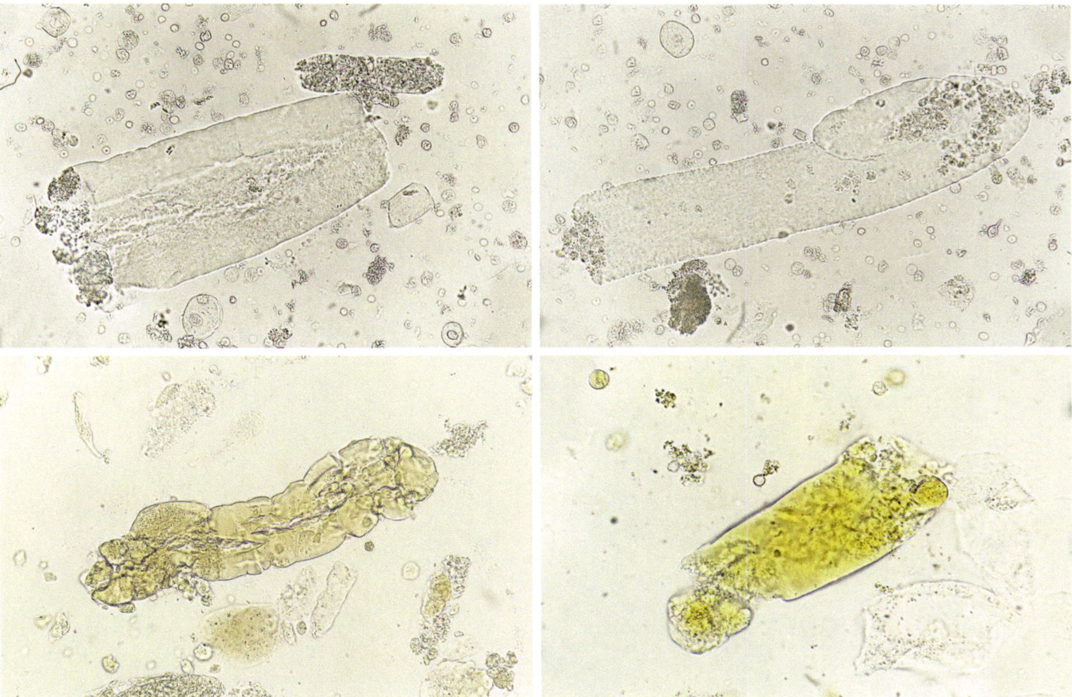

Fig. 3.43 Broad casts. Unstained, bright field, ×400

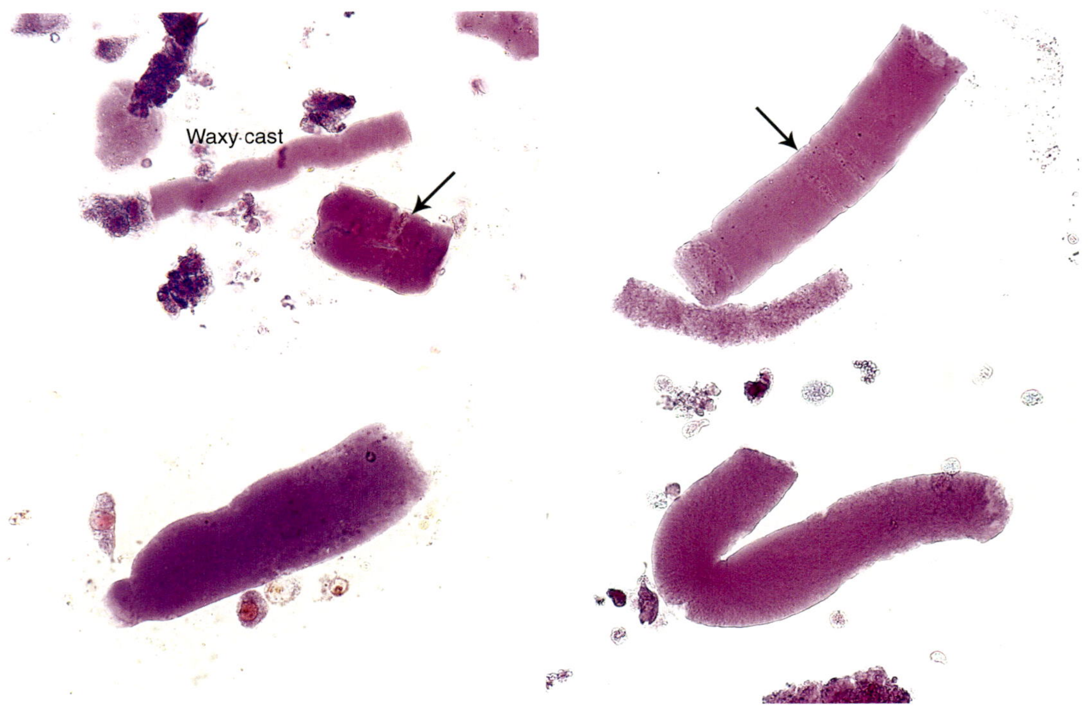

Fig. 3.44 Broad casts (↑). SM stain, ×400

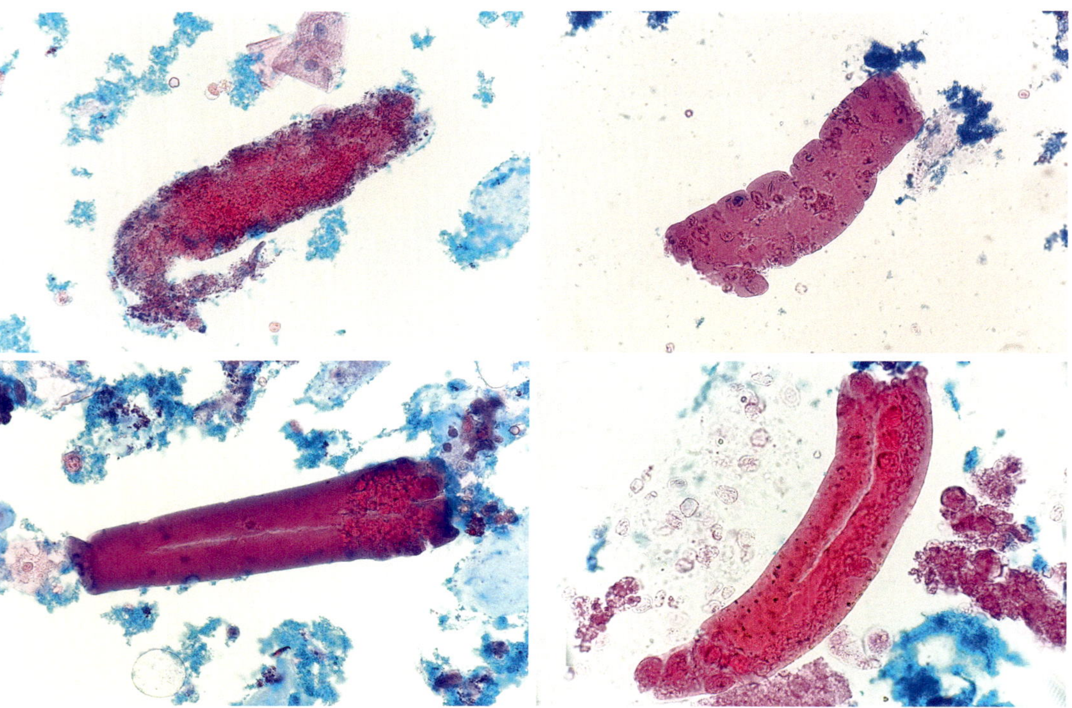

Fig. 3.45 Broad casts. S stain, ×400

3.11 Crystal Casts

3.11.1 Composition

Crystal casts consist of amorphous salts, calcium oxalate crystals, bilirubin crystals, drug crystals and other types of crystals within the cast matrix. These casts need to be differentiated from pseudocasts formed by salt crystals.

3.11.2 Unstained

The cast matrix appears transparent, and various forms of crystals can be observed within it, differing slightly in quantity and size (Fig. 3.46). Under phase contrast and dark field microscopy, the cast matrix appears transparent, while the crystals exhibit strong refractivity (Fig. 3.47).

The matrix of the leucine crystal casts is transparent, dark yellow leucine crystals can be seen within it (Fig. 3.48), and they turn green after the addition of CuSO4 (Fig. 3.49), which indicates that the patient has a serious hepatobiliary system disease.

Bilirubin casts, which appear orange-yellow, are observed in cases of bilirubinuria. The quantity of bilirubin crystals can vary, and they may present in a variety of shapes such as granular and small rod-like or in the form of needle bundles (Fig. 3.50).

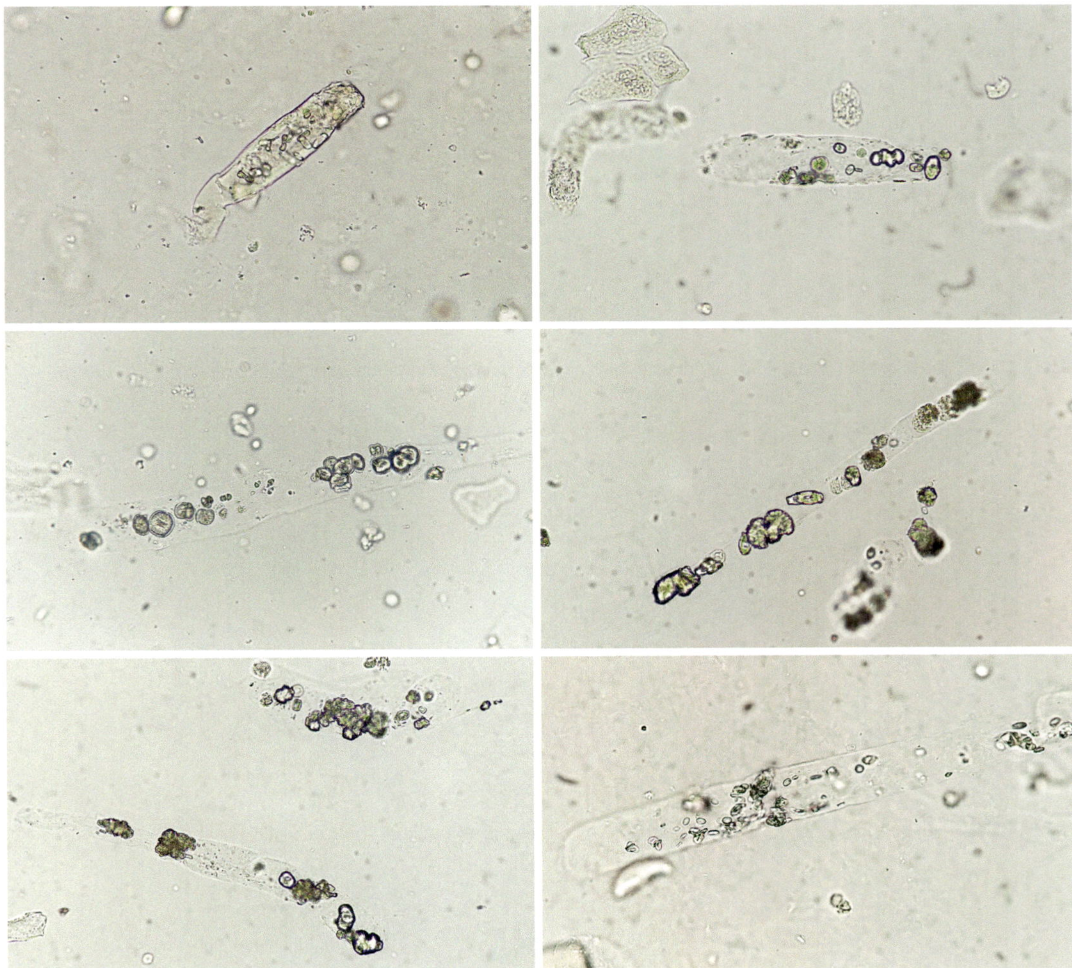

Fig. 3.46 Crystal casts. The matrix is transparent, with crystals visible inside. Unstained, bright field, ×400

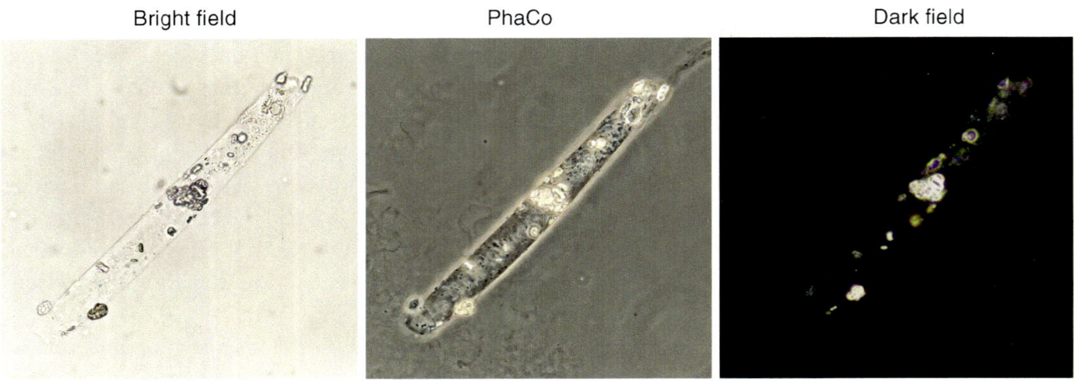

Fig. 3.47 Crystal casts. Unstained, ×400

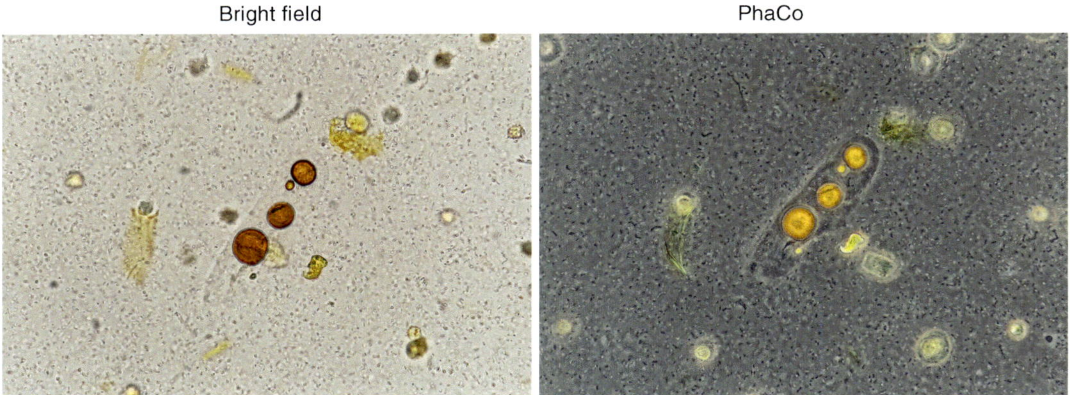

Fig. 3.48 Leucine crystal casts. The cast matrix is transparent, and the crystals have strong refractivity, ×400

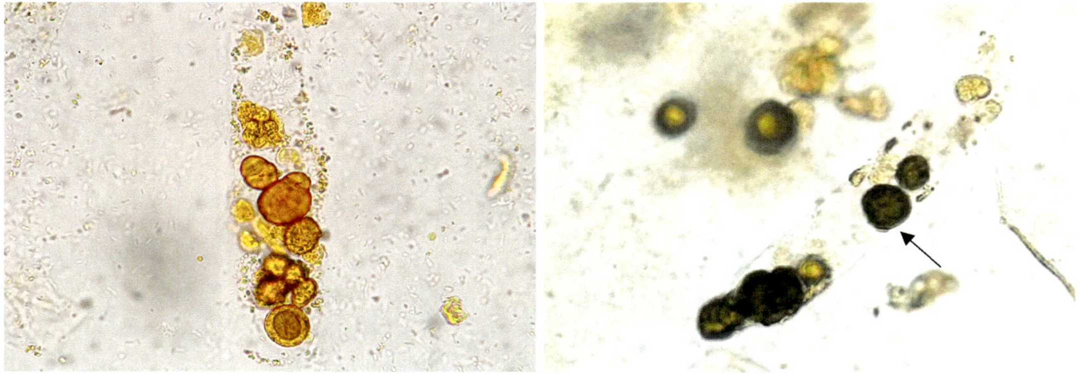

Fig. 3.49 Leucine crystal casts are yellow, and they turn green after the addition of $CuSO4$(↑), ×1000

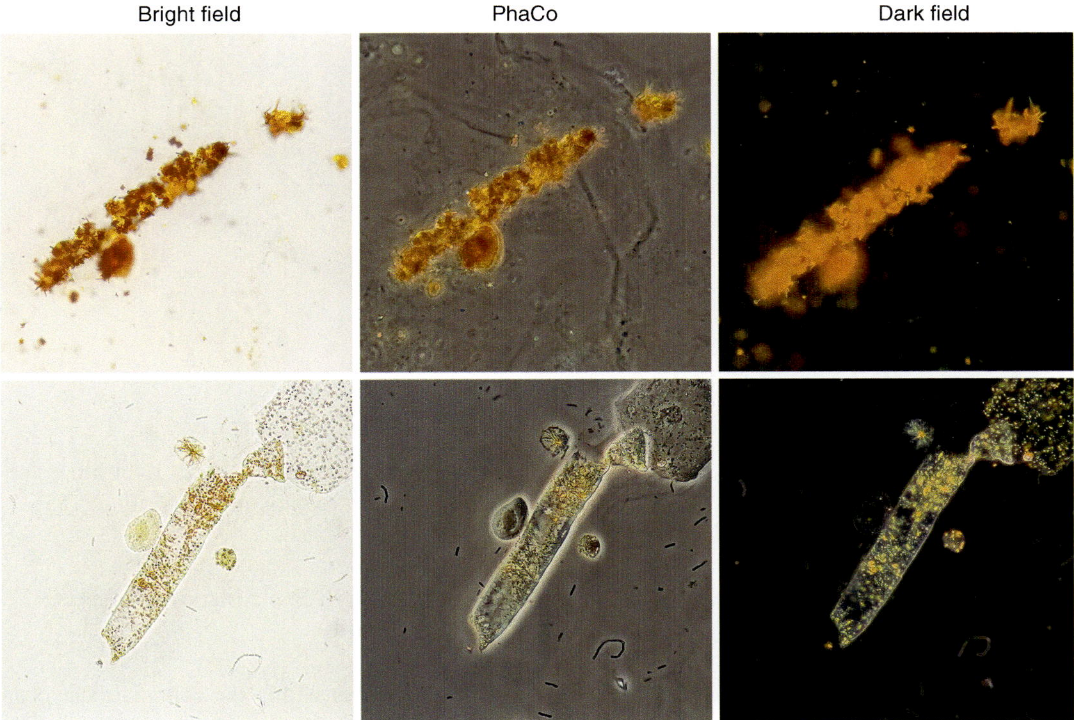

Fig. 3.50 Bilirubin crystal casts. Unstained, ×400

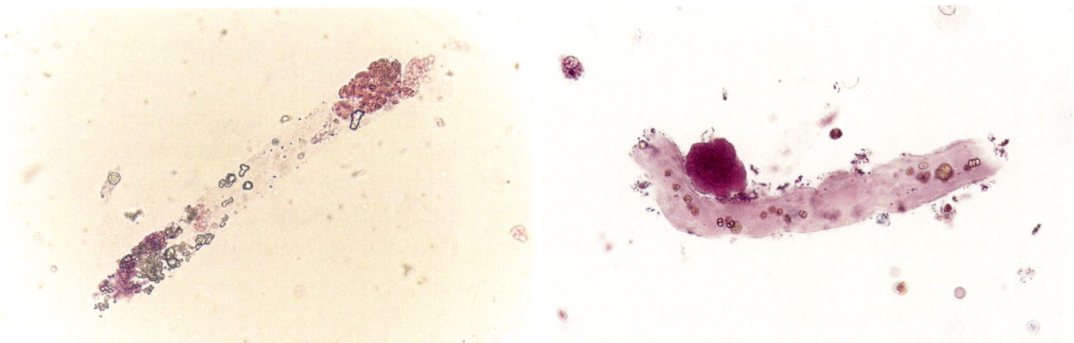

Fig. 3.51 Crystal casts. The matrix is pink, while the crystals remain unstained. SM stain, ×400

3.11.3 SM Stain or S Stain

Amorphous salt casts can be easily confused with granular casts, and they can be differentiated using staining methods. After SM staining, the cast matrix appears pink, while the crystals remain unstained (Fig. 3.51). Similarly, the cast matrix appears light blue, with the crystals unstained after S staining (Fig. 3.52).

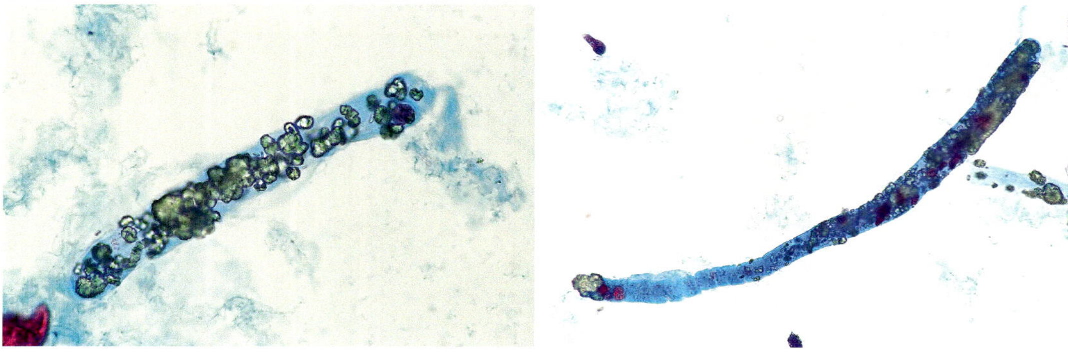

Fig. 3.52 Crystal casts. The matrix is blue, while the crystals unstained. S stain, ×400

3.11.4 Clinical Significance

The presence of crystal casts suggests the possibility of metabolic disorders or acute kidney injury caused by crystal deposition within the renal tubules. Calcium oxalate crystal casts may indicate oxalate nephropathy [10, 16].

3.12 Fatty Casts

3.12.1 Composition

Fatty casts contain numerous lipid droplets of varying sizes, derived from the breakdown of lipid-rich epithelial cells [2]. They are sometimes referred to as lipid casts.

3.12.2 Unstained

Fatty casts appear as varying-sized, highly refractile lipid droplets, with a pale yellow or yellow color (Fig. 3.53). Under contrast microscopy, the lipid droplets exhibit strong refractivity (Fig. 3.54). When the lipid droplets are large, Maltese crosses can be observed using polarized fluorescence microscopy.

3.12.3 SM Stain and S Stain

The cast matrix appears pink after SM stain, while the lipid droplets remain unstained after S staining, the cast matrix appears light blue, and the lipid droplets remain unstained (Fig. 3.55).

3.12.4 Sudan III Staining or Oil Red O Staining

The lipid droplets within the cast matrix appear orange-yellow after Sudan III staining (Fig. 3.56), and they appear orange-red after Oil Red O staining (Fig. 3.57).

3.12.5 Clinical Significance

Fatty casts are not normally present in the urine of healthy individuals. They are most commonly observed in nephrotic syndrome but can also be seen in diabetic nephropathy, hypothyroidism and certain chronic kidney diseases [14].

3.12.6 Identifying Fatty Casts from Similar Casts

Unstained fatty casts can sometimes be challenging to differentiate from protein casts and RBC casts. The size, color, and refractive properties of the contents within the cast matrix are the main factors for determining the type of casts (Figs. 3.56 and 3.58).

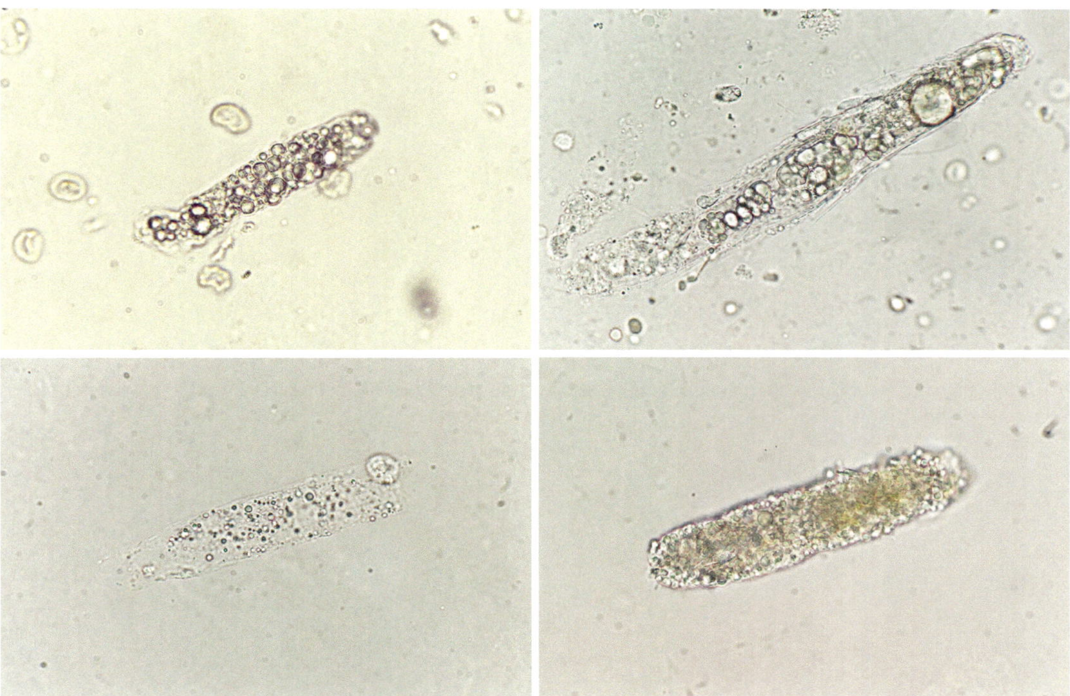

Fig. 3.53 Fatty casts. The matrix contains lipid droplets of varying size and number, exhibiting strong refractivity. Unstained, ×400

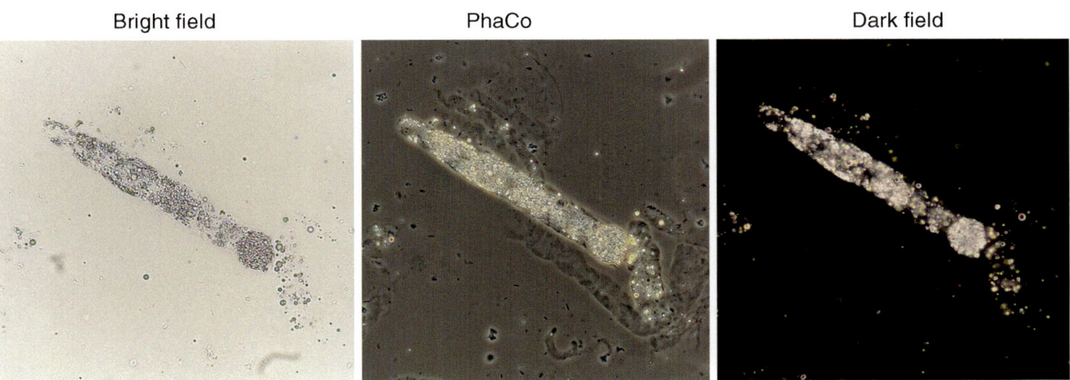

Fig. 3.54 Fatty casts. Lipid droplets exhibit strong refractivity under phase contrast microscopy and dark field. Unstained, ×400

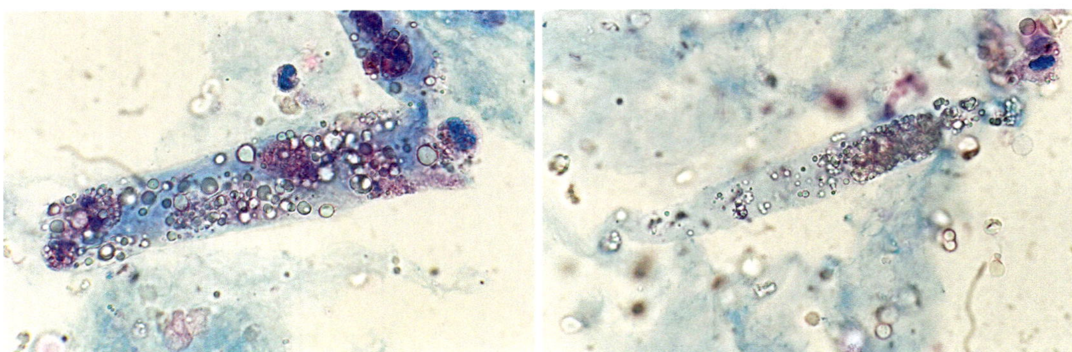

Fig. 3.55 Fatty casts. The cast matrix appears light blue, the lipid droplets unstained. And they exhibit strong refractive properties. S stain, ×400

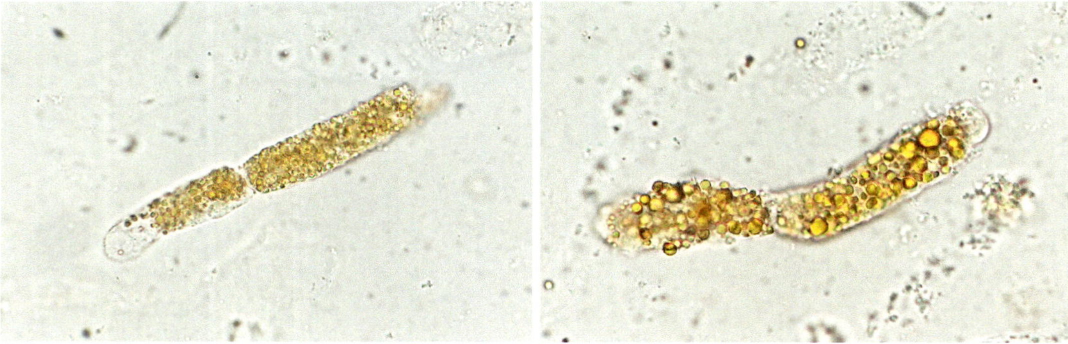

Fig. 3.56 Fatty casts. The lipid droplets within the matrix vary in size and appear orange-yellow. Sudan III staining, ×400

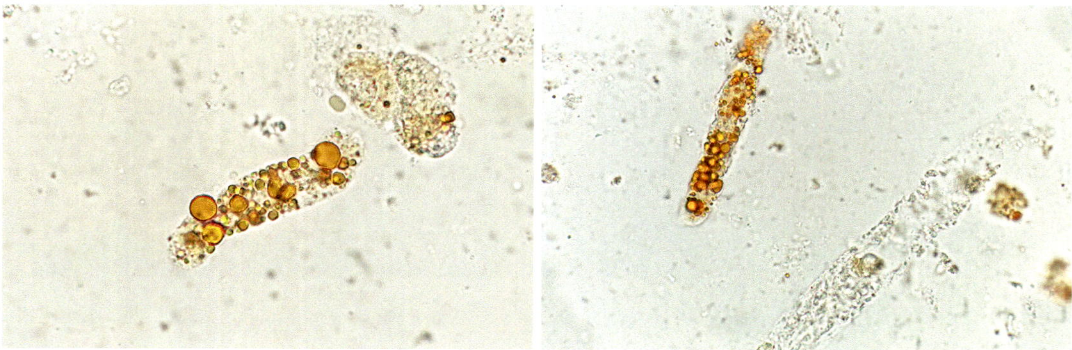

Fig. 3.57 Fatty casts. The lipid droplets within the matrix are large and appear orange-red. Oil Red O staining, ×400

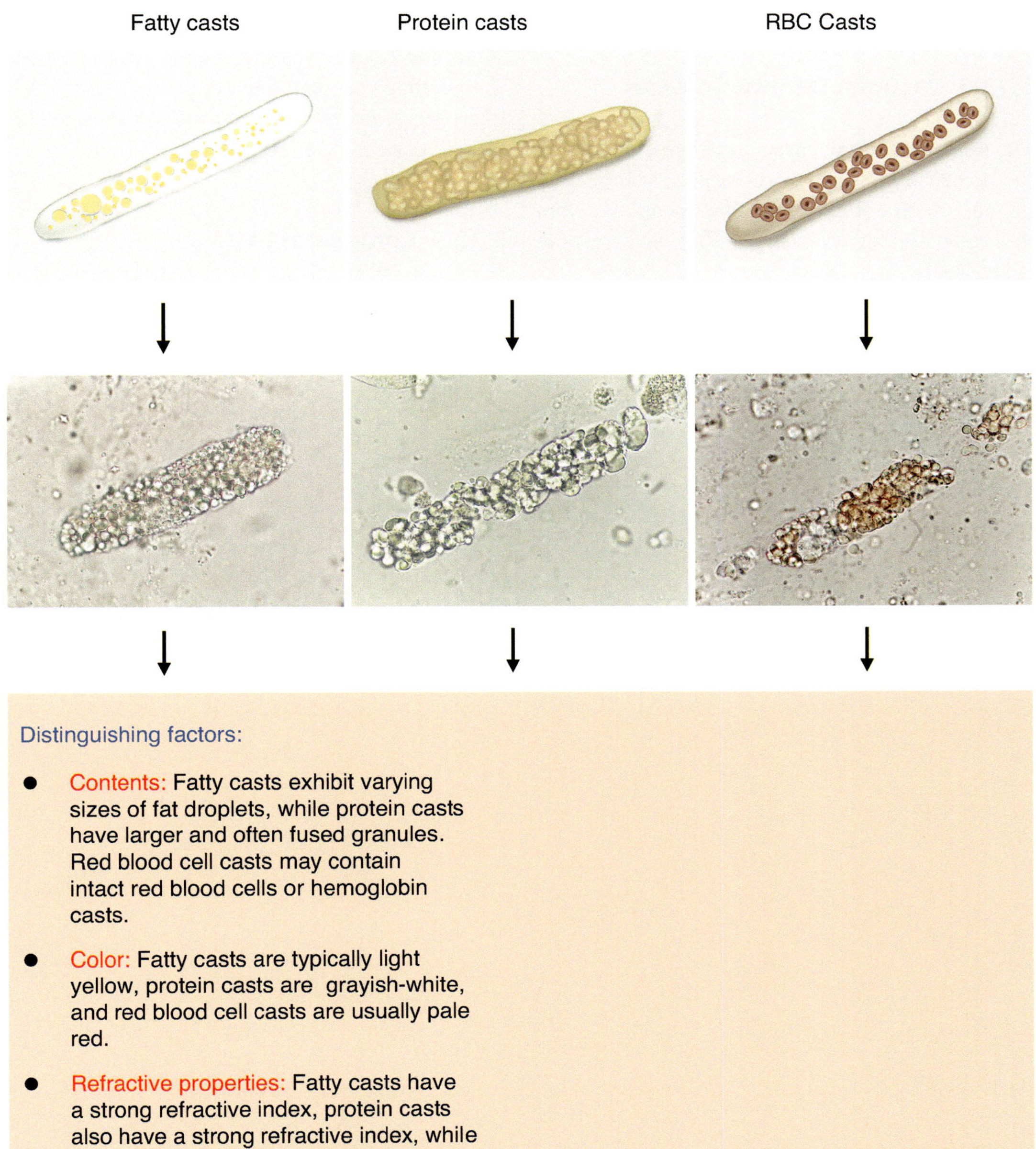

Fig. 3.58 Key distinguishing points between fatty casts, protein casts and RBC casts. Unstained, ×400

3.13 Other Special Casts

3.13.1 Vacuolar Denatured Casts

Vacuolar denatured casts are characterized by the presence of vacuoles of varying sizes within the cast matrix (Fig. 3.59). The vacuoles within the casts are lightly stained after SM staining (Fig. 3.60).

These casts are commonly found in more severe cases of diabetic nephropathy but can also be seen in chronic kidney failure and nephrotic syndrome caused by other factors. Studies have shown that vacuolar denatured casts are more likely to be detected in the urine of patients with acute kidney failure [10, 17].

3.13.2 Composite Casts

Two or more casts are arranged side by side. Each cast retains its distinct boundaries and can

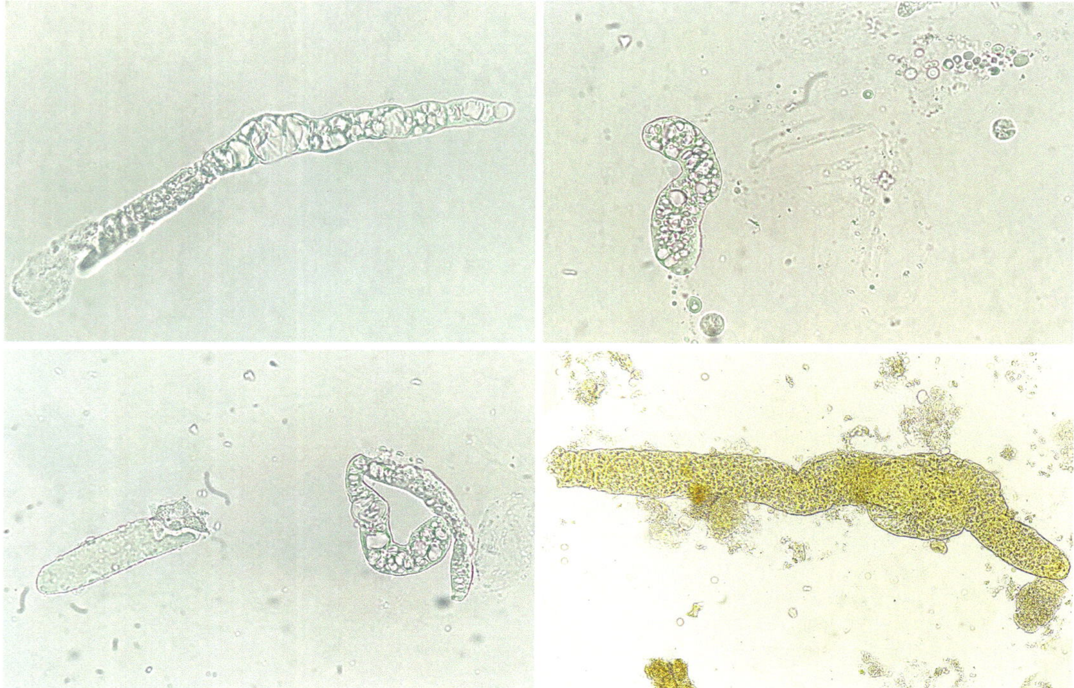

Fig. 3.59 Vacuolar denatured casts. The matrix contains vacuoles of varying sizes. Unstained, ×400

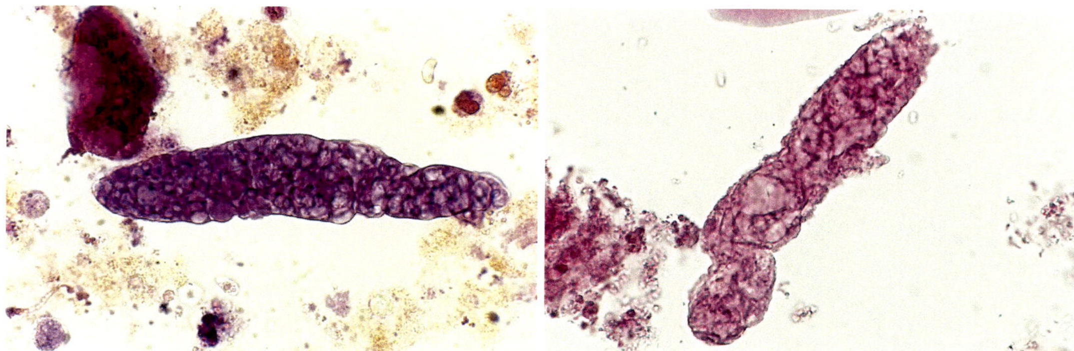

Fig. 3.60 The vacuoles within the casts are lightly stained. SM stain, ×1000

consist of the same or different types of casts (Fig. 3.61). The structure becomes more defined after supravital staining (Figs. 3.62 and 3.63). Typically, these casts are wider in appearance. The clinical significance is similar to the respective category of casts.

3.13.3 Nested Casts

Two casts nested or enveloped within each other. The inner cast has a distinct border, and the two casts can be of different types (Fig. 3.64). These casts become more defined under dark field

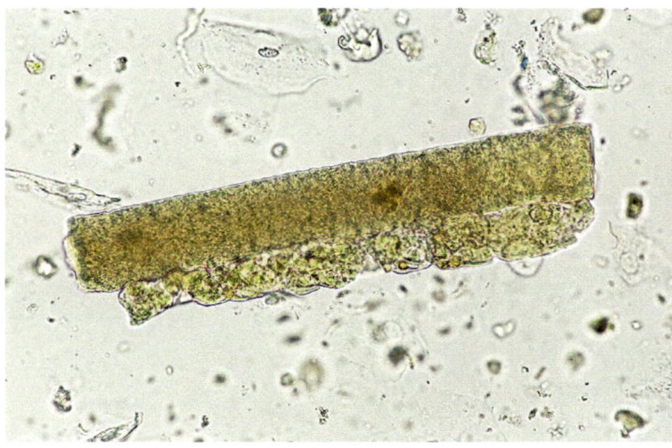
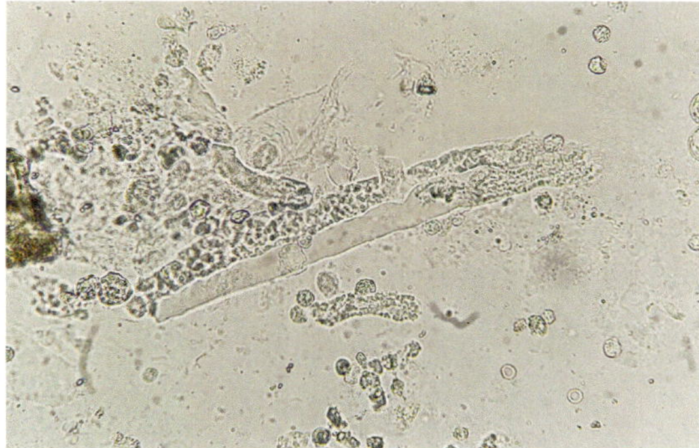

Fig. 3.61 Composite casts. Unstained, ×400

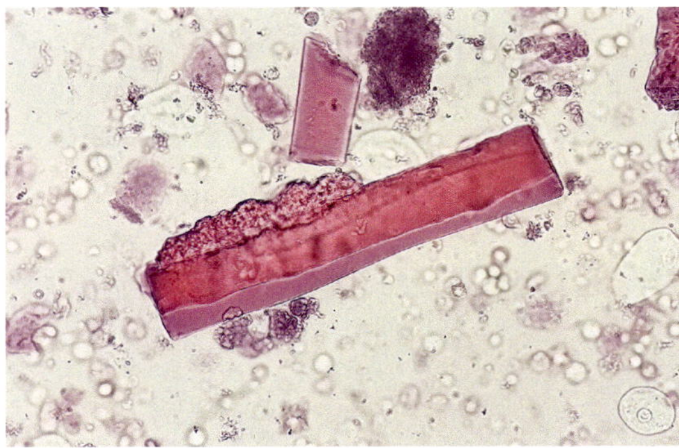
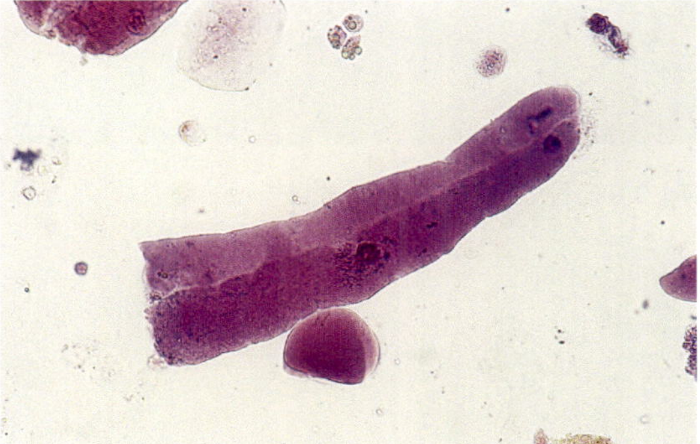

Fig. 3.62 Composite casts. SM stain, ×400

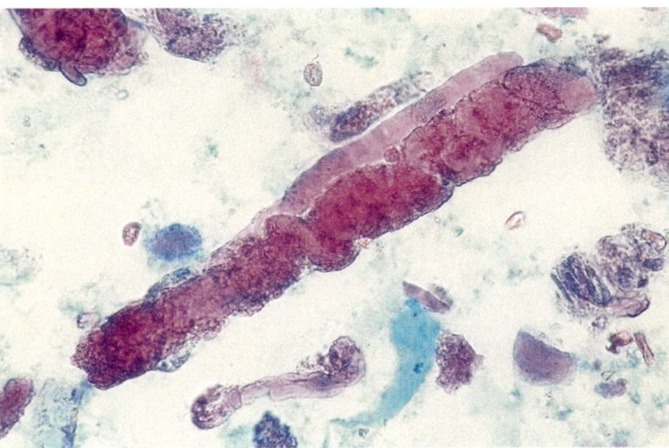
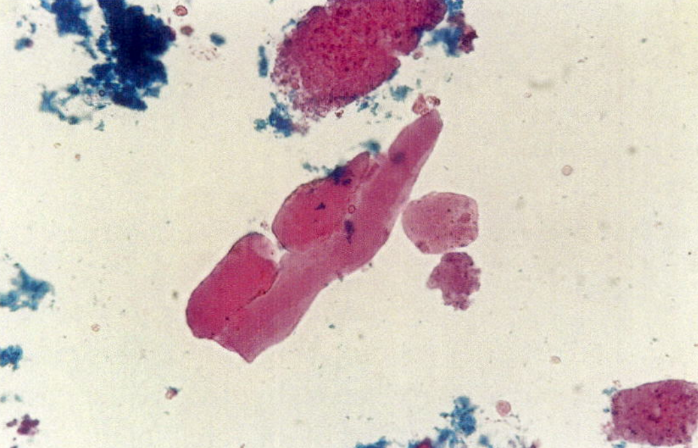

Fig. 3.63 Composite casts. S stain, ×400

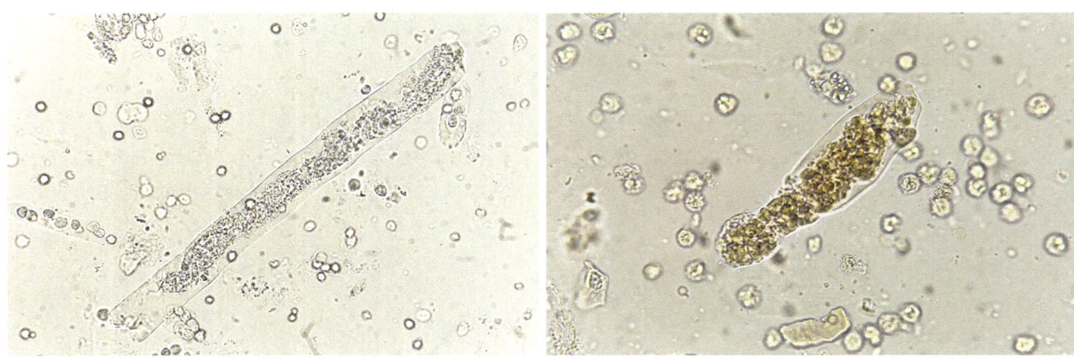

Fig. 3.64 Nested casts. They form nested structures. Unstained, ×400

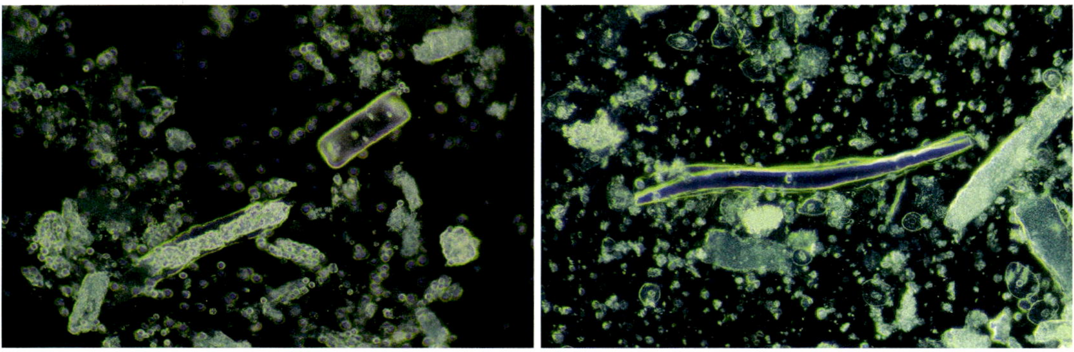

Fig. 3.65 Nested casts. Dark field, ×400

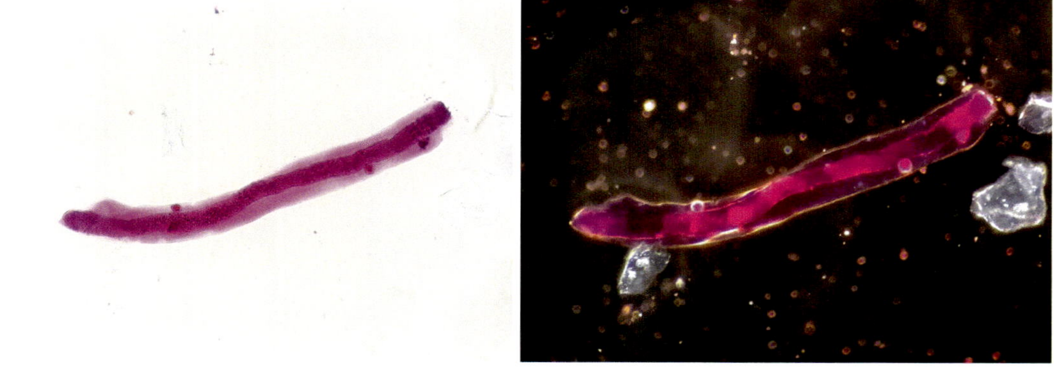

Fig. 3.66 Nested casts. SM stain, bright field and dark field, ×400

(Fig. 3.65) or after staining (Fig. 3.66). This phenomenon may occur when a slightly smaller cast is formed at the upper end of the renal tubule and then, with the flow of urine, moves down to the larger distal end of the tubule, where it becomes surrounded by another cast.

3.13.4 Hemosiderin Casts

Hemosiderin casts contain a large amount of hemosiderin granules. When unstained, the hemosiderin granules inside the cast appear golden yellow or dark yellow (Fig. 3.67), making them difficult to distinguish from granular casts or blood casts, which can lead to missed detection. The casts appear orange-yellow and have refractivity under dark field (Fig. 3.68). After iron staining, the granules turn deep blue (Fig. 3.69).

This type of cast is mainly observed in acute hemolytic anemia, post-transfusion reactions due to incompatible blood types, paroxysmal nocturnal hemoglobinuria, severe intravascular hemolysis, and other conditions that cause hemoglobinuria.

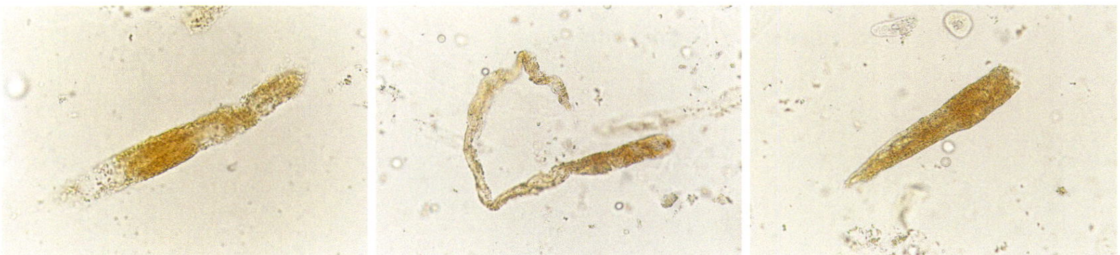

Fig. 3.67 Hemosiderin casts. The granules appear golden yellow. Unstained, ×400

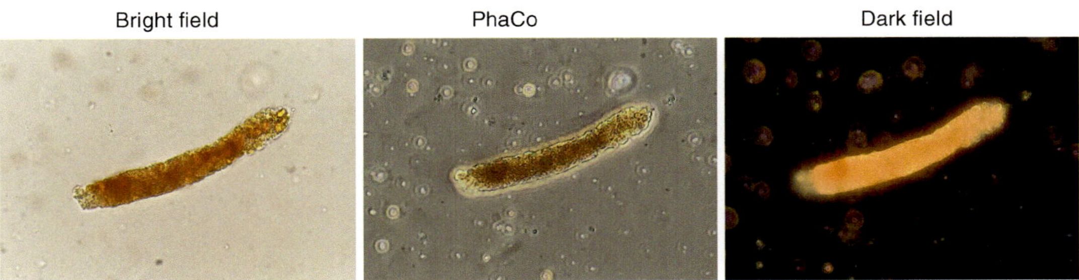

Fig. 3.68 Hemosiderin casts. Unstained, ×400

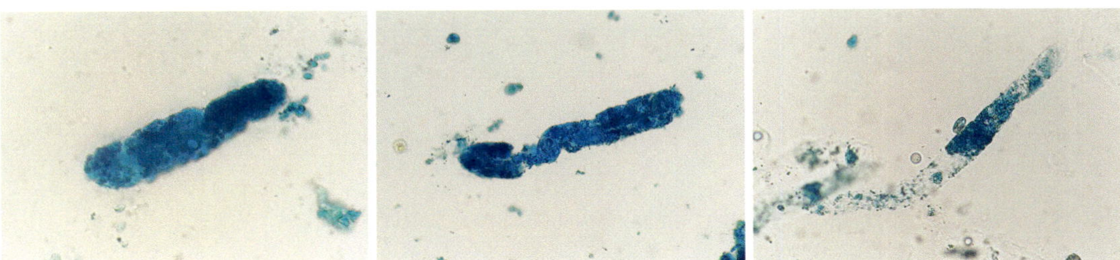

Fig. 3.69 Hemosiderin casts. The granules within the casts appear dark blue after iron staining, ×400

3.13.5 Mixed Casts

Mixed casts contain a combination of various substances (such as RBCs, WBCs, RTE cells, crystals, or fat bodies) enclosed within a protein matrix. When the cast contains two or more types of cells, it is referred to as a mixed-cell cast (Fig. 3.70). The substances within the matrix can be easily recognized after supravital staining (Figs. 3.71 and 3.72). The cells or other substances within the casts can be clearly identified under a contrast microscope (Fig. 3.73). They are commonly seen in conditions such as glomerulonephritis and nephrotic syndrome [18].

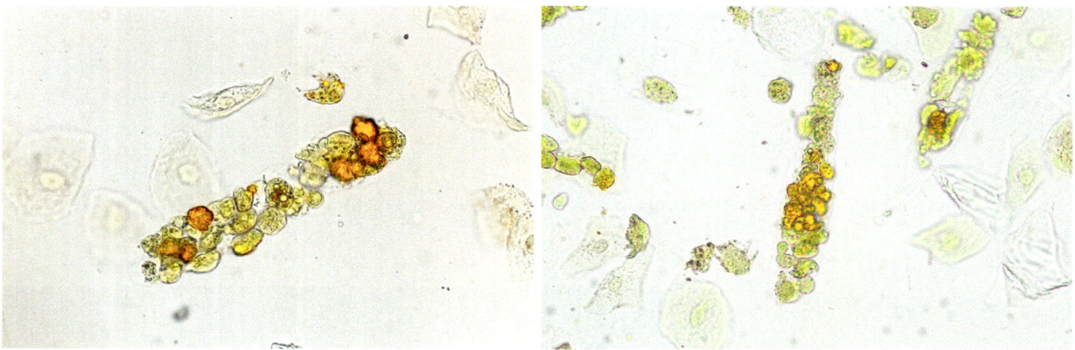

Fig. 3.70 Mixed casts. The casts contain RTE cells and leucine crystals. Bilirubinuria. Unstained, ×400

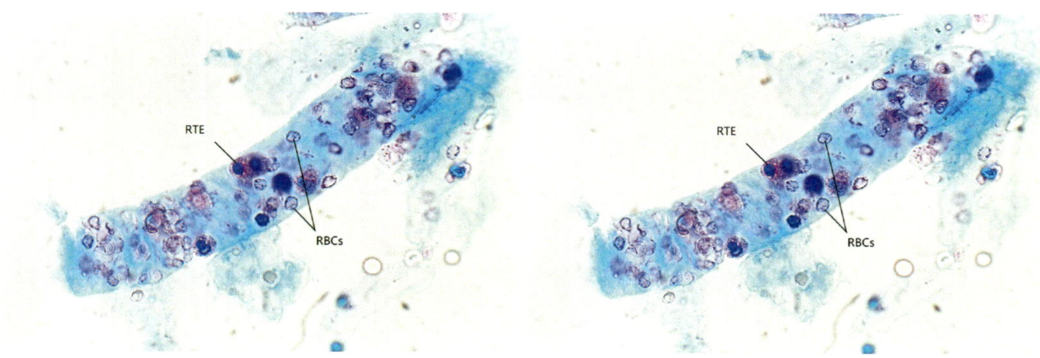

Fig. 3.71 Mixed casts. The casts contained both RBCs and RTE cells. S stain, ×400

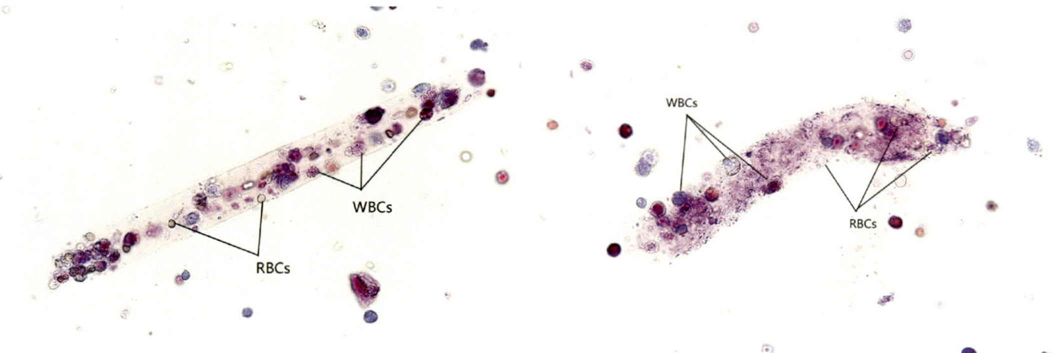

Fig. 3.72 Mixed casts. The casts contained both RBCs and WBCs. SM stain, ×400

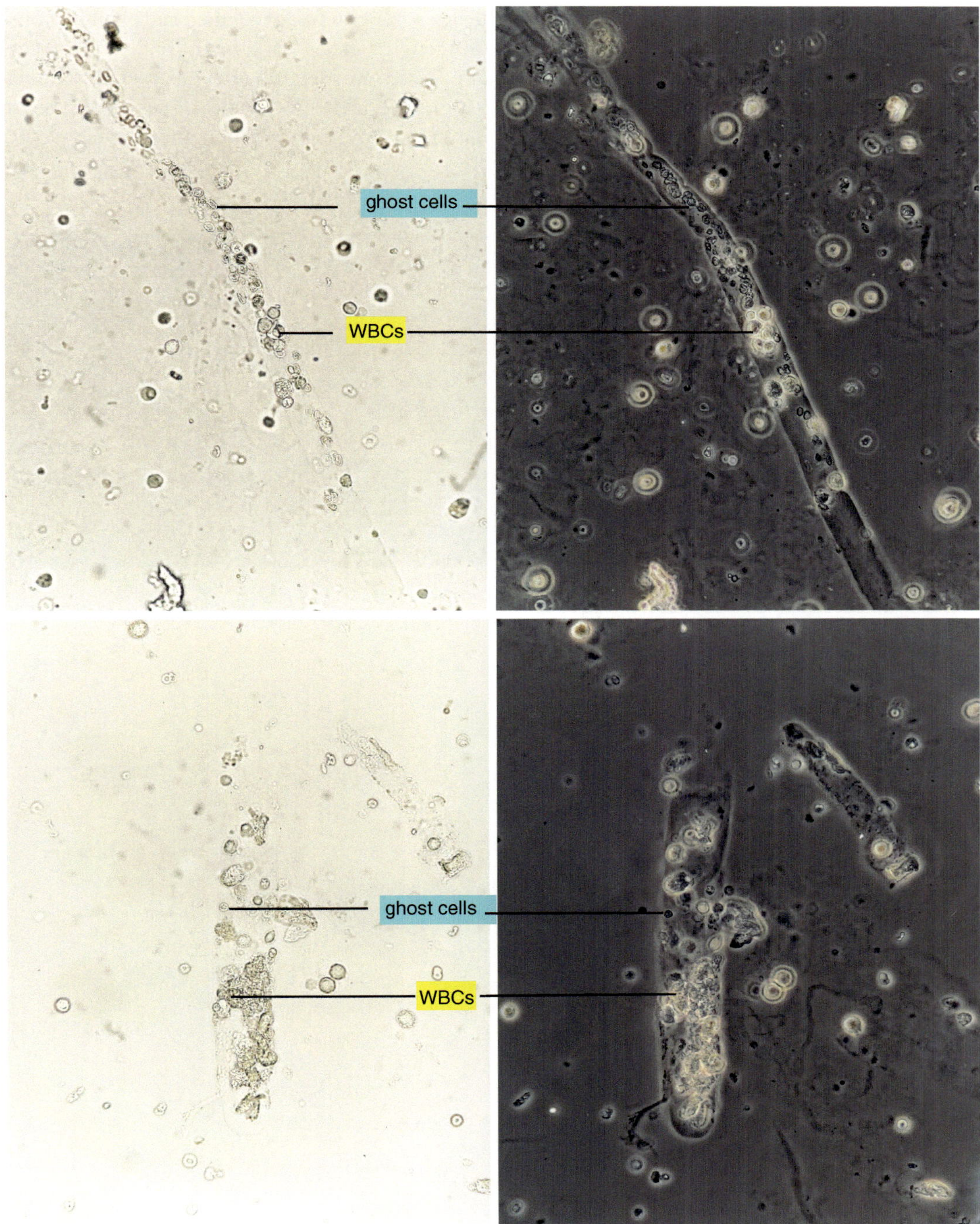

Fig. 3.73 Mixed casts. Unstained, ×400

3.13.6 Protein Casts

The cast matrix is composed of large molecular proteins, such as Bence-Jones proteins. The granules within the cast are coarse and resemble frog eggs, often fused together, and exhibit strong refractivity under dark field (Fig. 3.74). They are easier to identify after supravital staining (Figs. 3.75 and 3.76). Bence-Jones protein casts are frequently observed in multiple myeloma.

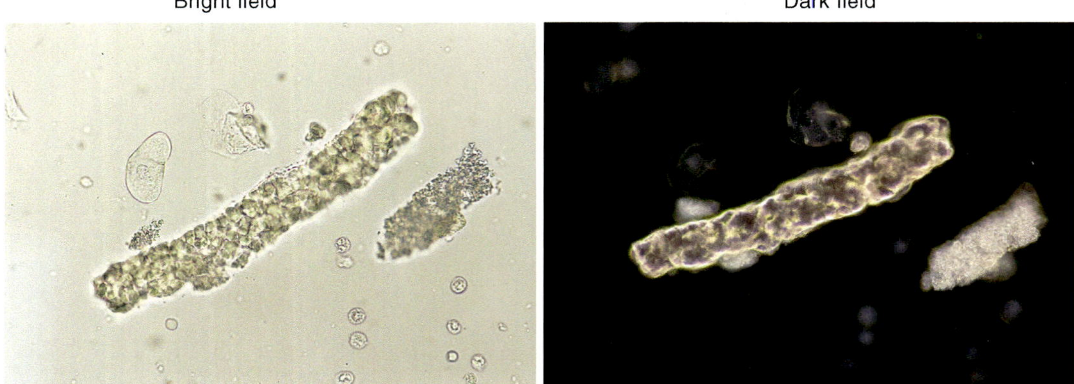

Fig. 3.74 Protein casts. Unstained, ×400

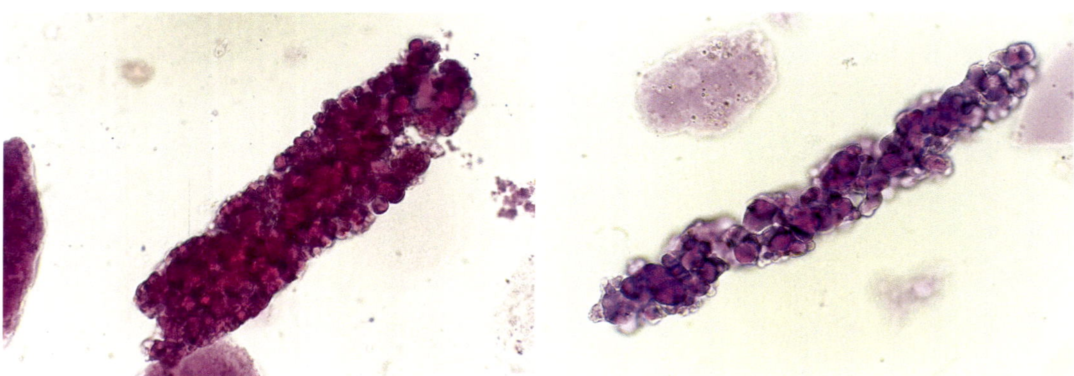

Fig. 3.75 Protein casts. SM stain, ×400

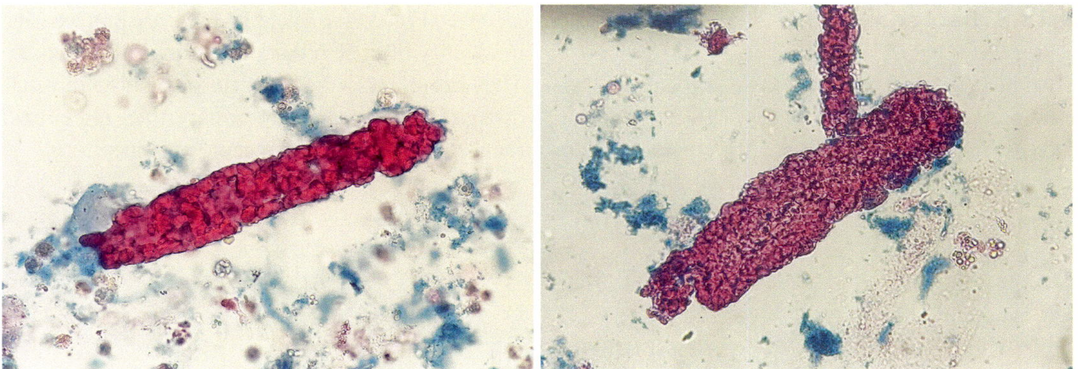

Fig. 3.76 Protein casts. S stain, ×400

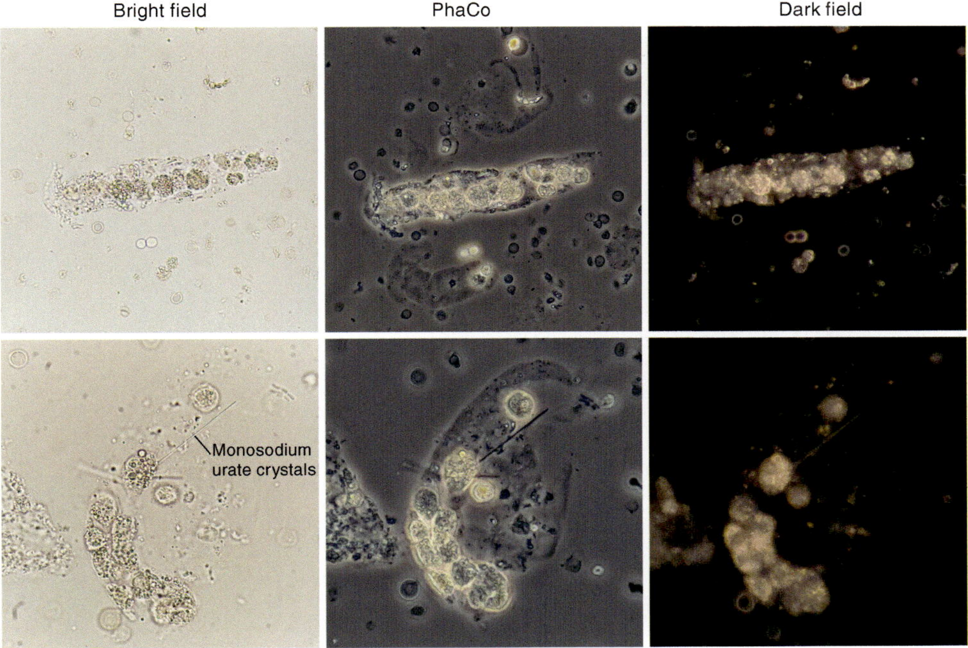

Fig. 3.77 Oval fat body casts. Unstained, ×400

3.13.7 Oval Fat Body Casts

Oval fat body casts contain one or multiple oval fat bodies within the matrix(which are cells with fat droplets). The size of the fat droplets varies, and they have a pale-yellow color and strong refractivity (Fig. 3.77). The lipid droplets remain unstained after supravital staining (Figs. 3.78 and 3.79). This type of cast is commonly observed in nephrotic syndrome and some chronic kidney diseases.

3.13.8 Bacterial Casts

Hyaline casts containing variable amounts of bacteria are known as bacterial casts. Bacteria within the cast matrix can be scattered or concentrated in a specific area of the cast matrix, resembling granular casts (Fig. 3.80). Bacterial casts are much easier to identify in PhaCo than in the bright field mode. They are commonly found in patients with renal diseases accompanied by urinary tract infections, renal septic conditions, or acute pyelonephritis.

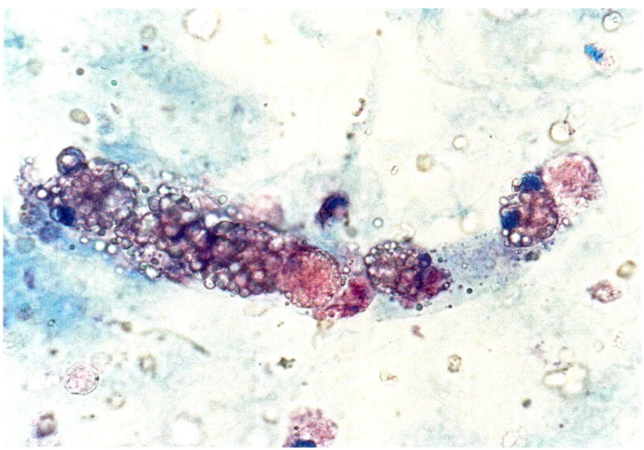

Fig. 3.78 Oval fat body casts. S stain, ×1000

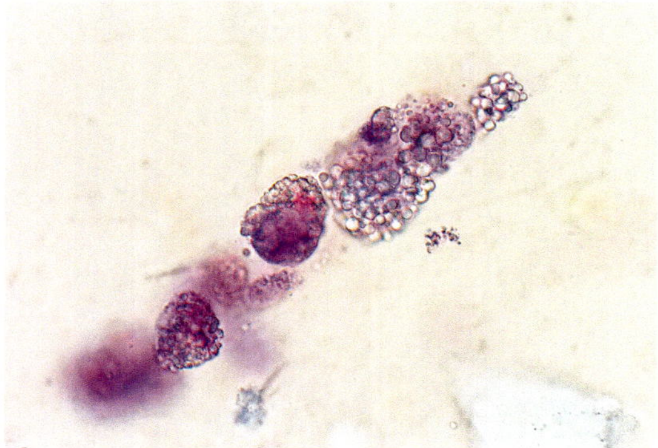

Fig. 3.79 Oval fat body casts. SM stain, ×1000

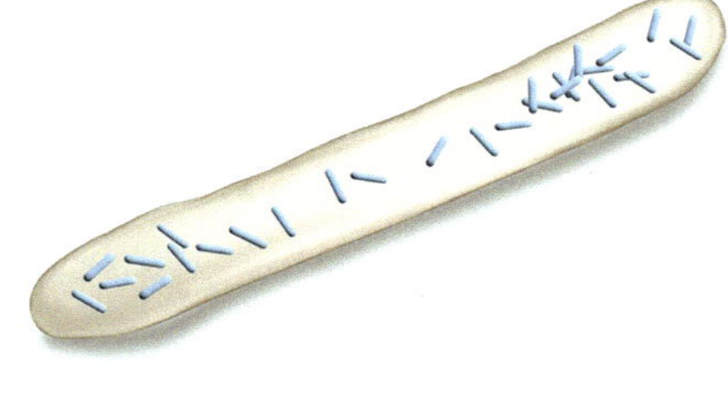

Fig. 3.80 Illustration of bacterial casts

3.14 Some Case About Casts

3.14.1 Case 1 (Fig. 3.81)

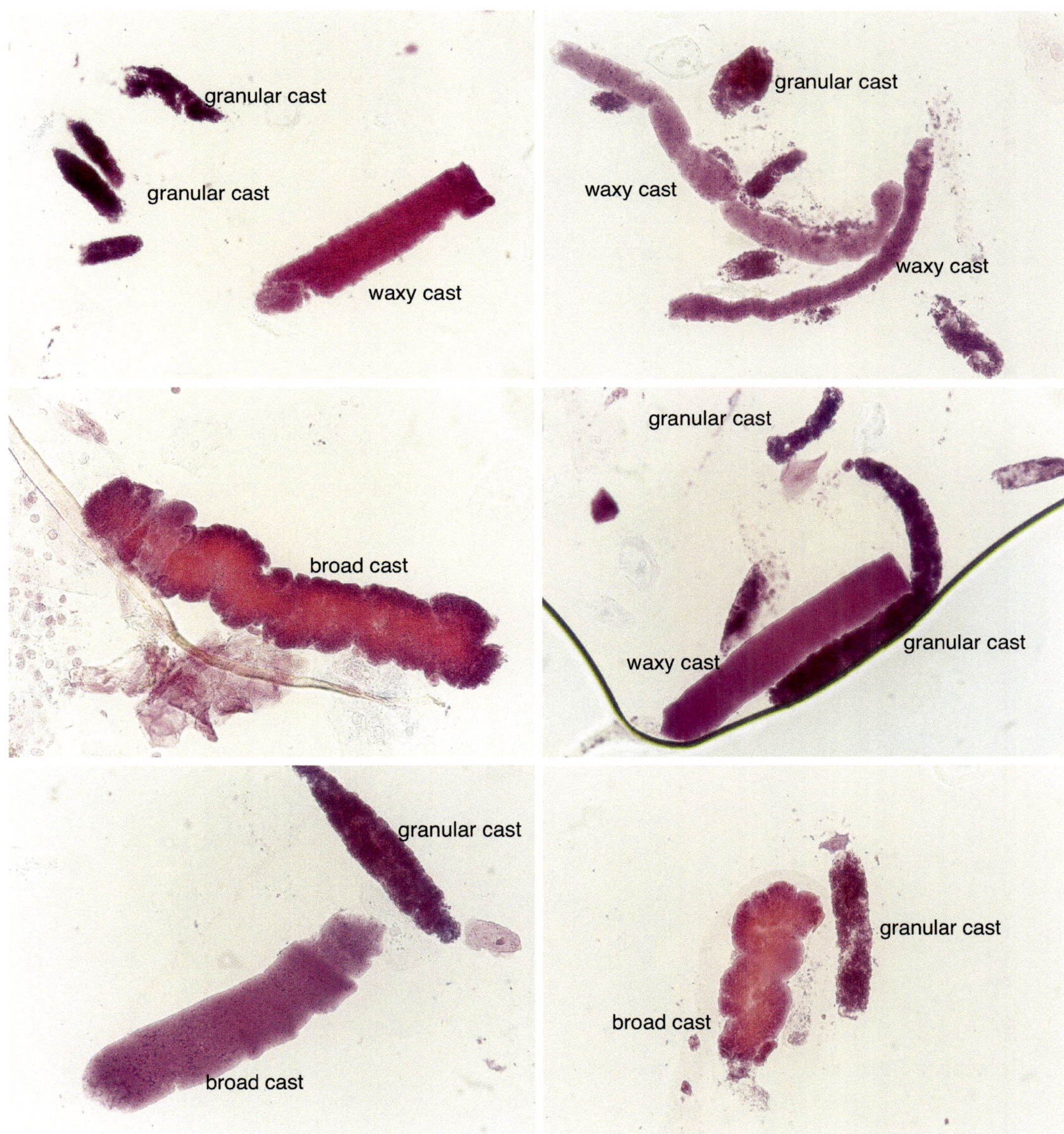

Fig. 3.81 The patient in the image was diagnosed with chronic kidney disease 1 year ago. Urinalysis shows a protein level of +++, and microscopic examination of the urine sediment reveals various forms of casts. The cast structures are clear after SM staining, with slight variations in width and color. Granular casts appear darker in color compared to other types. Based on the color, content and width of the casts, it is possible to distinguish granular casts, waxy casts and broad casts. SM stain, ×400

3.14.2 Case 2 (Fig. 3.82)

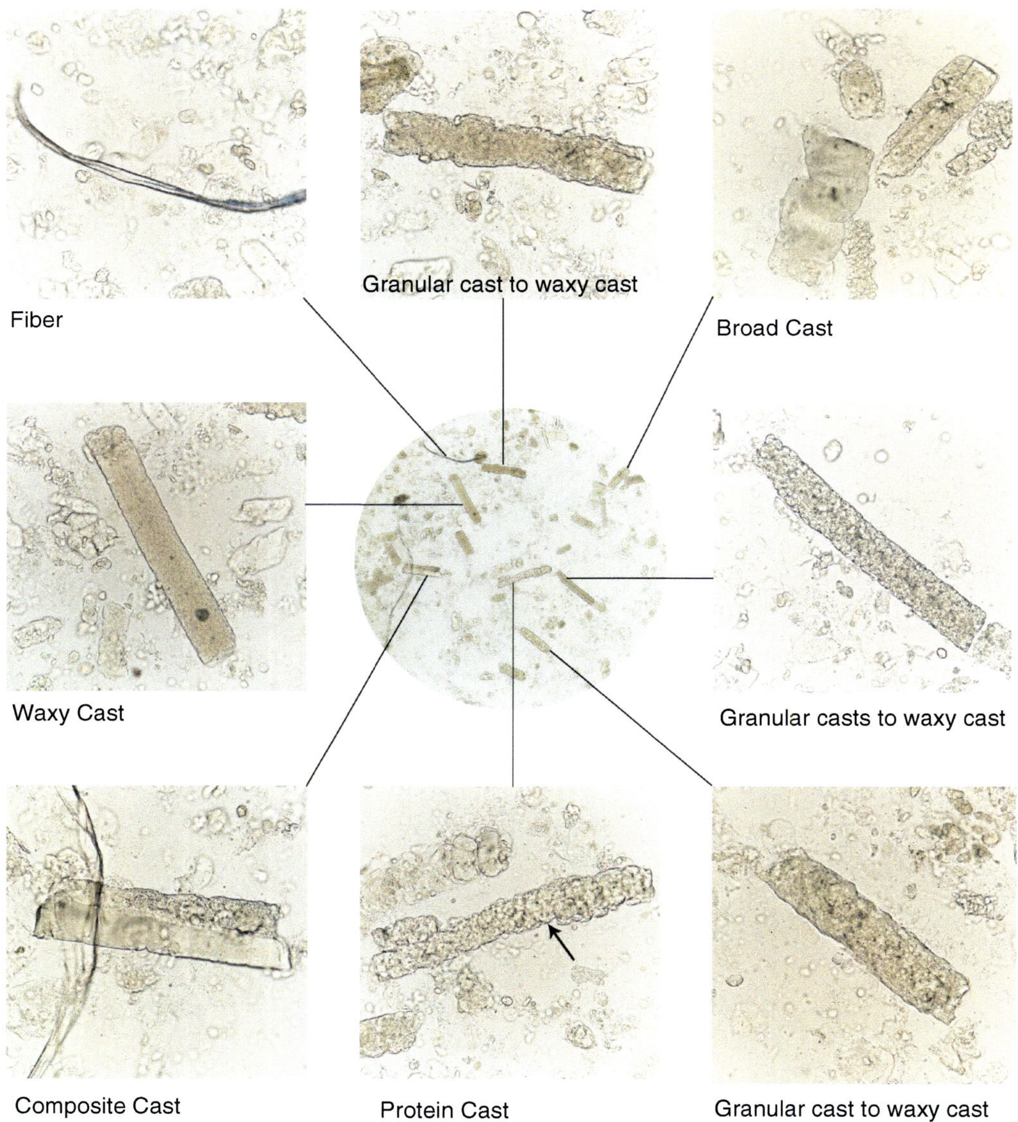

Fig. 3.82 The patient, a male, experienced acute kidney injury due to hemorrhagic shock caused by trauma. Urine analysis shows a high level of protein (3+) and the presence of various types of casts in the urine, including numerous broad casts. Unstained, bright field, ×400

References

1. Cavanaugh C, Perazella MA. Urine sediment examination in the diagnosis and management of kidney disease: core curriculum 2019. Am J Kidney Dis. 2019;73(2):258–72.
2. Caleffi A, Lippi G. Cylindruria. Clin Chem Lab Med. 2015;53(s2):s1471–7.
3. Cohen AJLI. Morphology of renal tubular hyaline casts. Lab Invest. 1981;44(3):280–7.
4. Adachi M, Hoshi M, Ushimaru S, Hayashi A, Nakamoto K, Kanbe A, et al. Clinical significance of hyaline casts in the new CKD risk classification (KDIGO 2009). Rinsho Byori. 2013;61(2):104–11.
5. Brunzel NA. Fundamentals of urine and body fluid analysis. Elsevier Health Sciences; 2021.
6. Strasinger SK, Di Lorenzo MS. Urinalysis and body fluids. FA Davis; 2014.
7. Xu D, Li J, Wang S, Tan Y, Liu Y, Zhao M. The clinical and pathological relevance of waxy casts in urine sediment. Ren Fail. 2022;44(1):1038–44.
8. Spinelli D, Consonni D, Garigali G, Fogazzi GB. Waxy casts in the urinary sediment of patients with different types of glomerular diseases: results of a prospective study. Clin Chim Acta. 2013;424:47–52.
9. Rivera M, Velez J. Urinary waxy casts are associated with greater severity of acute tubular injury. J Investig Med. 2020;68(2):672.
10. Neuendorf J. Description of urinary sediment constituents. In: Urine sediment. Cham: Springer International Publishing; 2020. p. 29–45.
11. Zhou Y, Zhou H. Automatic classification and recognition of particles in urinary sediment images. Dordrecht; 2012.
12. Fogo AB, Cohen AH, Colvin RB, Jennette JC, Alpers CE, Fogo AB, et al. Calcineurin inhibitor toxicity, polyomavirus, and recurrent disease. In: Fundamentals of renal pathology. 2014. p. 217–24.
13. Kanbay M, Kasapoglu B, Perazella MA. Acute tubular necrosis and pre-renal acute kidney injury: utility of urine microscopy in their evaluation-a systematic review. Int Urol Nephrol. 2010;42:425–33.
14. Perazella MA. The urine sediment as a biomarker of kidney disease. Am J Kidney Dis. 2015;66(5):748–55.
15. Simerville JA, Maxted WC, Pahira JJ. Urinalysis: a comprehensive review. Am Fam Physician. 2005;71(6):1153–62.
16. Ridley JW. Fundamentals of the study of urine and body fluids. Berlin/Heidelberg: Springer; 2018.
17. Fogazzi GB, Garigali G. The clinical art and science of urine microscopy. Curr Opin Nephrol Hypertens. 2003;12(6):625–32.
18. Graber M, Lane B, Lamia R, Pastoriza-Munoz E. Bubble cells: renal tubular cells in the urinary sediment with characteristics of viability. J Am Soc Nephrol. 1991;1(7):999–1004.

4 Crystals

Lizhi Yan, Jiancheng Xu, Aijun Duan, Yonghui Guo, Hong Kong, Jinlong Yao, Junjie Huang, Huixian Luo, and Zhiliang Cai

4.1 Crystal: Overview

Many human metabolites are excreted in urine. As the concentration of certain salts increases, exceeding the solubility of the solute, crystals of a specific structure may form under a certain condition of pH and temperature, which are referred to as urinary crystals [1].

Various kinds of crystals can be found in urine samples, and the same kind of crystals may show different forms, which can be distinguished according to urine pH, the color of sediments, microscopic morphological characteristics, and solubility. Uric acid crystals, monosodium urate crystals, and amorphous urates can be seen in acidic urine, while phosphatase crystals, calcium phosphate crystals, struvite crystals, and amorphous phosphates can be seen in alkaline urine (Table 4.1).

Crystalluria is a marker of urine supersaturation with substances deriving from metabolic disorders, inherited diseases, or drugs [2]. There are all varieties of crystal in urine, which may sometimes reflect the problems of the organism. These crystals can be intervened by diet, drinking water, lifestyle changes, etc., and some medical inter-

L. Yan (✉)
Department of Laboratory Medicine, Nanfang Hospital, Southern Medical University, Guangzhou, China

J. Xu
Department of Laboratory Medicine, First Hospital of Jilin University, Changchun, China
e-mail: xjc@jlu.edu.cn

A. Duan
Department of Laboratory Medicine, Henan Xinhe Hospital, Xinyang, Henan, China

Y. Guo
Department of Laboratory Medicine, Zhujiang Hospital, Southern Medical University, Guangzhou, China

H. Kong
Department of Laboratory Medicine, Shengjing Hospital of China Medical University, Liaoning Clinical Research Center for Laboratory Medicine, Shenyang, China

J. Yao
Department of Clinical Laboratory, Jiangkou County Hospital of Traditional Chinese Medicine, Jiangkou, Guizhou, China

J. Huang
Department of Laboratory Medicine, Nanfang Hospital, Southern Medical University, Guangzhou, China

H. Luo
Department of Laboratory Medicine, Zhujiang Hospital, Southern Medical University, Guangzhou, China

Z. Cai
Department of Laboratory Medicine, Nanfang Hospital, Guangzhou, China

L. Zheng et al. (eds.), *Urine Formed Elements*, https://doi.org/10.1007/978-981-99-7739-0_4

Table 4.1 Characteristics of normal urine crystals

Types	Characteristics	Diagram
Calcium oxalate crystals	• Colorless; yellow color in bilirubinuria • Octahedral or polyhedral structure, spherical, dumbbell-shaped, drumstick-shaped, or irregular • Soluble in HCl	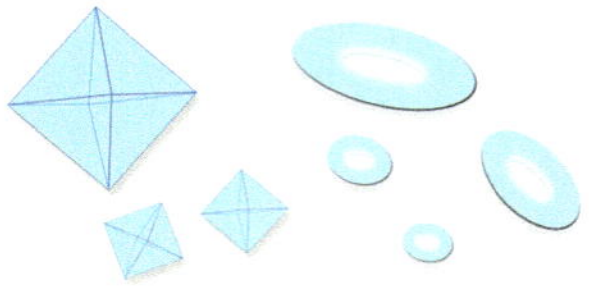
Uric acid crystals	• Yellow or dark yellow • Diamonds, hexagons, spheres, dumbbells, cubes, or irregularities • Clustered into patterns or tubular shapes • Soluble in alkali	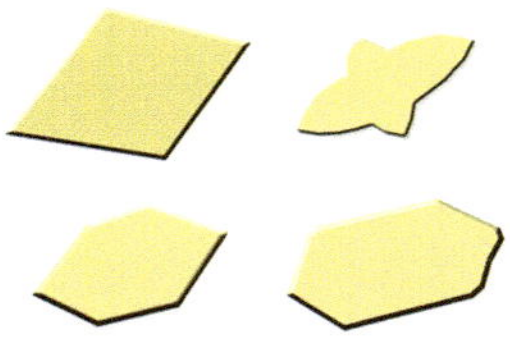
Monosodium urate crystals	• Light yellow • Needle-like or slender rod-shaped • Aggregate into bundles or patterns • Soluble in alkali	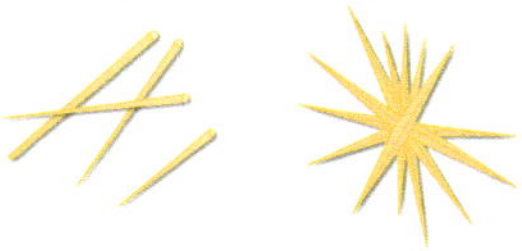
Amorphous urates	• Yellow to yellow-orange • The sediment is pink • Amorphous granules or small spheres • Soluble in alkali • Dissolves upon heating	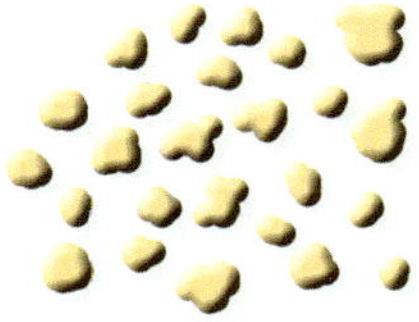
Ammonium biurate crystals	• Yellow-brown • Soluble in acetic acid, HCl, and alkali • Root-shaped, dumbbell-shaped, or spherical • Soluble at 60 °C	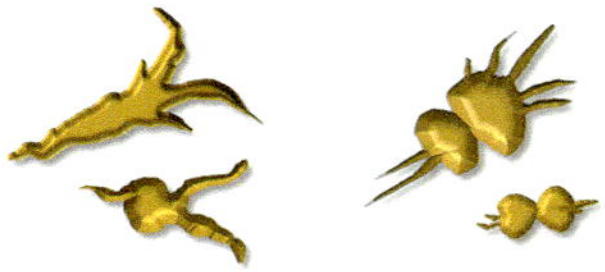
Struvite/triple phosphate	• Colorless transparent • Roof-shaped, envelope-shaped, cube, diamond, or irregular • Soluble in acetic acid and HCl	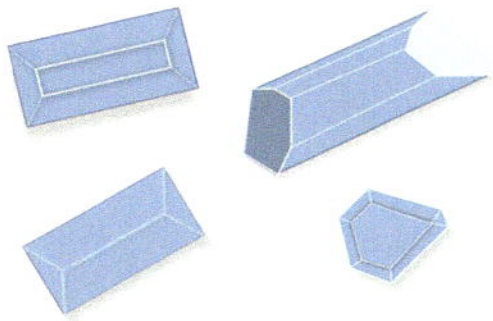
Calcium phosphate crystals	• Colorless • Flaky, firewood-like, dumbbell-shaped, chrysanthemums-like, or form bundles • Soluble in acetic acid and HCl	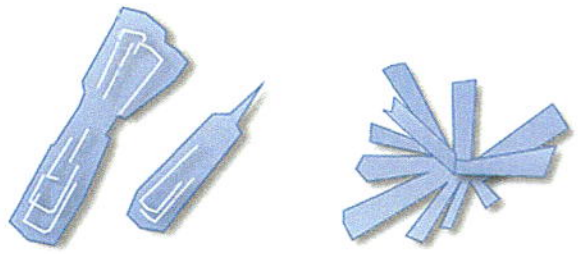
Amorphous phosphates	• Colorless • Amorphous granular • Soluble in acetic acid and HCl	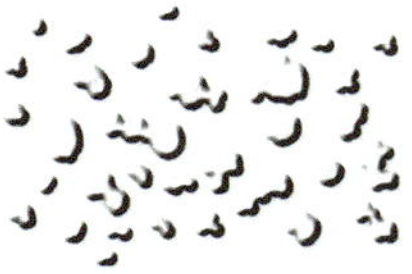
Calcium carbonate crystals	• Yellow-brown • Opaque root-shape, dumbbell-shaped, or spherical with needle-like protrusion • Soluble in acetic acid, HCl, and alkali • Soluble at 60 °C	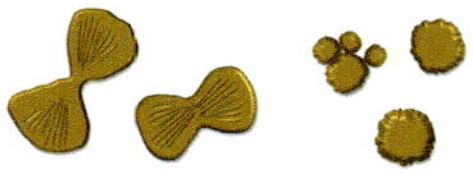

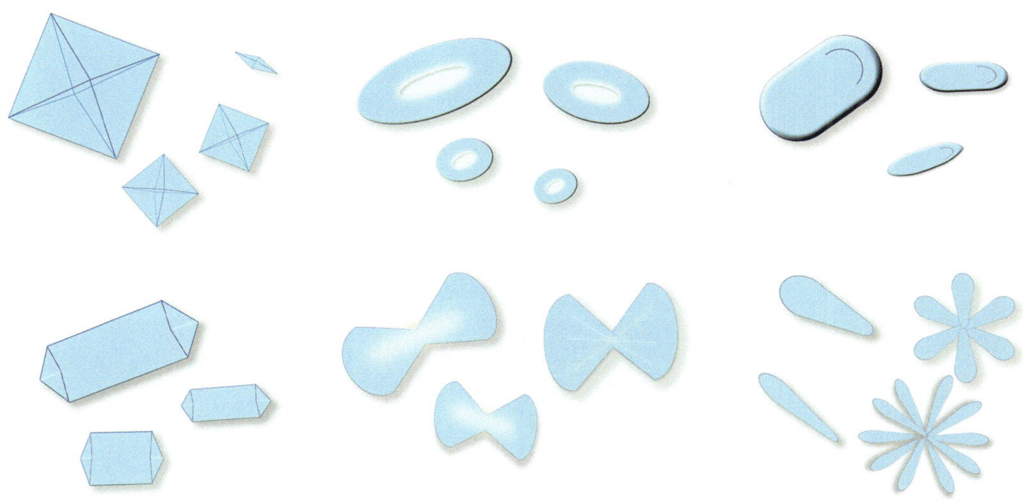

Fig. 4.1 Appearance of calcium oxalate crystals

ventions may be performed in more severe cases. Research evidence in recent years shows that the incidence and prevalence of kidney stones have an upward trend worldwide, and dietary patterns may be a key factor [3]. Deposition of supersaturated crystals in the kidneys increases the risk of kidney stones [4]. Therefore, understanding these crystals is of great clinical importance for disease diagnosis.

Due to the unequal size of crystals, some crystals have a huge volume, while others can only be observed under high magnification or oil immersion microscope. The figures in the book are all annotated with the magnification factor for reference purposes only.

4.2 Calcium Oxalate Crystals

4.2.1 Characteristics

Calcium oxalate (CO) crystals are classified into CO monohydrate (COM, whewellite) and CO dihydrate (COD, weddellite) [5]. Calcium oxalate crystals are generally colorless and transparent and have strong refraction, which may appear yellow in bilirubinuria. The appearance of calcium oxalate crystals includes octahedral or polyhedral structure, oval, spherical, dumbbell-shaped, drumstick-shaped, or irregular (Fig. 4.1). COD morphology is octahedral or polyhedral structure, and COM is oval, spherical, dumbbell-shaped, drumstick-shaped, or irregular [2].

4.2.2 Differential

Calcium oxalate crystals often occur in acidic, neutral, or alkaline urine. The crystals can be dissolved in HCl but are insoluble in acetic acid and 10% KOH, and they are insoluble upon heating. Round calcium oxalate crystals are similar to RBC in morphology. RBCs are dissolved after addition of acetic acid, while calcium oxalate crystals are insoluble.

These crystals have strong refractivity when observed under phase contrast and dark field microscopy (Fig. 4.2). Calcium oxalate crystals are typically colorless and exhibit diverse forms under bright field microscopy (Figs. 4.3, 4.4, 4.5, 4.6, 4.7, 4.8, 4.9, 4.10, 4.11, 4.12, and 4.13). However, they can appear pale yellow or yellow in bilirubinuria (Figs. 4.14, 4.15, and 4.16).

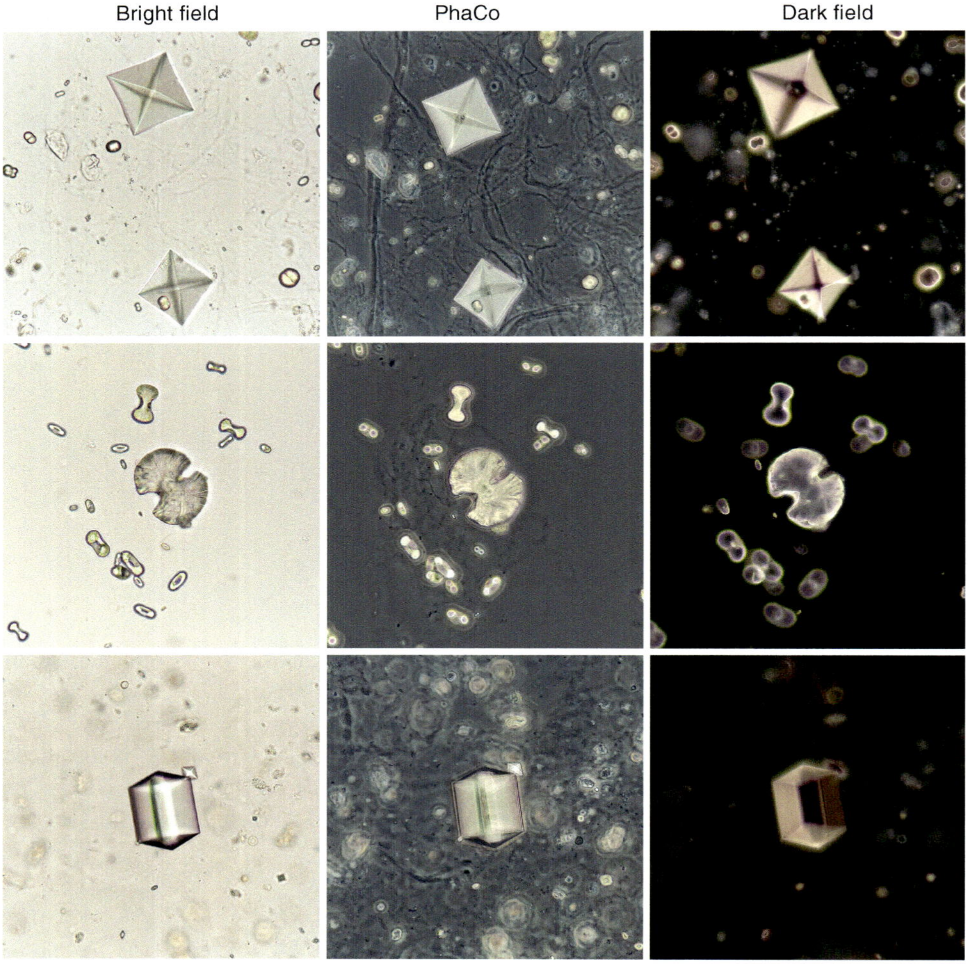

Fig. 4.2 Calcium oxalate crystals. These crystals have diverse forms and varying in size and exhibit strong refractivity, ×400

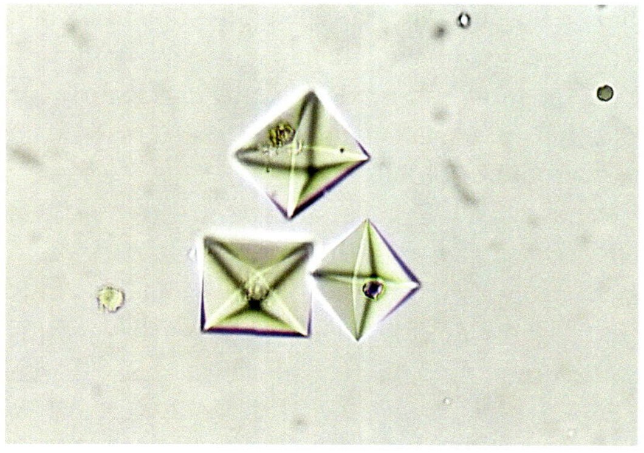

Fig. 4.3 Calcium oxalate crystals, octahedral. Unstained, bright field, ×400

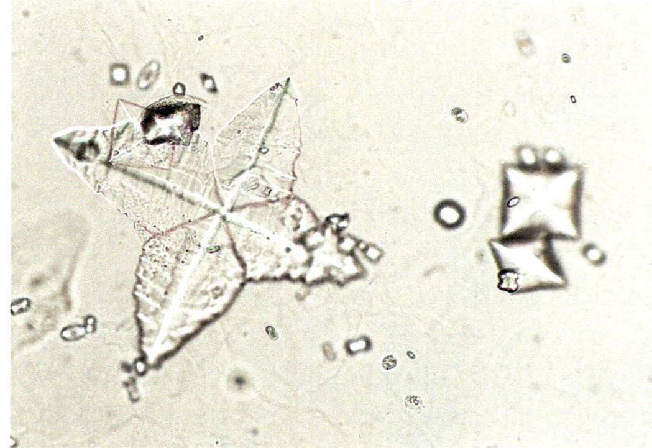

Fig. 4.4 Calcium oxalate crystals, polyhedral, large volume. Unstained, bright field, ×400

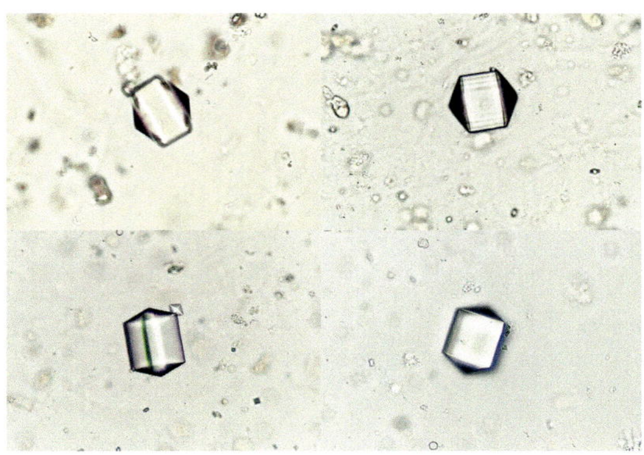

Fig. 4.5 Calcium oxalate crystals, colorless and transparent, polyhedral. Unstained, bright field, ×400

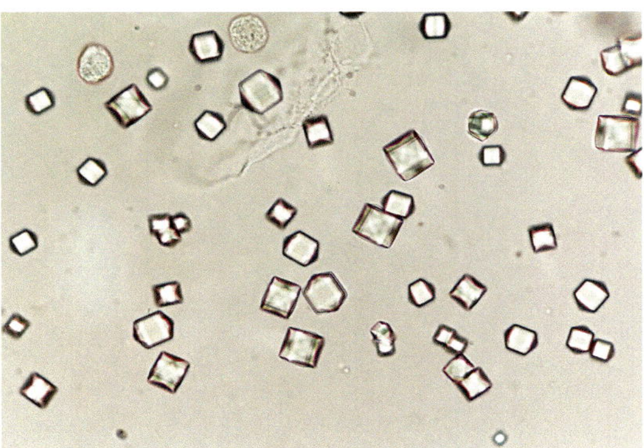

Fig. 4.6 Calcium oxalate crystals, polyhedral. Unstained, bright field, ×400

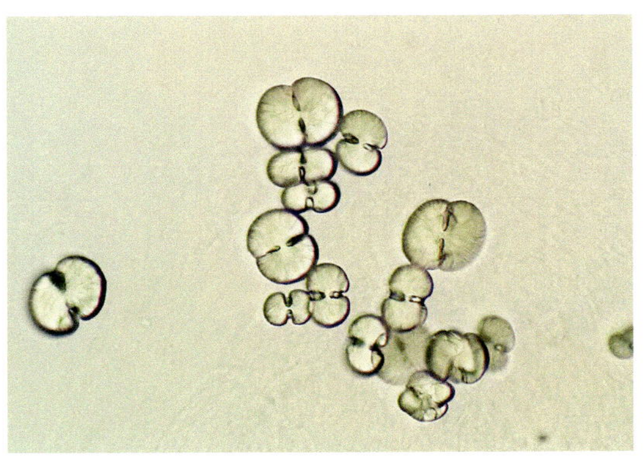

Fig. 4.7 Calcium oxalate crystals, dumbbell-shaped. Unstained, bright field, ×400

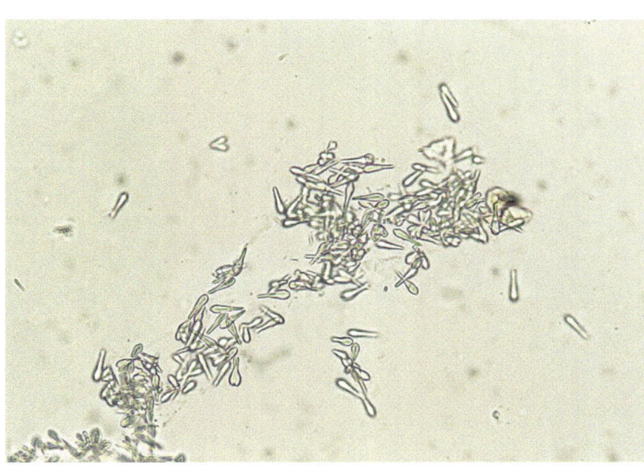

Fig. 4.8 Calcium oxalate crystals, drumstick-shaped. Unstained, bright field, ×400

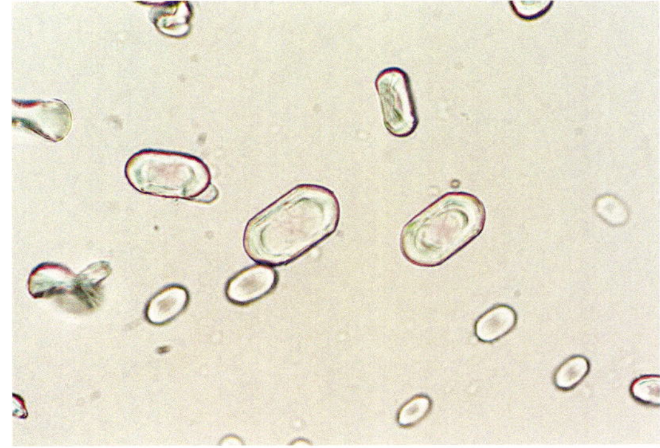

Fig. 4.9 Calcium oxalate crystals, track-like. Unstained, bright field, ×400

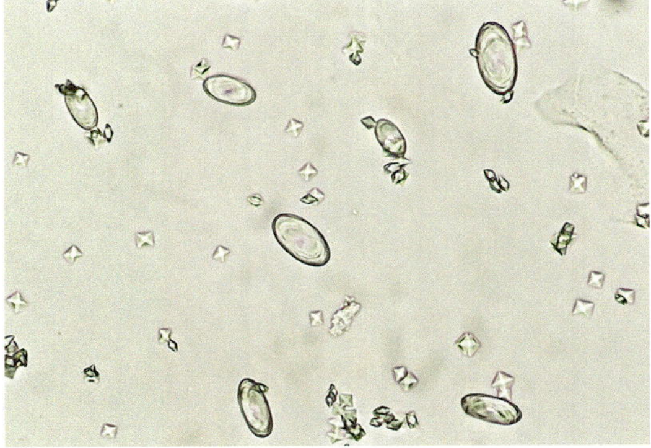

Fig. 4.10 Calcium oxalate crystals, oval or small octahedral structures. Unstained, bright field, ×400

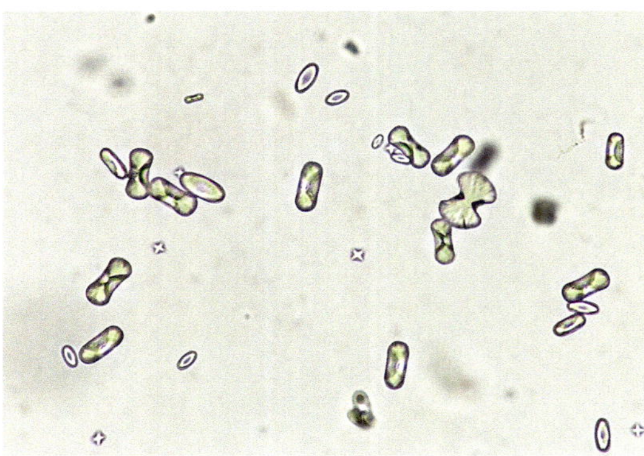

Fig. 4.11 Calcium oxalate crystals, oval. Unstained, bright field, ×400

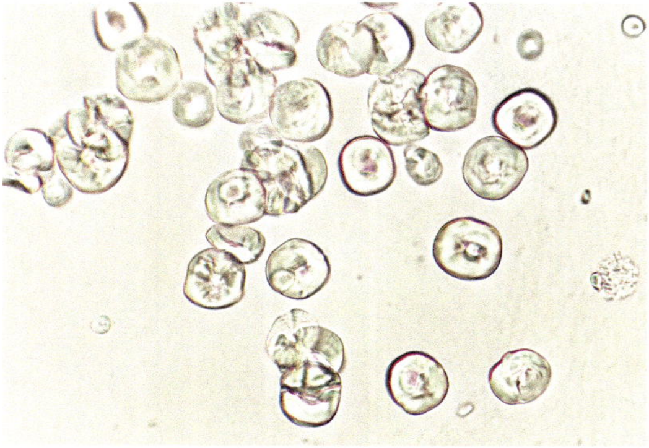

Fig. 4.12 Calcium oxalate crystals, round-shaped, and their central area is sunken. Unstained, bright field, ×400

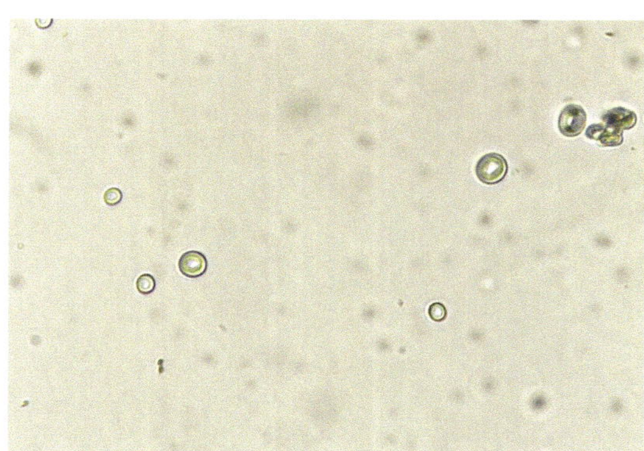

Fig. 4.13 Calcium oxalate crystals, like red blood cells, vary in size, and exhibit strong refractivity. Unstained, bright field, ×400

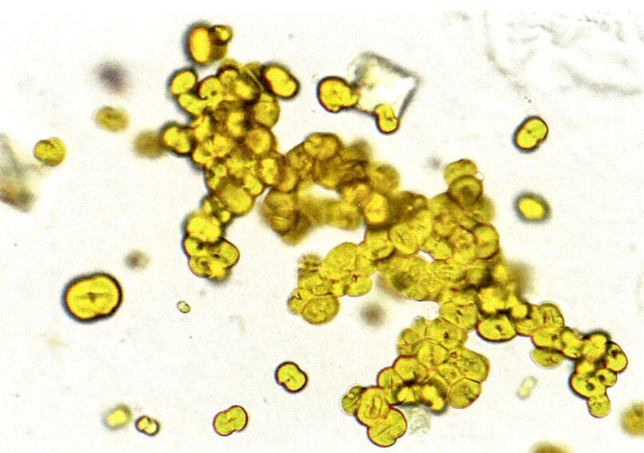

Fig. 4.14 Calcium oxalate crystals, yellow, bilirubinuria. Unstained, bright field, ×400

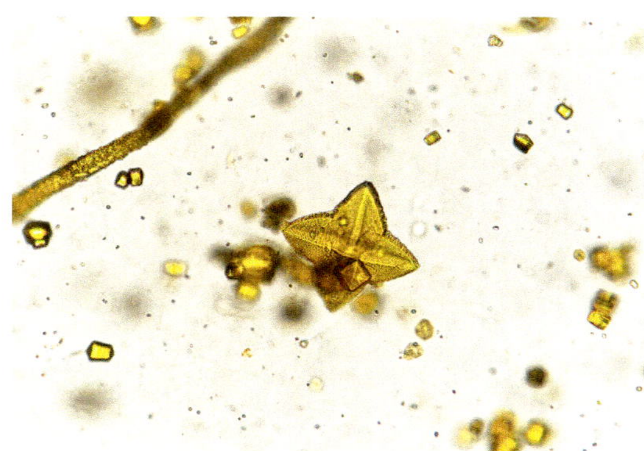

Fig. 4.15 Calcium oxalate crystals, yellow, polyhedral. Bilirubinuria, bright field, ×400

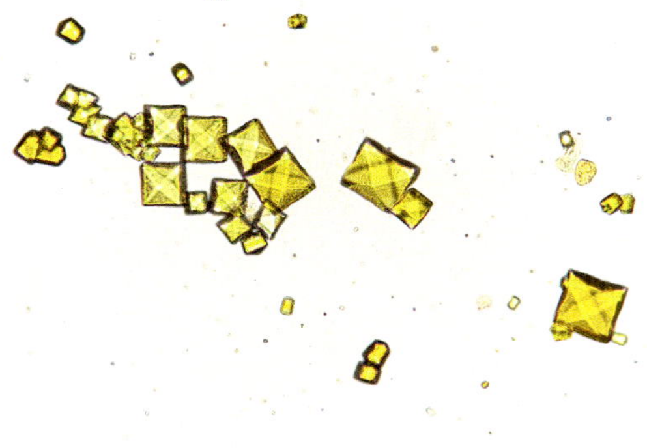

Fig. 4.16 Calcium oxalate crystals, yellow, octahedral structure. Bilirubinuria, bright field, ×400

4.2.3 Clinical Significance

Calcium oxalate crystals are one of the most common crystals found in urine and generally have no clinical significance. If they persist and appear in large quantities in fresh urine, it may suggest a risk of urinary calculi. An analysis of calcium oxalate crystals in urine showed that the COD was present in healthy subjects and stone formers, whereas the COM, which is thermodynamically more stable and constitutes the core of most calcium oxalate stones, was present in stone formers only. Some scholars have shown that hyperoxaluria can cause oxalate nephropathy [6] or other kidney diseases through multiple mechanisms, including tubular obstruction from calcium oxalate crystals, sterile inflammation, and tubular epithelial cell injury. Hyperoxaluria is also observed in individuals with diabetes mellitus and obesity, which are in turn risk factors for chronic kidney disease [7].

4.3 Uric Acid Crystals

4.3.1 Characteristics

Uric acid crystals generally are yellow, light yellow, or dark yellow. The appearance of uric acid crystals has various forms, diamonds, hexagons, spheres, dumbbells, cubes, or irregularities, and the crystals can be clustered into patterns or tubular shapes (Fig. 4.17). These crystals exhibit strong refractivity under phase contrast or dark field microscopy (Fig. 4.18). Uric acid crystals exhibit diverse forms, and they are typically dispersed individually, but they can also aggregate together, forming flower-like patterns under bright field microscopy (Figs. 4.19, 4.20, 4.21, 4.22, 4.23, 4.24, 4.25, 4.26, 4.27, 4.28, 4.29, 4.30, 4.31, 4.32, 4.33, 4.34, 4.35, 4.36, 4.37, 4.38, 4.39, 4.40, 4.41, 4.42, 4.43, 4.44, 4.45, 4.46, 4.47, and 4.48).

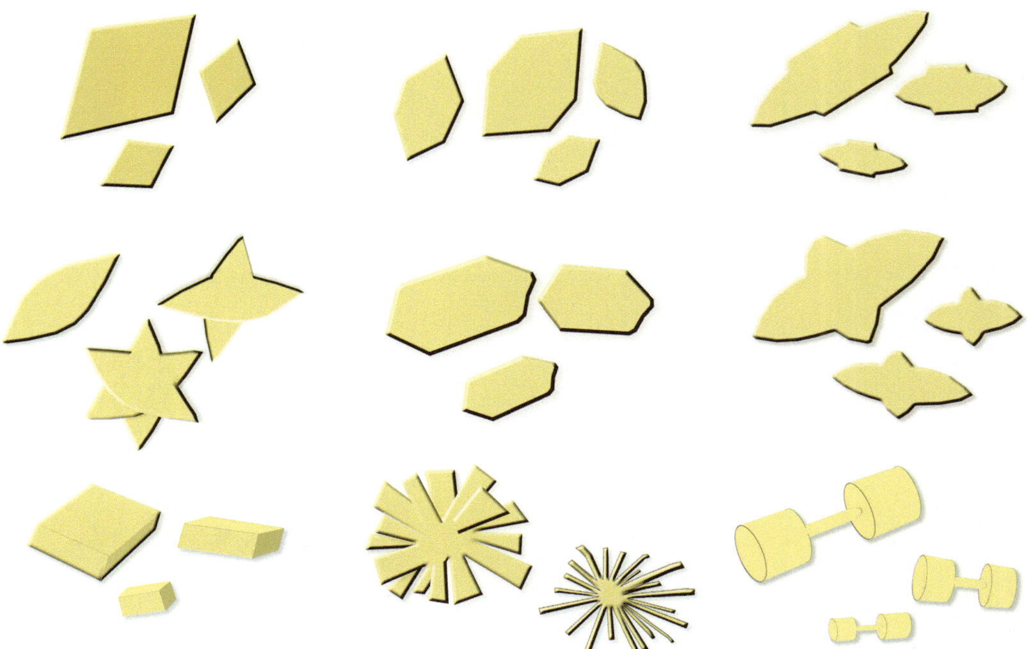

Fig. 4.17 Appearance of uric acid crystals

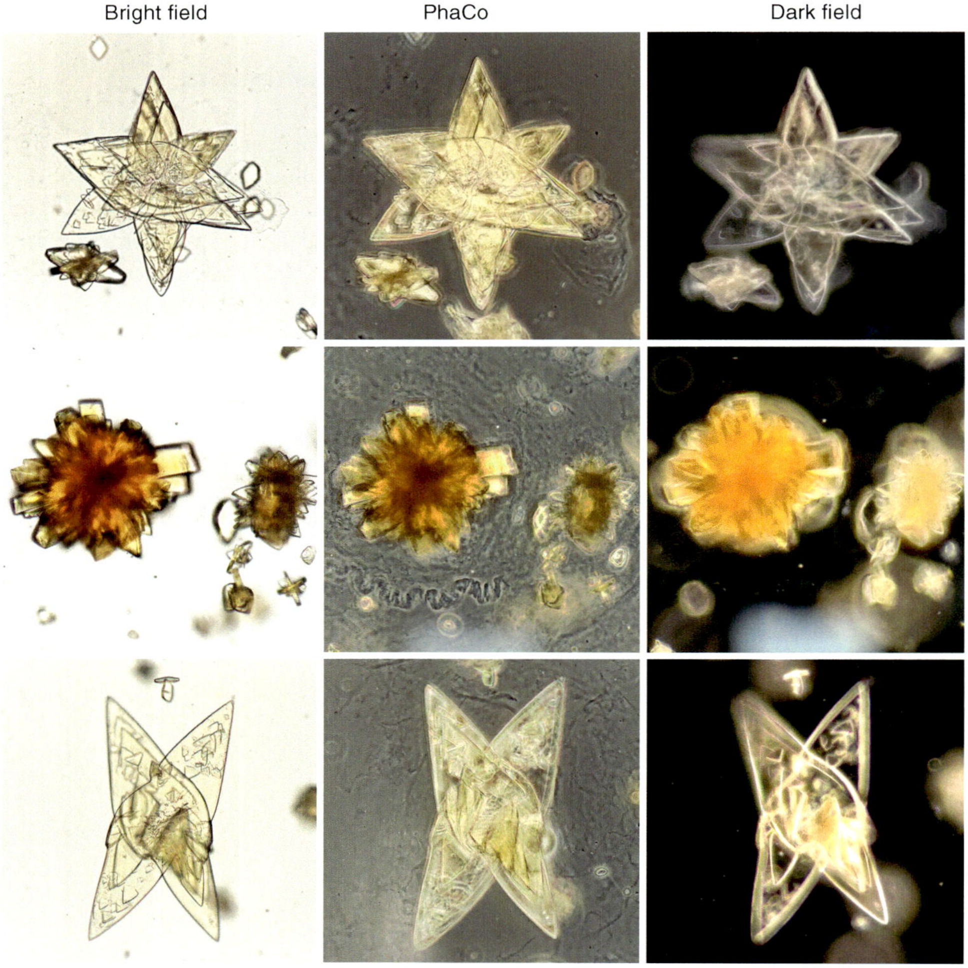

Bright field PhaCo Dark field

Fig. 4.18 Uric acid crystals. These crystals are large in size and exhibit strong refractivity. Unstained, ×400

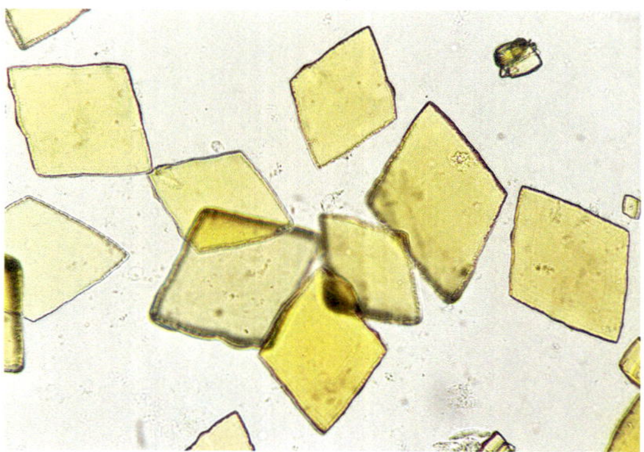

Fig. 4.19 Uric acid crystals, diamond-shaped, yellow. Unstained, bright field, ×400

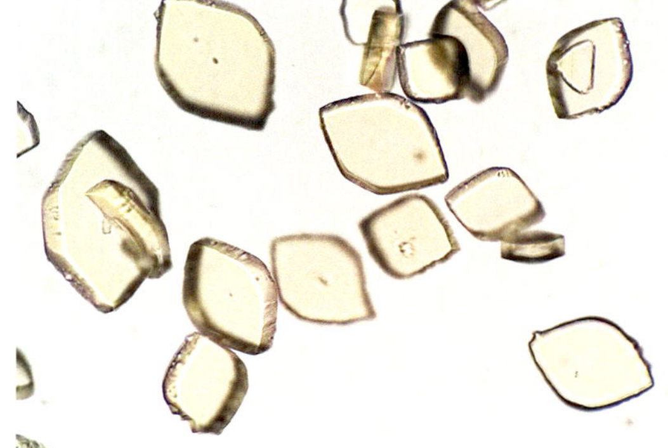

Fig. 4.20 Uric acid crystals, diamond-shaped or hexagon. Unstained, bright field, ×400

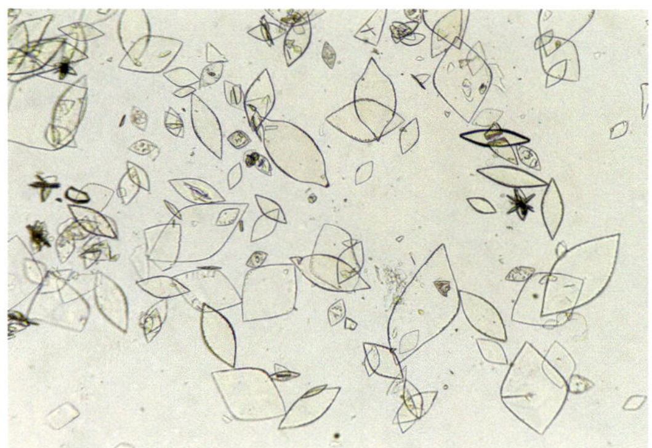

Fig. 4.21 Uric acid crystals, approximately diamond-shaped. Unstained, bright field, ×200

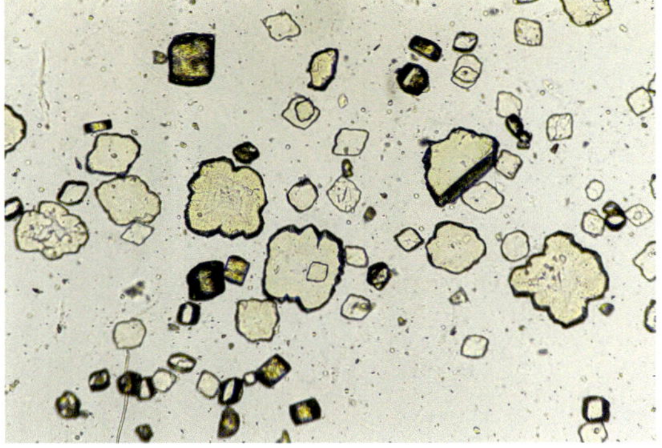

Fig. 4.22 Uric acid crystals, the volume size varies, irregular shape. Unstained, bright field, ×200

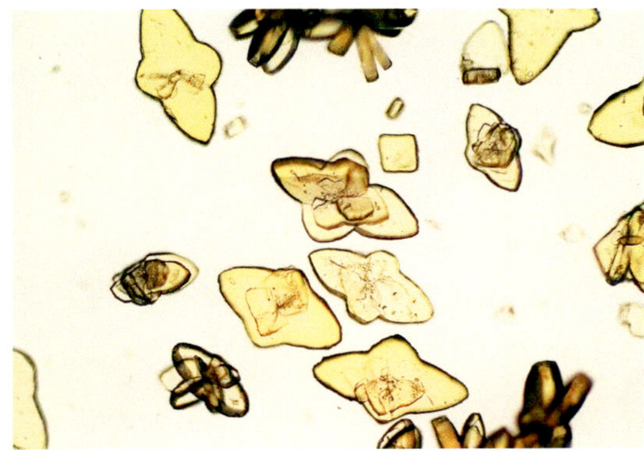

Fig. 4.23 Uric acid crystals, irregular shape. Unstained, bright field, ×400

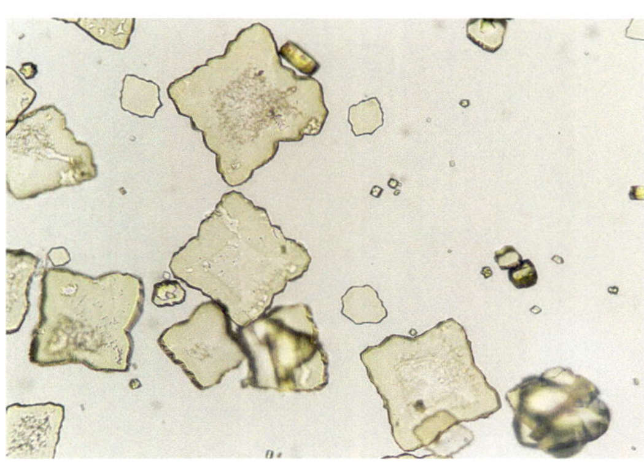

Fig. 4.24 Uric acid crystals, approximately square. Unstained, bright field, ×400

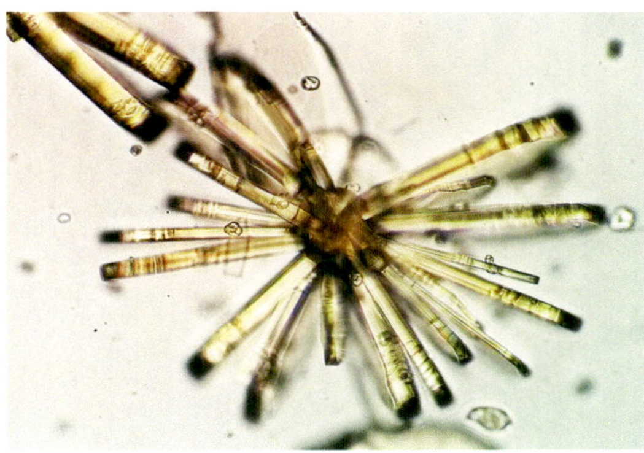

Fig. 4.25 Uric acid crystals, gathered into patterns. Unstained, bright field, ×400

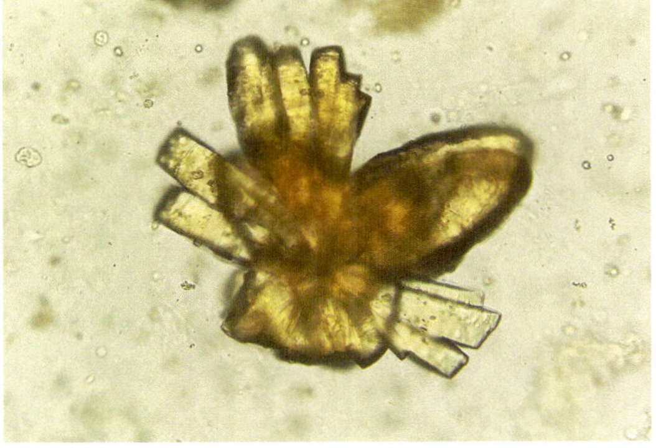

Fig. 4.26 Uric acid crystals, yellow, gathered into patterns. Unstained, bright field, ×400

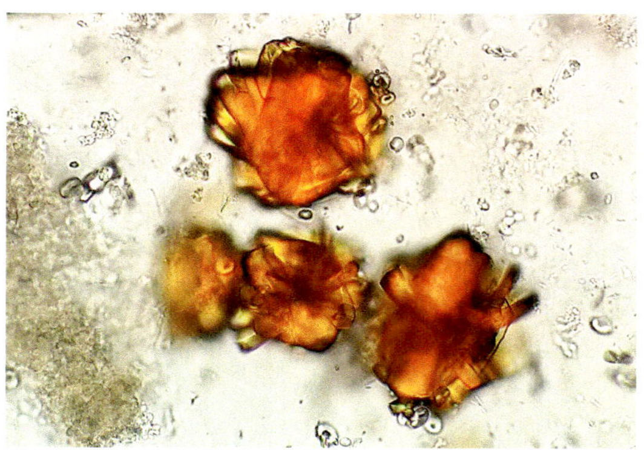

Fig. 4.27 Uric acid crystals, dark yellow, irregular. Unstained, bright field, ×400

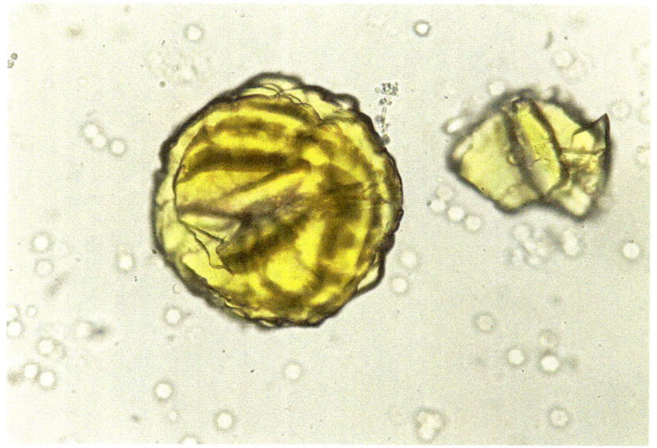

Fig. 4.28 Uric acid crystals, yellow, irregular. Unstained, bright field, ×400

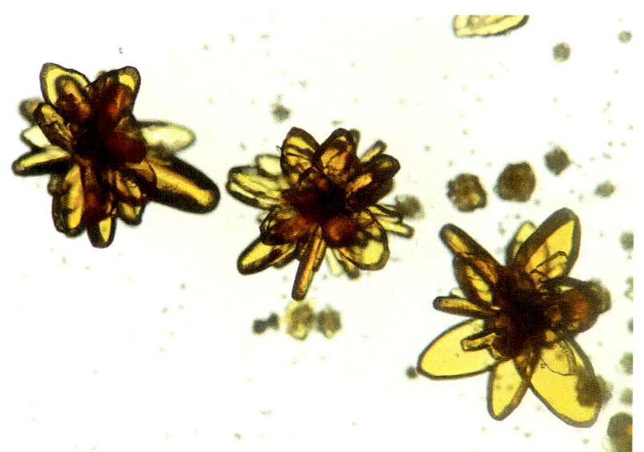

Fig. 4.29 Uric acid crystals, yellow, flower-like. Unstained, bright field, ×400

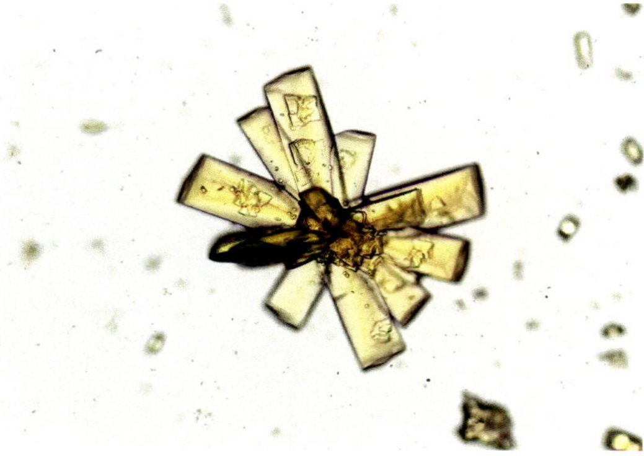

Fig. 4.30 Uric acid crystals, they aggregate into flower-like patterns. Unstained, bright field, ×400

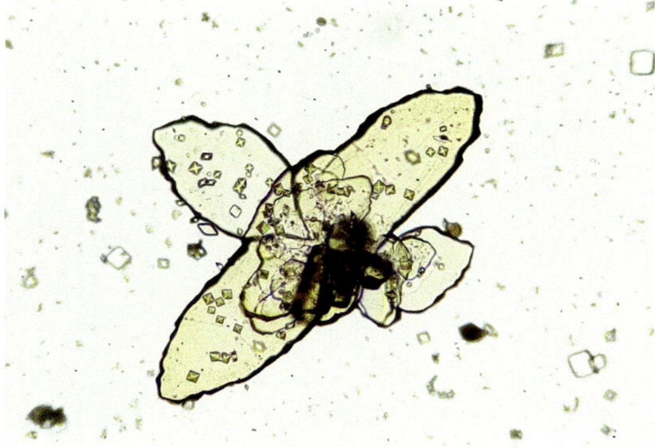

Fig. 4.31 Uric acid crystals, calcium oxalate crystals attached to the surface. Unstained, bright field, ×400

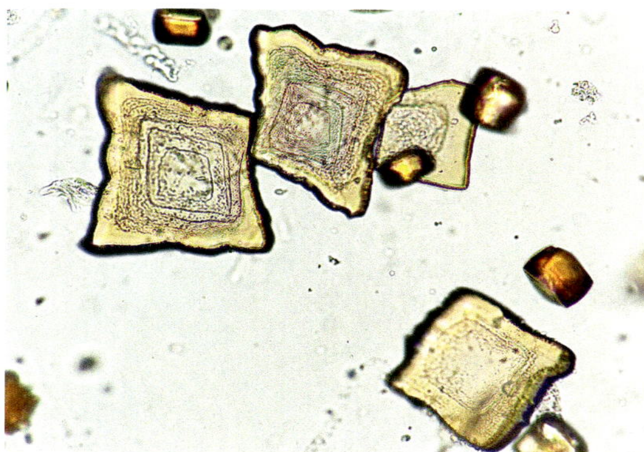

Fig. 4.32 Uric acid crystals. Unstained, bright field, ×400

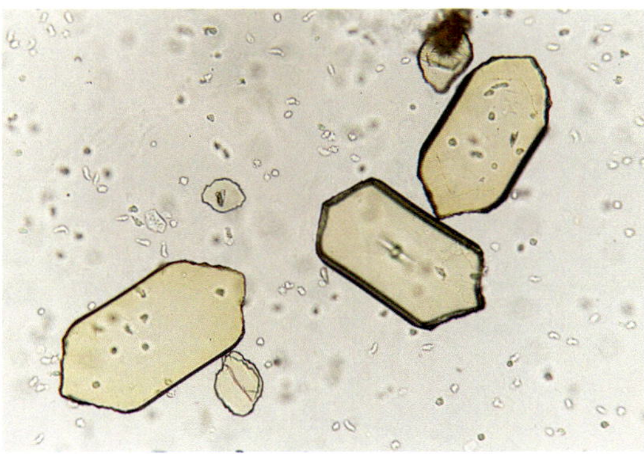

Fig. 4.33 Uric acid crystals, hexagon. Unstained, bright field, ×400

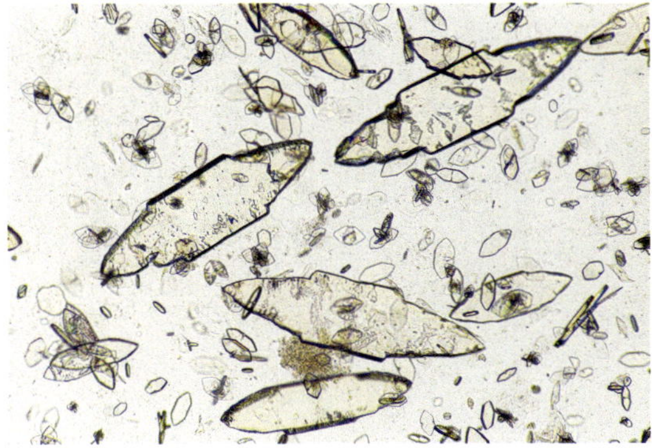

Fig. 4.34 Uric acid crystals, some crystals are very large. Unstained, bright field, ×400

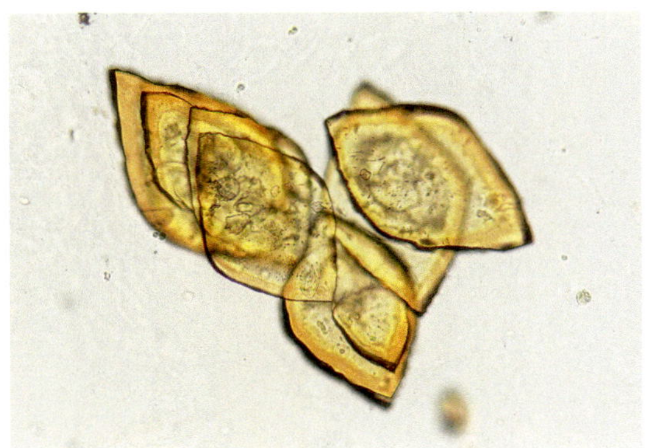

Fig. 4.35 Uric acid crystals, dark yellow, they stack together. Unstained, bright field, ×400

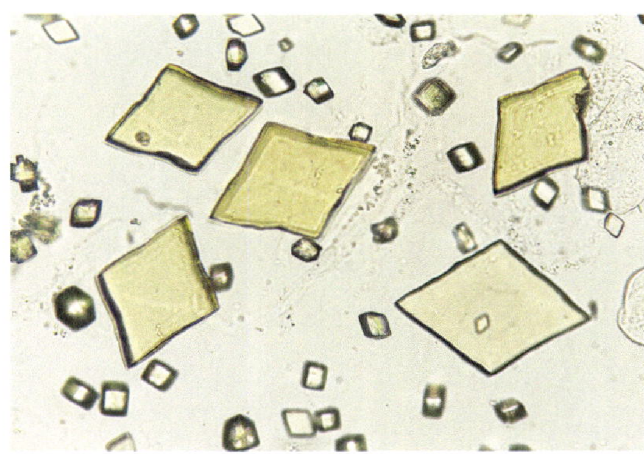

Fig. 4.36 Uric acid crystals, they vary in size. Unstained, bright field, ×400

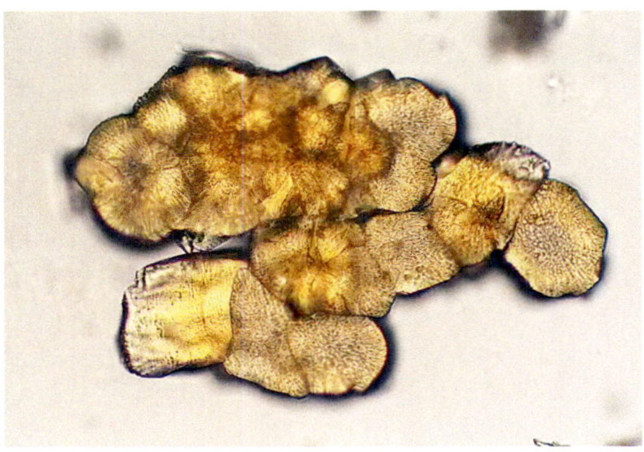

Fig. 4.37 Uric acid crystals, integrate with each other. Unstained, bright field, ×400

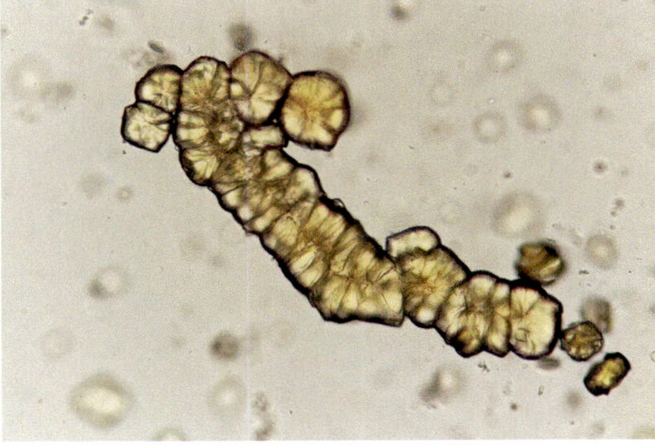

Fig. 4.38 Uric acid crystals. Unstained, bright field, ×400

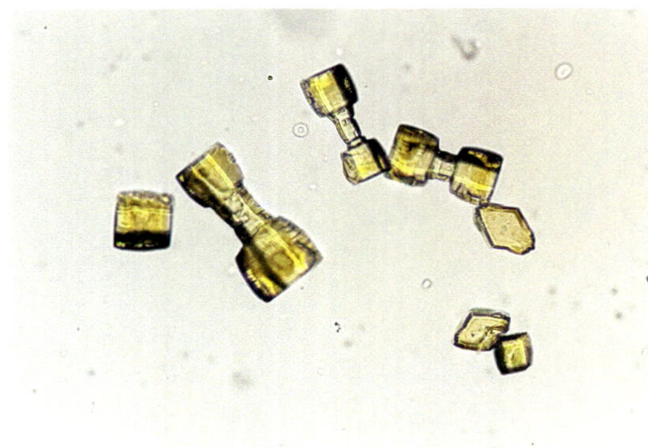

Fig. 4.39 Uric acid crystals, yellow, dumbbell-shaped. Unstained, bright field, ×400

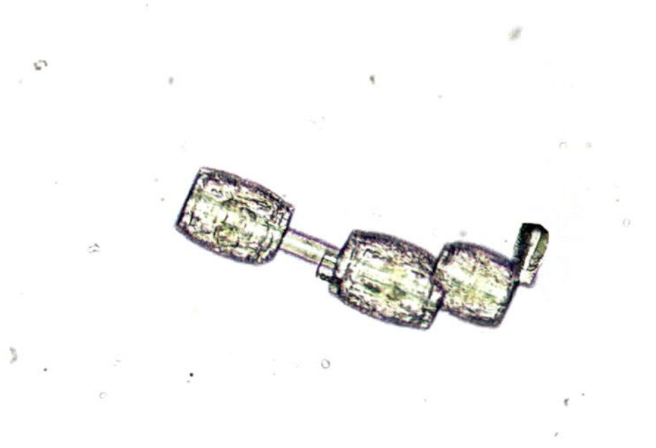

Fig. 4.40 Uric acid crystals, dumbbell-shaped. Unstained, bright field, ×400

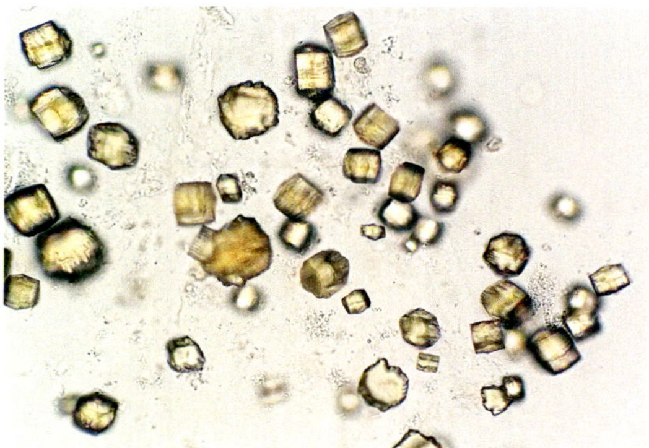

Fig. 4.41 Uric acid crystals, three-dimensional structure. Unstained, bright field, ×400

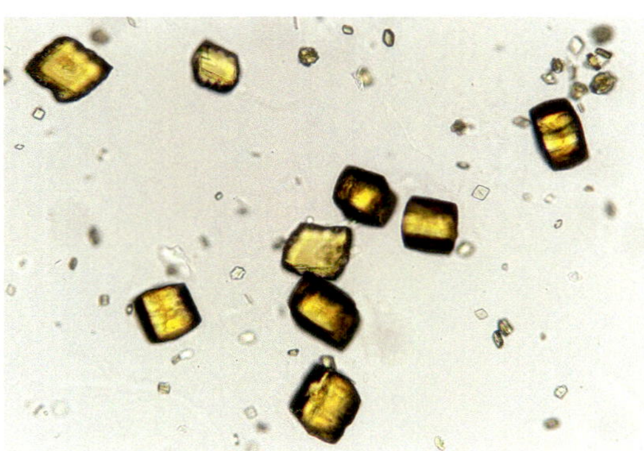

Fig. 4.42 Uric acid crystals, dark yellow, cube shape. Unstained, bright field, ×400

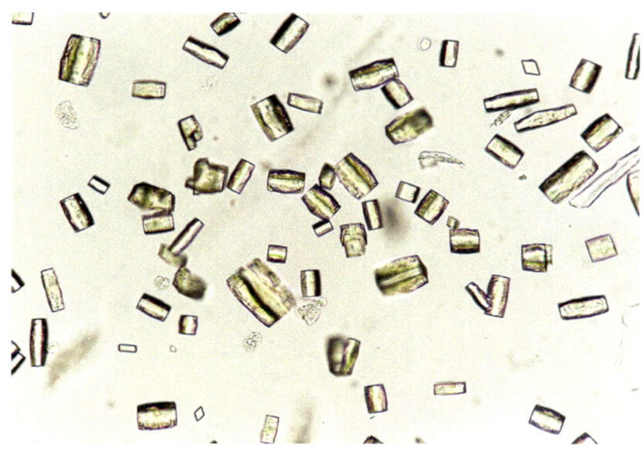

Fig. 4.43 Uric acid crystals. Unstained, bright field, ×400

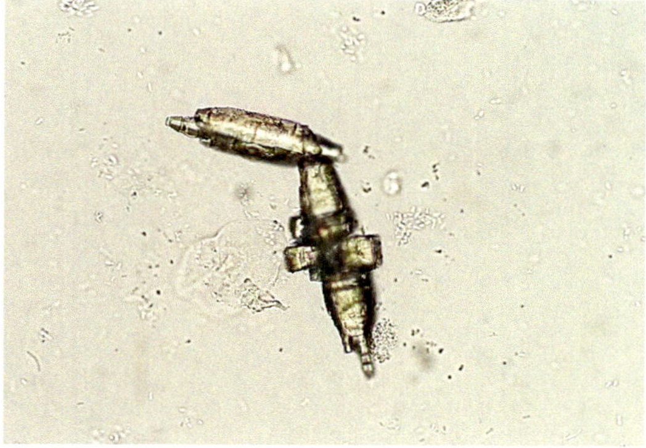

Fig. 4.44 Uric acid crystals. Irregular, unstained, bright field, ×400

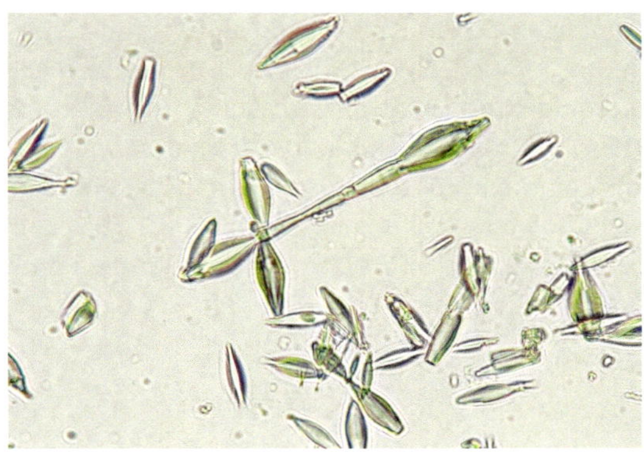

Fig. 4.45 Uric acid crystals, pale yellow, tapered. Unstained, bright field, ×400

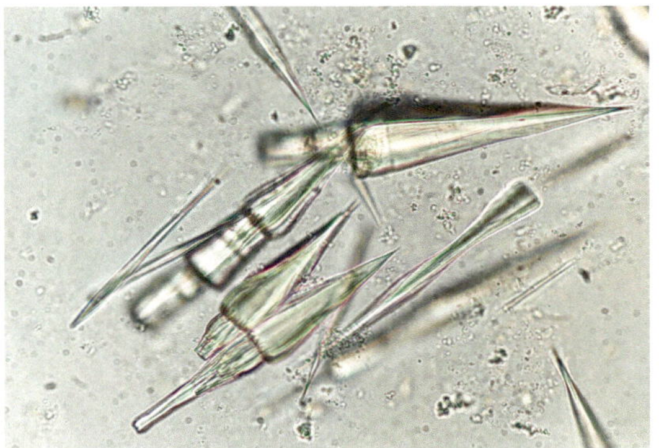

Fig. 4.46 Uric acid crystals. They resemble the tip of a calligraphy brush. Unstained, bright field, ×400

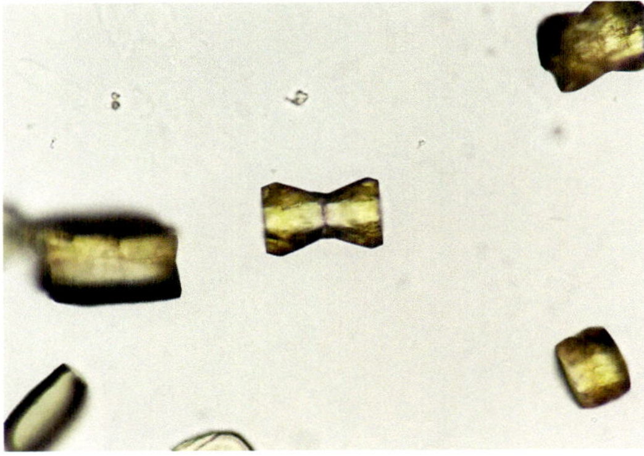

Fig. 4.47 Uric acid crystals, drum-like shape. Unstained, bright field, ×400

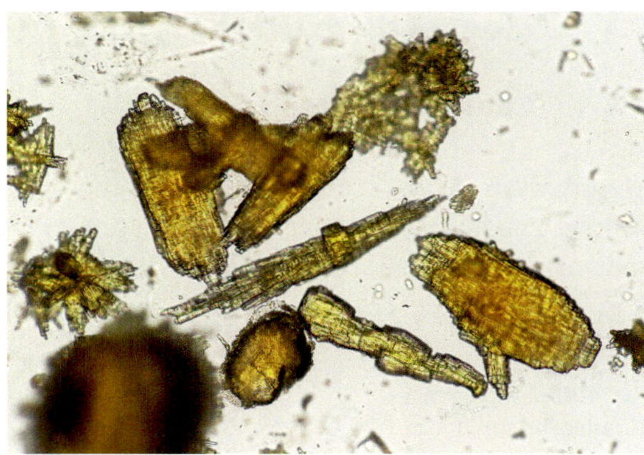

Fig. 4.48 Uric acid crystals. They are large in size and have irregular shapes. Unstained, bright field, ×200

Under certain conditions, uric acid crystals can be broken down or converted to other forms of urate. Uric acid crystals are commonly found in acidic urine, dissolved in 10% KOH solution, and insoluble in acetic acid and hydrochloric acid. The sediment after centrifugation is dark yellow or brick red.

4.3.2 Clinical Significance

Uric acid crystals are one of the most common crystals in urine, which can be seen after a high-purine diet, as well as in the urine of gout patients [8] and interstitial nephritis, high uric acid nephropathy, and leukemia patients and children with acute fever [9]. Long-term deposition of uric acid crystals can form uric acid stones in the urinary system, which may be related to lower urinary pH, lower uric acid fractional excretion, and higher serum uric acid [10]. Uric acid stone formation is frequently associated with metabolic syndrome, obesity, type 2 diabetes, and so on [11]. If uric acid crystals are deposited in the renal tubules for a long time, they can block the renal tubules and lead to glomerular dysfunction.

4.4 Monosodium Urate Crystals

4.4.1 Characteristics

Monosodium urate crystals are pale yellow or yellow, needle-like, or slender rod-shaped [12] and may aggregate into bundles or patterns (Fig. 4.49). These crystals are pale yellow and vary in thickness and length under bright field microscopy (Fig. 4.50). Their structure appears more distinct under dark field microscopy (Figs. 4.51 and 4.52). Monosodium urate crystals are commonly observed in acidic urine and can be dissolved when it is heated to 60 °C. They can be converted to uric acid crystals after the addition of HCl.

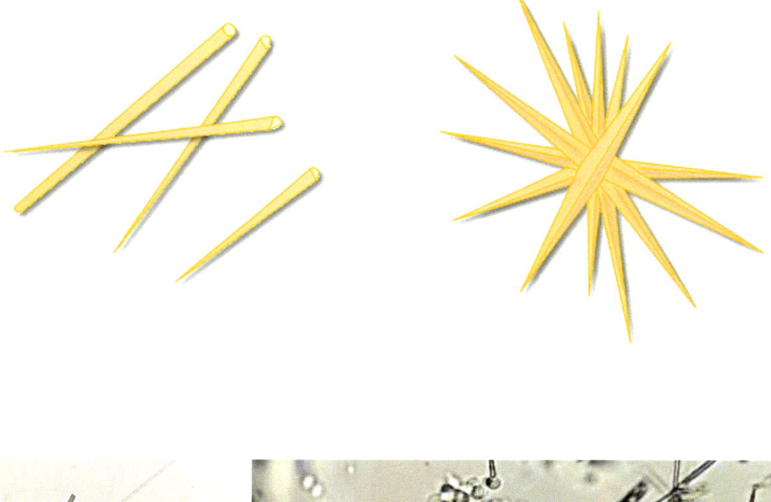

Fig. 4.49 Appearance of monosodium urate crystals

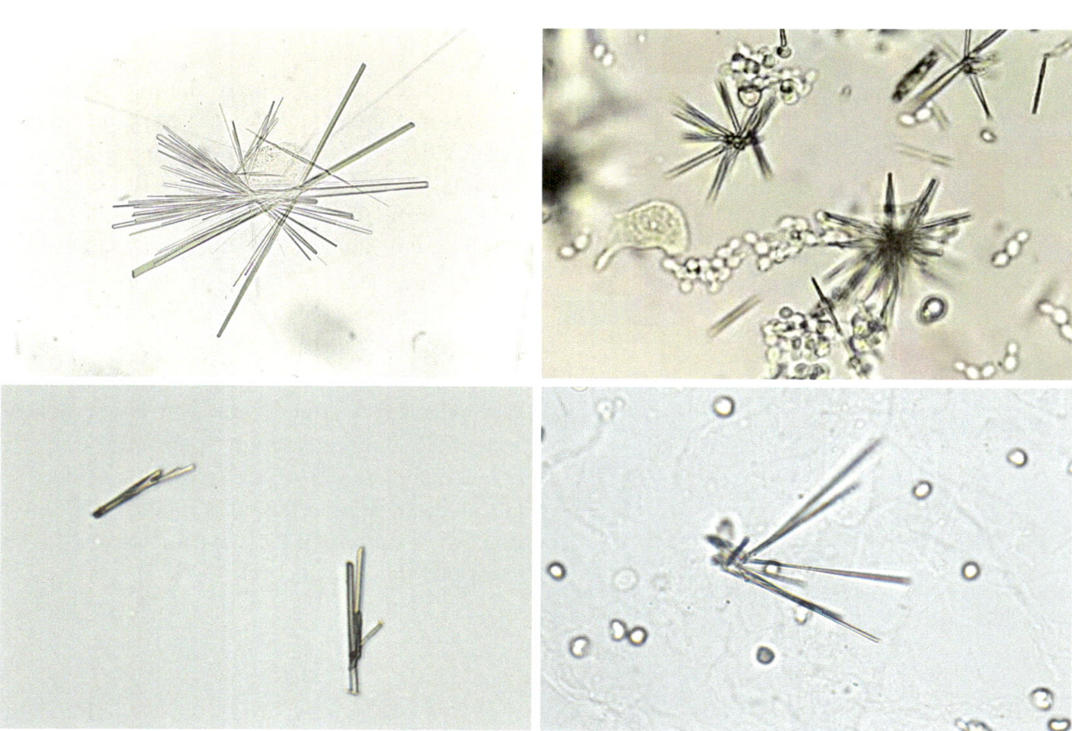

Fig. 4.50 Monosodium urate crystals, rod-shaped, some aggregated into bundles. Bright field, ×400

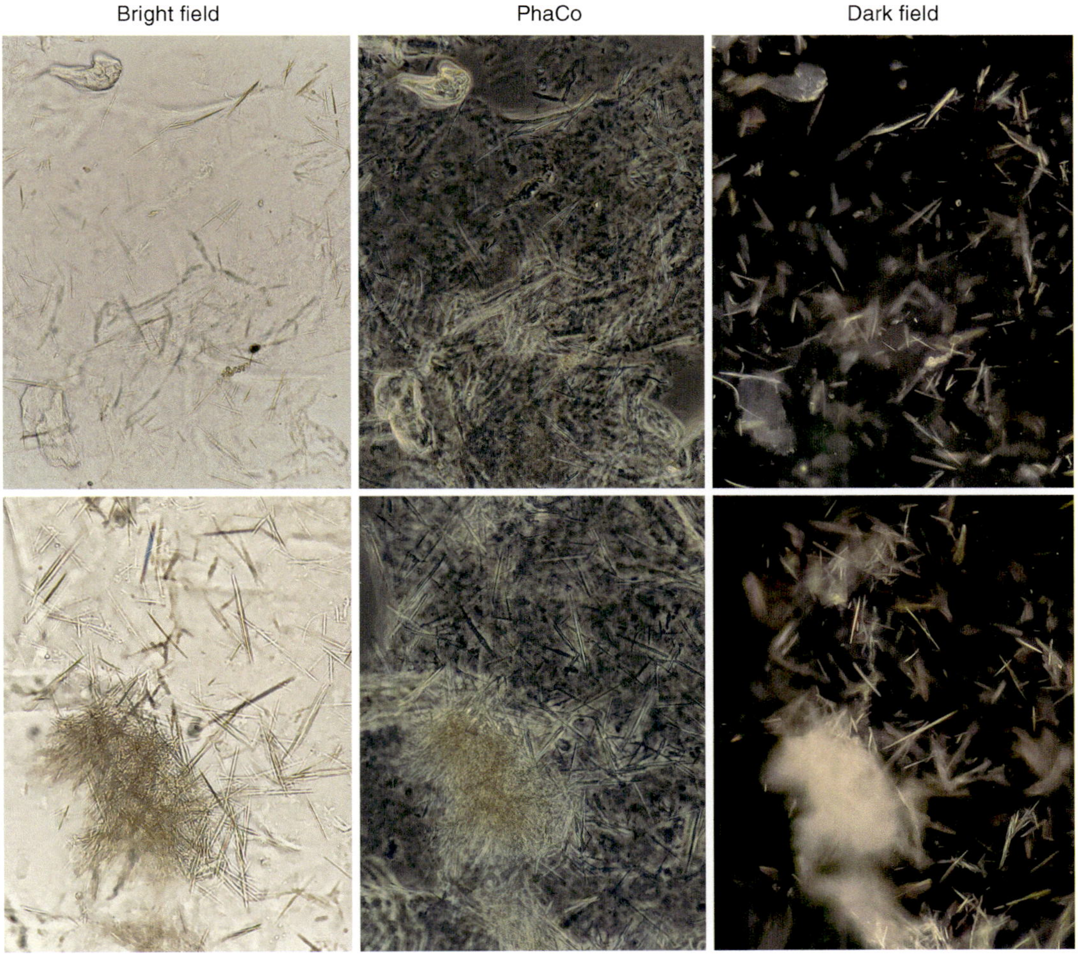

Bright field
PhaCo
Dark field

Fig. 4.51 Monosodium urate crystals. Pale yellow, needle-like bundles. Unstained, ×400

Bright field
PhaCo
Dark field

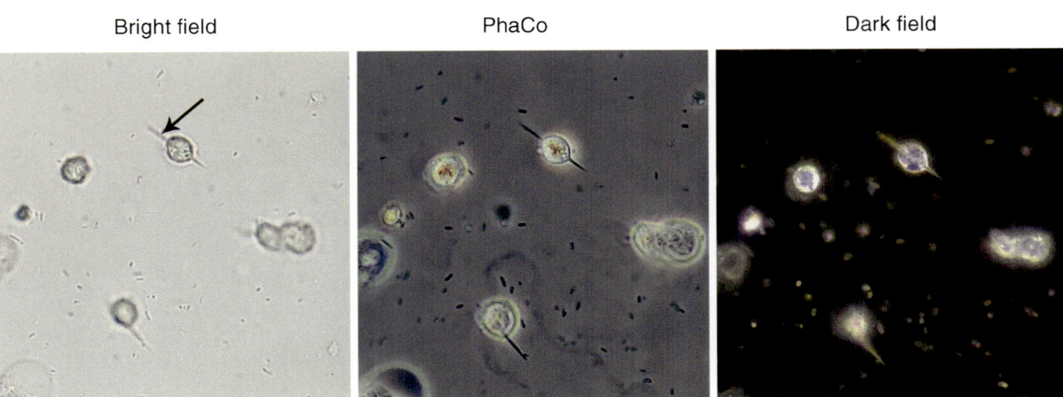

Fig. 4.52 Monosodium urate crystals (↑). The crystals are small in size and pass through white blood cells. Unstained, ×400

4.4.2 Clinical Significance

It has been suggested that monosodium urate crystals may participate in the formation of urinary calculi and may be seen in the urine of some patients with gout [13].

4.5 Amorphous Urates

4.5.1 Characteristics

Amorphous urates are granules or small spheres of different sizes (Fig. 4.53). These crystals appear yellow or orange, and the granule sizes vary under bright field microscopy (Figs. 4.54 and 4.55). The urine is cloudy and has a pH of ≤7.0. They dissolve when heated or upon the addition of 10% KOH, and the centrifuged sediments are mostly pale pink.

4.5.2 Clinical Significance

Amorphous urates can precipitate at lower temperatures or with longer sample retention time, which generally has no clinical significance. However, they can interfere with the analysis of other formed elements [14]. Amorphous urates can be dissolved by placing the sample in a water bath at 37 °C for 5–10 min [15].

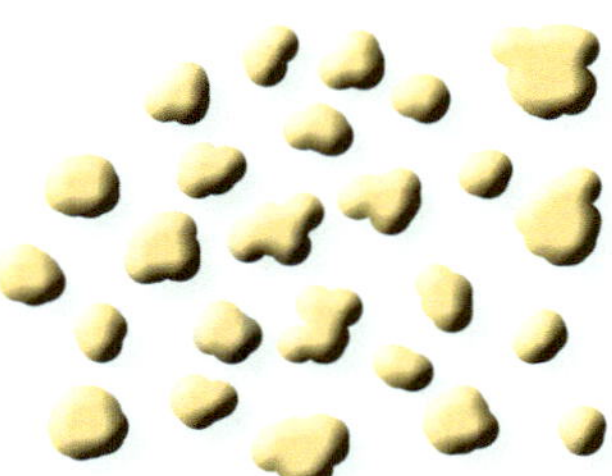

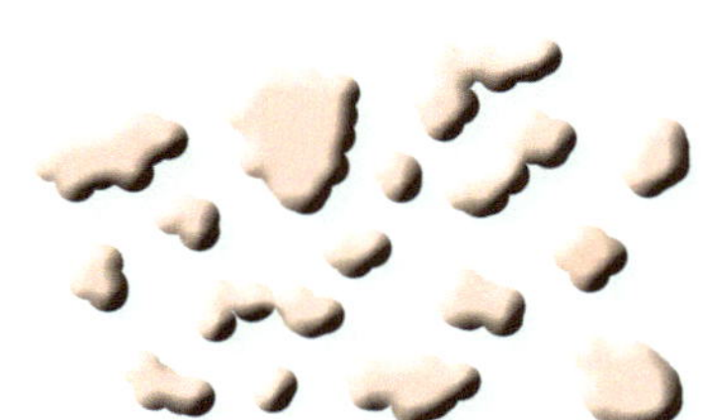

Fig. 4.53 Appearance of amorphous urates

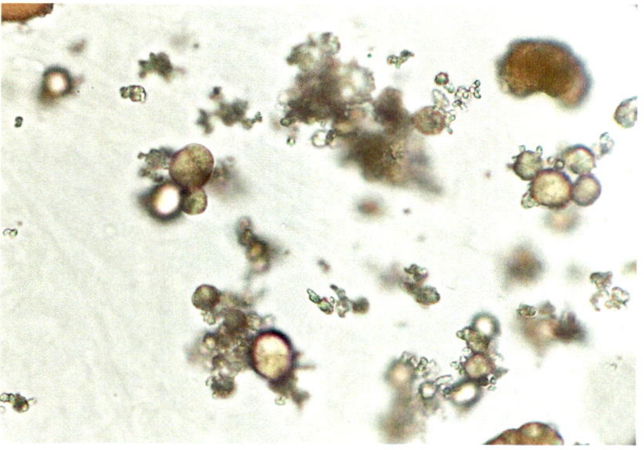

Fig. 4.54 Amorphous urates. The granules vary in size, yellow. Unstained, bright field, ×400

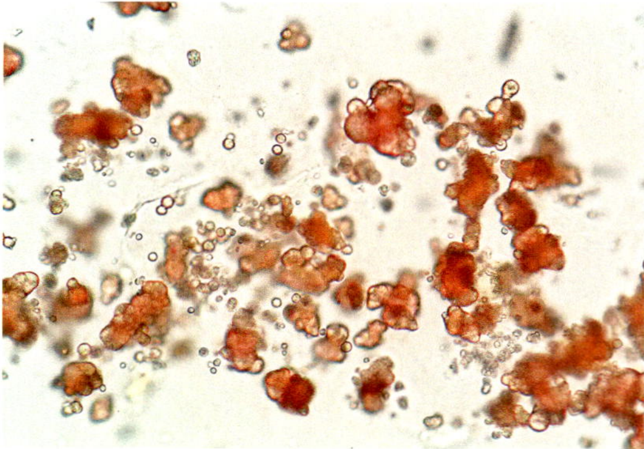

Fig. 4.55 Amorphous urates, orange, some granules aggregate together. Unstained, bright field, ×400

4.6 Ammonium Biurate Crystals

4.6.1 Characteristics

Ammonium biurate crystals are yellow-brown, have opaque appearance, and can exhibit a root-shaped, dumbbell-shaped, or spherical morphology with needle-like protrusions (Figs. 4.56, 4.57, 4.58, 4.59, 4.60, 4.61, 4.62, 4.63, 4.64, and 4.65). These crystals are unique among urate crystals as they are found in alkaline urine, although they may also occur in neutral or weakly acidic urine. Ammonium biurate crystals dissolve in HCl, acetic acid, and 10% KOH solution and can be dissolved by heating as well [16].

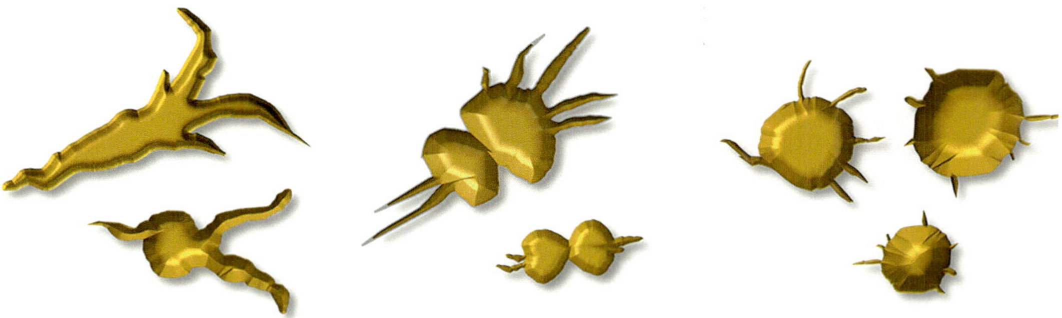

Fig. 4.56 Appearance of ammonium biurate crystals

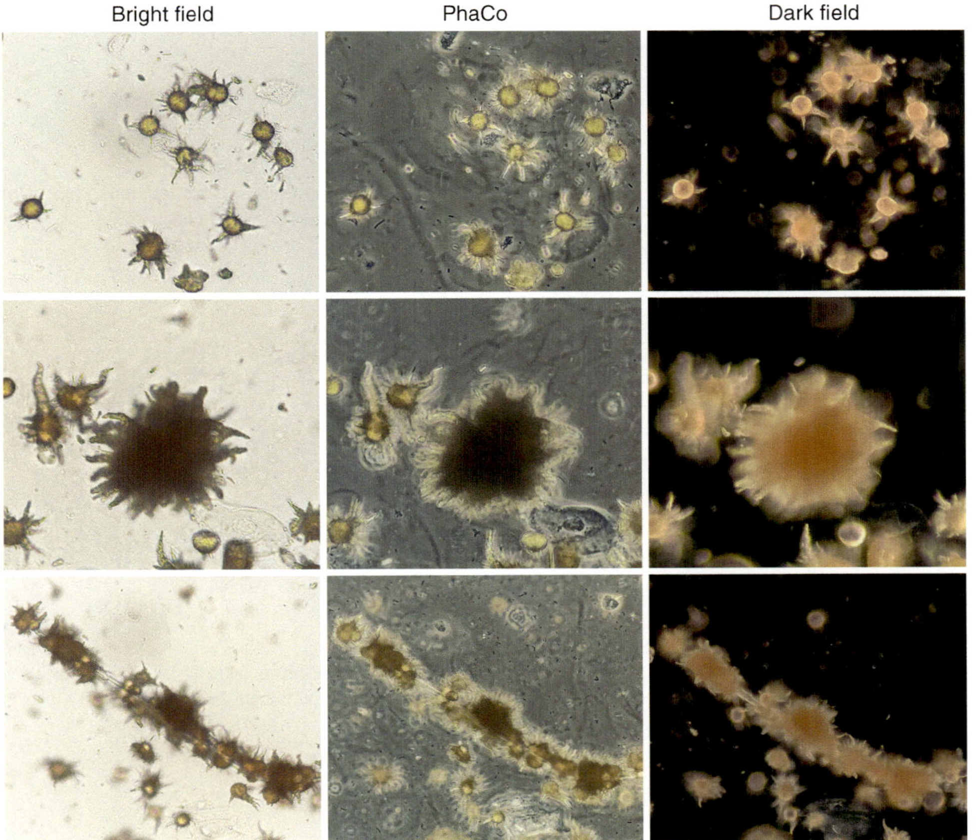

Fig. 4.57 Ammonium biurate crystals, ×400

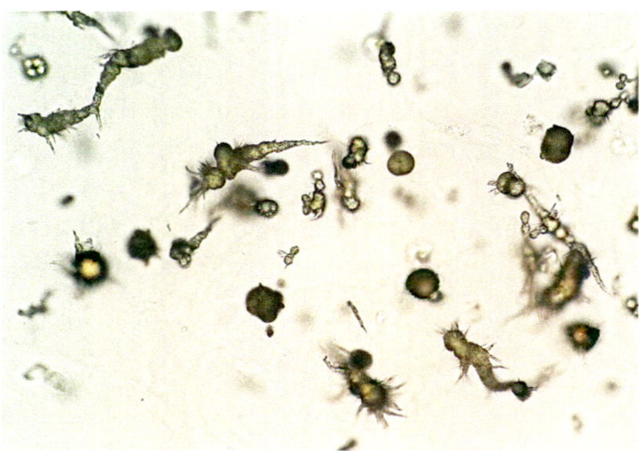

Fig. 4.58 Ammonium biurate crystals, brown, root-shaped or spherical. Unstained, bright field, ×400

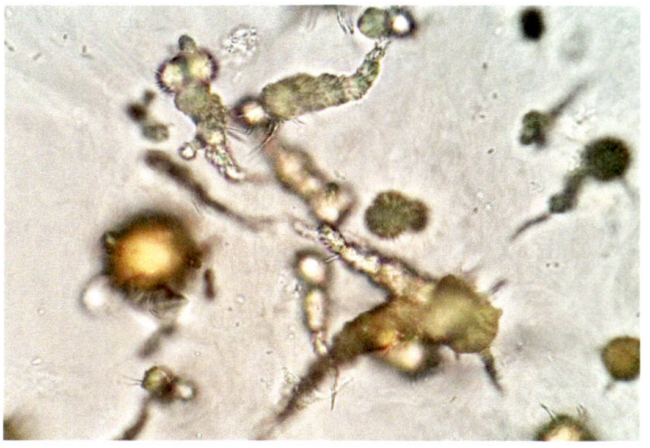

Fig. 4.59 Ammonium biurate crystals, brown-yellow, root-like. Unstained, bright field, ×400

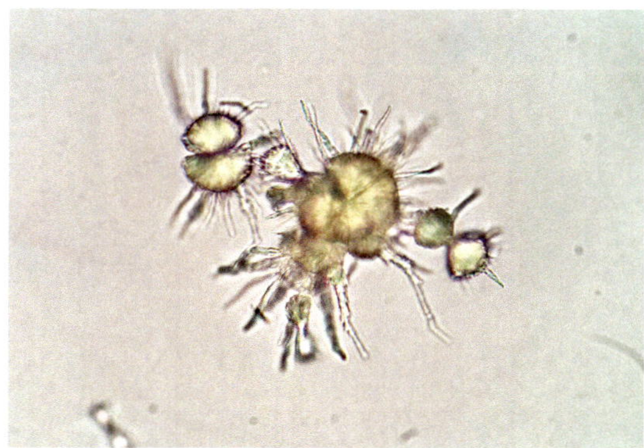

Fig. 4.60 Ammonium biurate crystals, yellow, dumbbell-shaped with burrs. Unstained, bright field, ×400

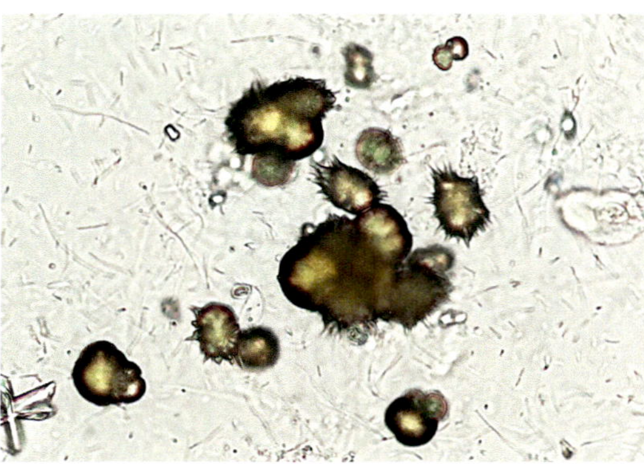

Fig. 4.61 Ammonium biurate crystals, brown-yellow, spherical, a few crystals with burrs. Unstained, bright field, ×400

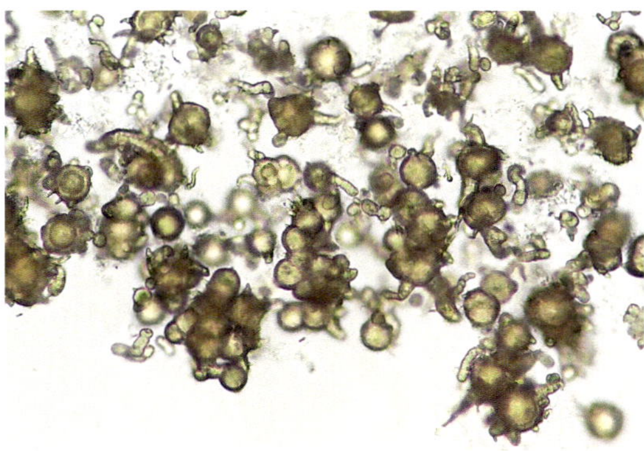

Fig. 4.62 Ammonium biurate crystals, brown-yellow, spherical. Unstained, bright field, ×400

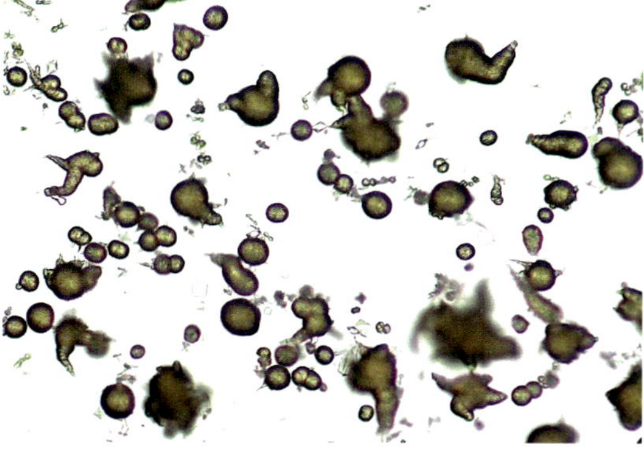

Fig. 4.63 Ammonium biurate crystals, brown-yellow, varying in size. Unstained, bright field, ×400

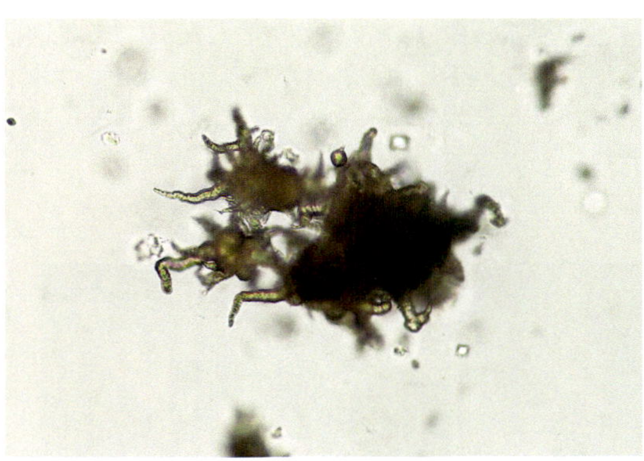

Fig. 4.64 Ammonium biurate crystals, brown, with root protuberances. Unstained, bright field, ×400

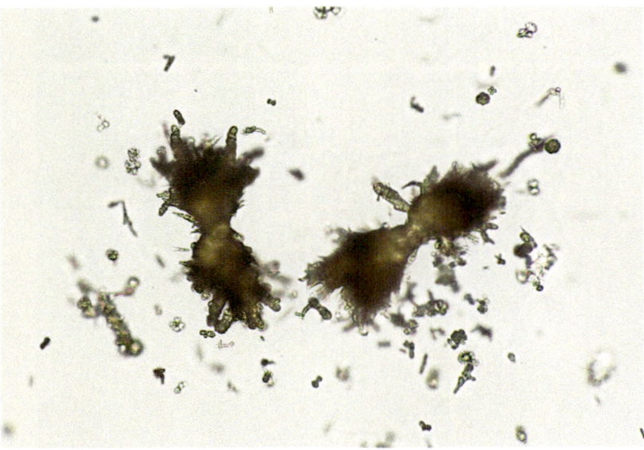

Fig. 4.65 Ammonium biurate crystals, brown, firewood-shaped. Unstained, bright field, ×400

4.6.2 Clinical Significance

Ammonium urate crystals are commonly found in bacterial urine, especially in children or infants. Additionally, they may also be observed in older urine. Abundant ammonium urate crystals in fresh urine suggest the presence of bacterial cystitis. Laxative abuse should be suspected whenever a woman has an ammonium urate renal calculus in sterile urine [17]. Ammonium urate stones were associated with hyperoxaluria and chronic diarrheal syndromes [18].

4.7 Struvite Crystals/Triple Phosphate Crystals

4.7.1 Characteristics

Struvite crystals/triple phosphate crystals are large, colorless, and transparent. They exhibit strong refraction and take on various appearances, including roof-shaped, envelope-shaped, cubic, diamond or irregular shapes, and so on (Fig. 4.66). The same urine sample may appear in different forms of struvite crystals. The common appearance of struvite crystals is depicted below. These crystals display strong refractivity under

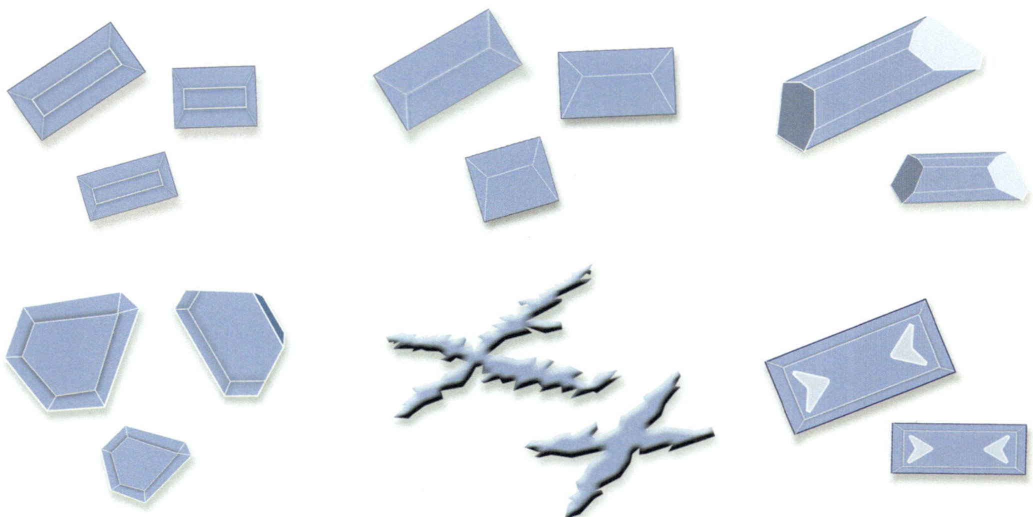

Fig. 4.66 Appearance of struvite crystals

phase contrast and dark field microscopy (Figs. 4.67, 4.68, 4.69, 4.70, 4.71, 4.72, and 4.73). These crystals are colorless and exhibit diverse forms when observed under bright field microscopy (Figs. 4.74, 4.75, 4.76, 4.77, 4.78, 4.79, 4.80, 4.81, 4.82, 4.83, 4.84, 4.85, 4.86, 4.87, 4.88, 4.89, 4.90, 4.91, 4.92, 4.93, 4.94, and 4.95).

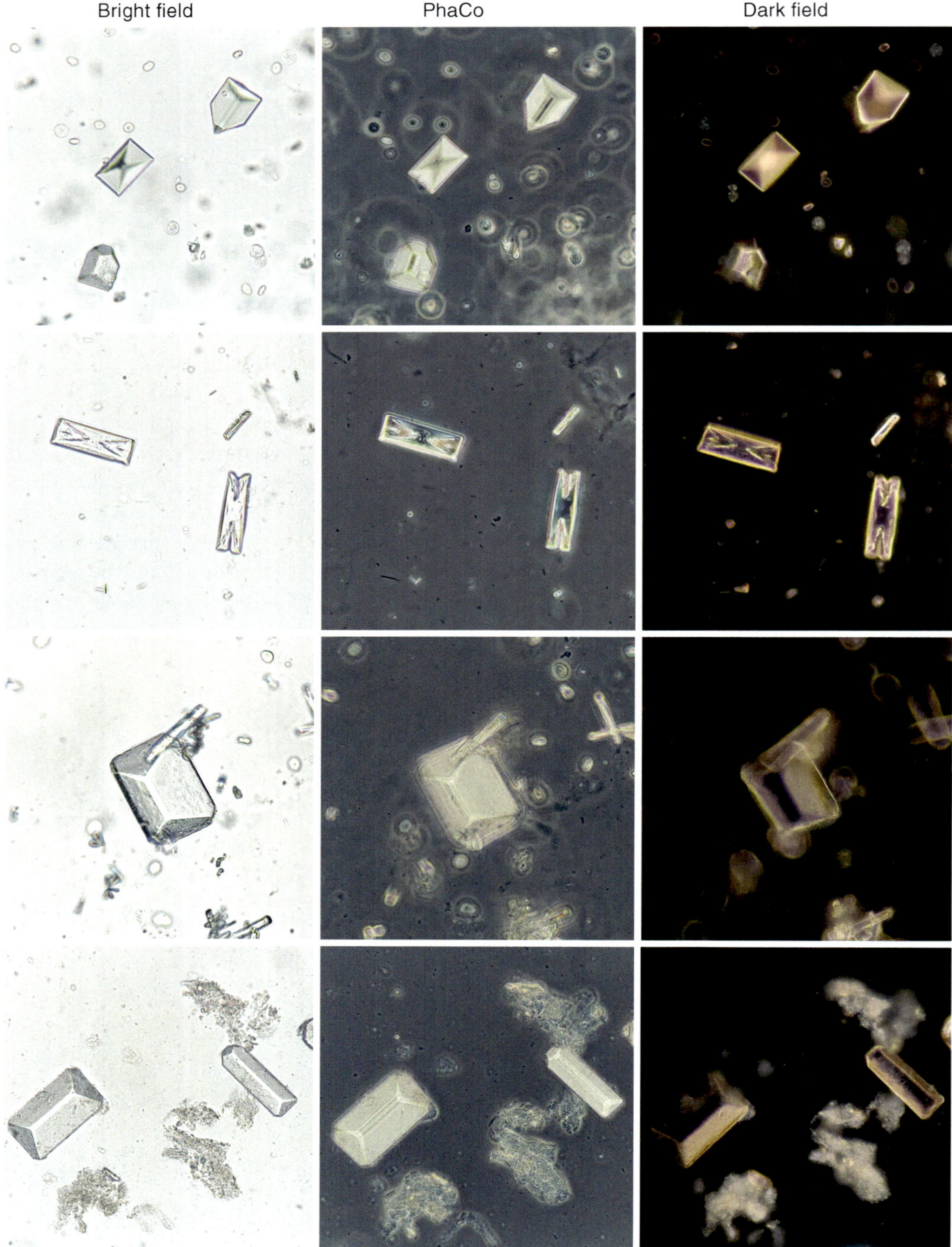

Fig. 4.67 Struvite crystals. They exhibit varying sizes and strong refractivity. Unstained, ×400

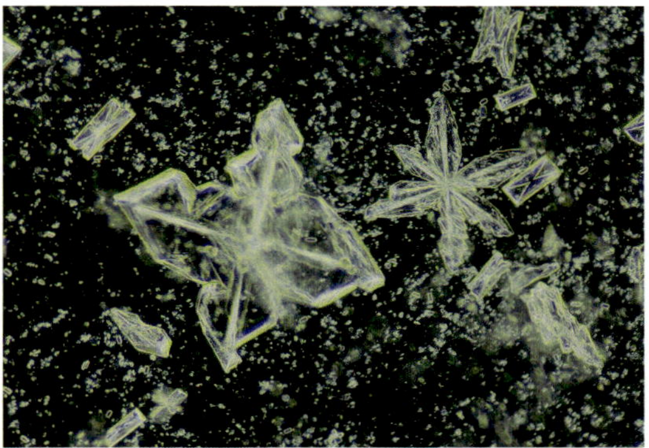

Fig. 4.68 Struvite crystals. These crystals vary in size. A large number of small granules of phosphate are visible in the background. Dark field, ×200

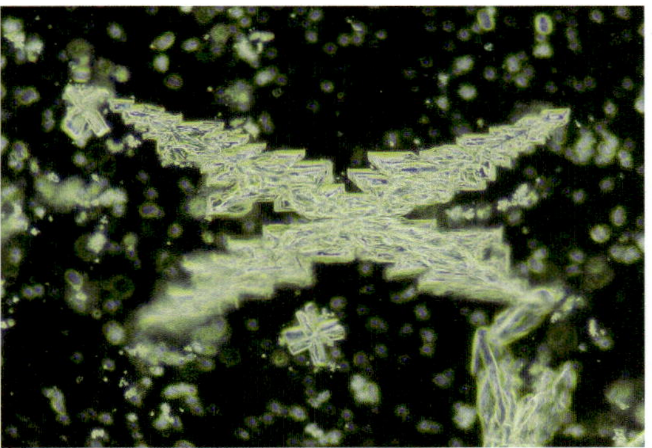

Fig. 4.69 Struvite crystals. They are significantly large in size, scissors-shaped. Dark field, ×200

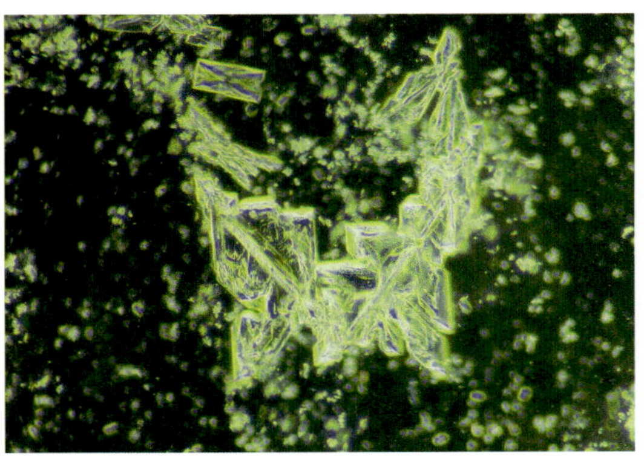

Fig. 4.70 Struvite crystals. They have a larger volume, irregular. Dark field, ×200

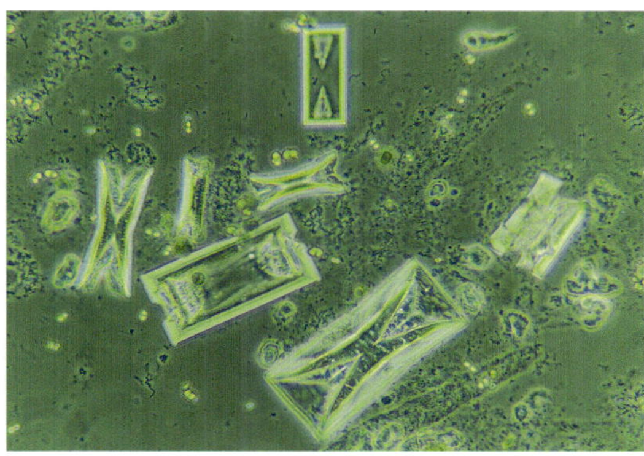

Fig. 4.71 Struvite crystals, various shapes and sizes, phase contrast microscope, ×400

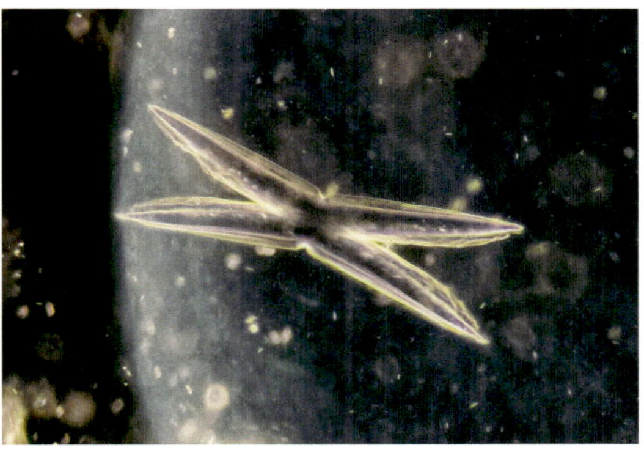

Fig. 4.72 Struvite crystals. Scissor-shaped. Dark field, ×200

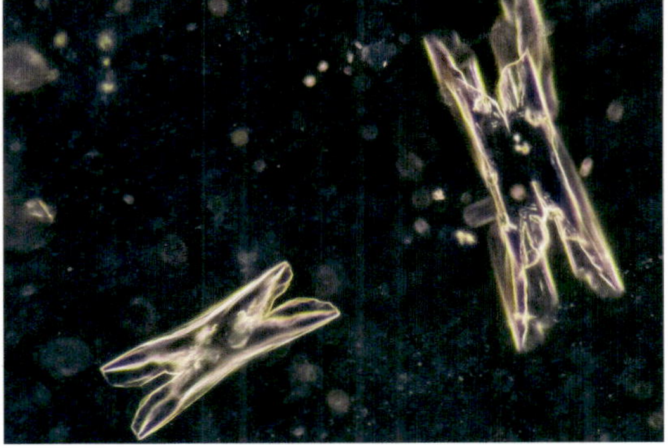

Fig. 4.73 Struvite crystals, irregular, strong refractivity. Dark field, ×200

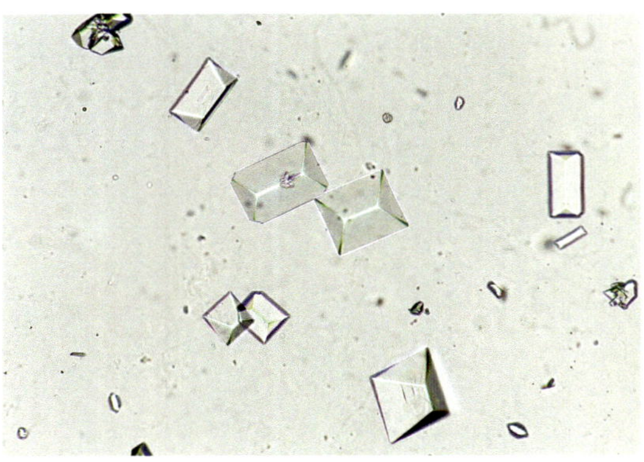

Fig. 4.74 Struvite crystals, colorless, transparent, roof-like. Unstained, bright field, ×400

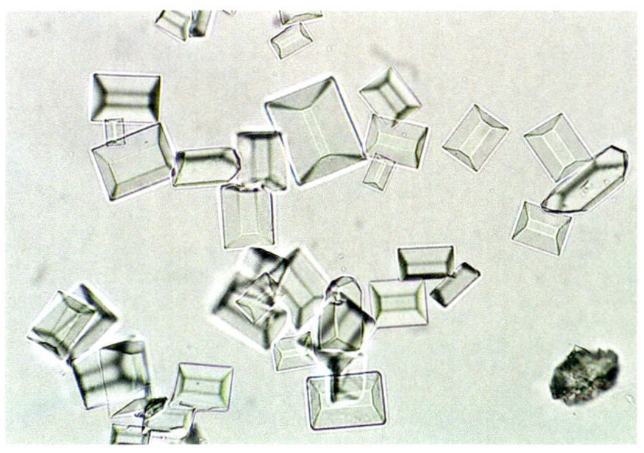

Fig. 4.75 Struvite crystals, roof-like. Unstained, bright field, ×400

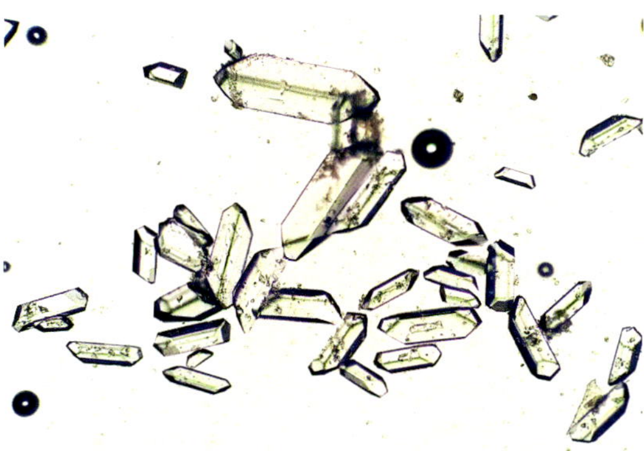

Fig. 4.76 Struvite crystal. They have an irregular polyhedral structure. Unstained, bright field, ×400

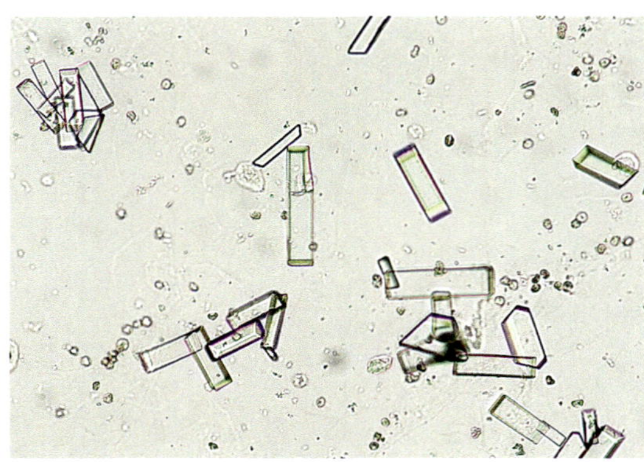

Fig. 4.77 Struvite crystals, lid-like. Unstained, bright field, ×400

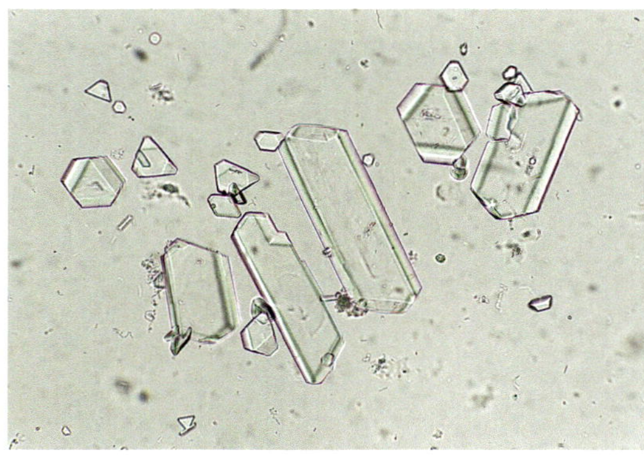

Fig. 4.78 Struvite crystals, irregular. Unstained, bright field, ×400

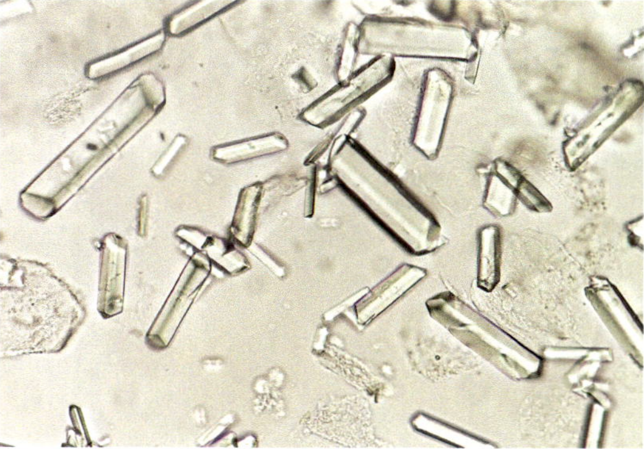

Fig. 4.79 Struvite crystals, long strip. Unstained, bright field, ×400

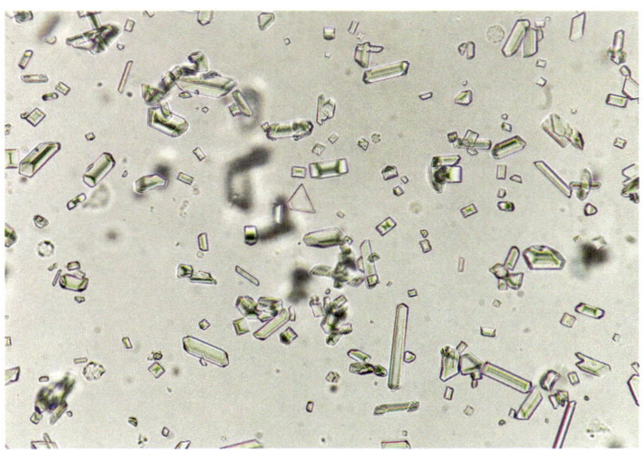

Fig. 4.80 Struvite crystals, multiple shapes appear at once. Unstained, ×200

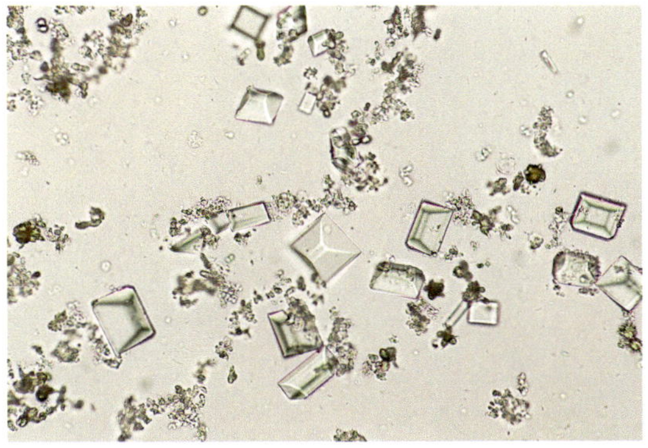

Fig. 4.81 Struvite crystals vary in size and exhibit diverse forms. There are a large number of amorphous phosphates in the background. Unstained, bright field, ×400

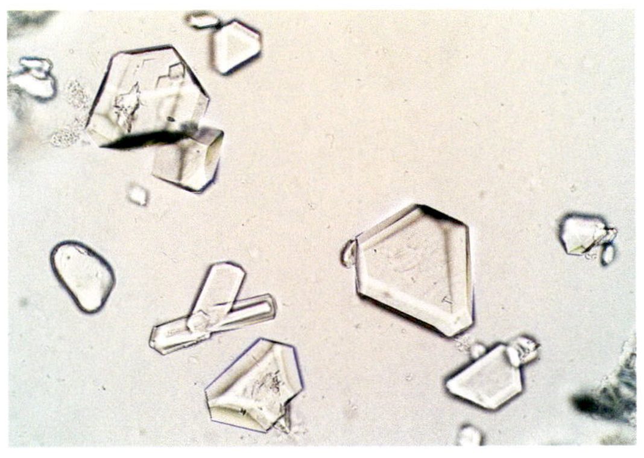

Fig. 4.82 Struvite crystals with various forms. Unstained, bright field, ×400

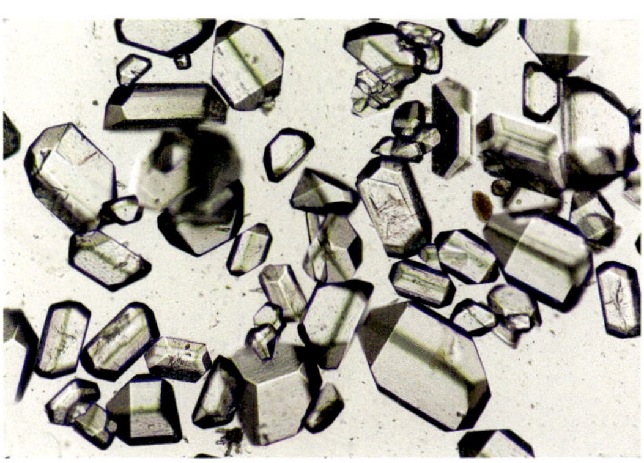

Fig. 4.83 Struvite crystals of various sizes and shapes. Unstained, bright field, ×400

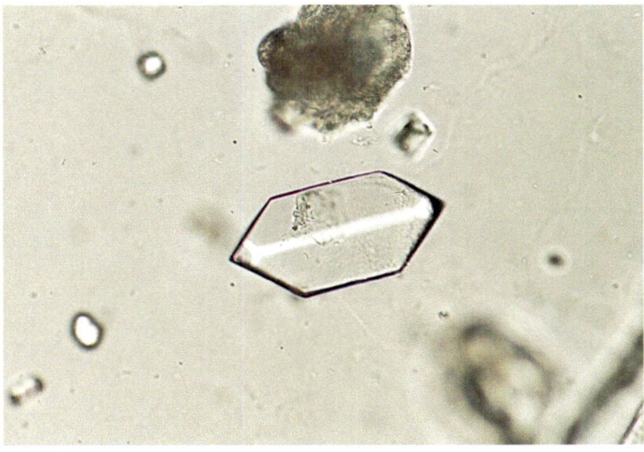

Fig. 4.84 Struvite crystals, irregular. Unstained, bright field, ×400

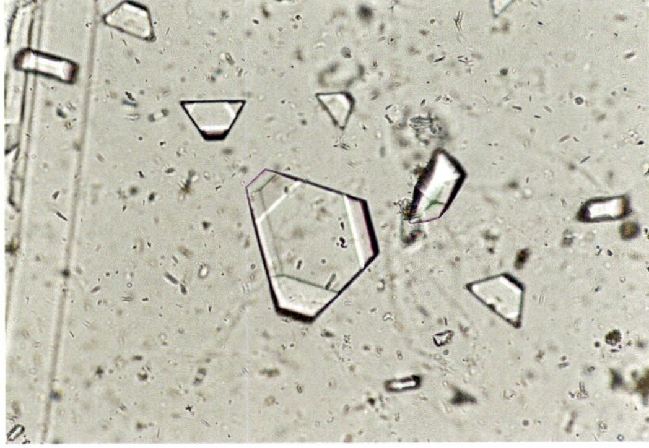

Fig. 4.85 Struvite crystals, irregular polyhedral structure. Unstained, bright field, ×400

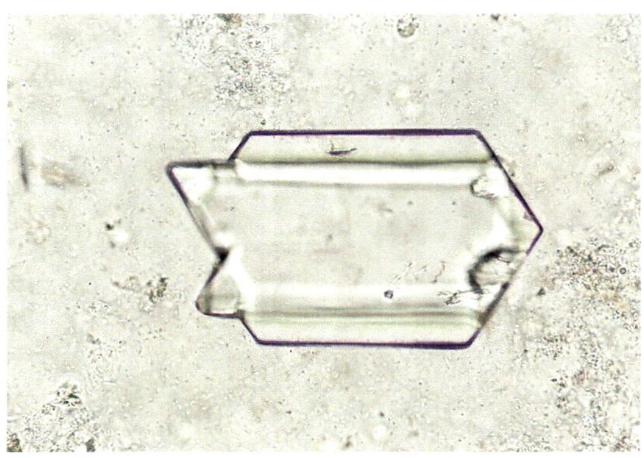

Fig. 4.86 Struvite crystals are large in size and exhibit an irregular shape. Unstained, bright field, ×400

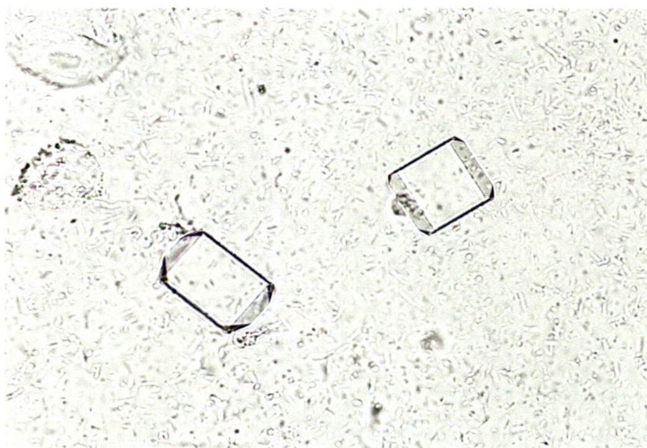

Fig. 4.87 Struvite crystals, colorless, transparent. Large numbers of bacteria can be seen in the background. Unstained, bright field, ×400

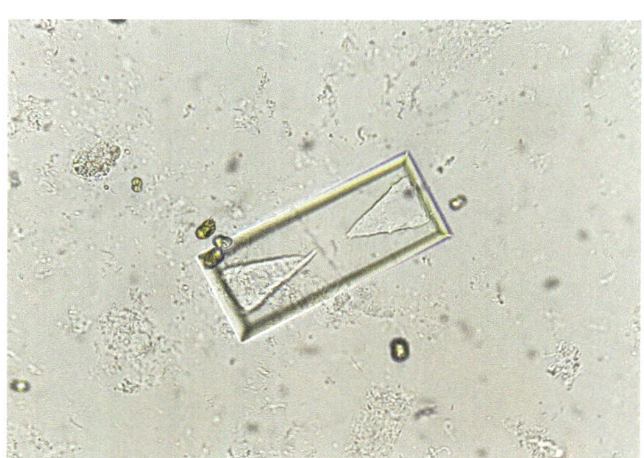

Fig. 4.88 Struvite crystals, colorless, transparent. Unstained, bright field, ×400

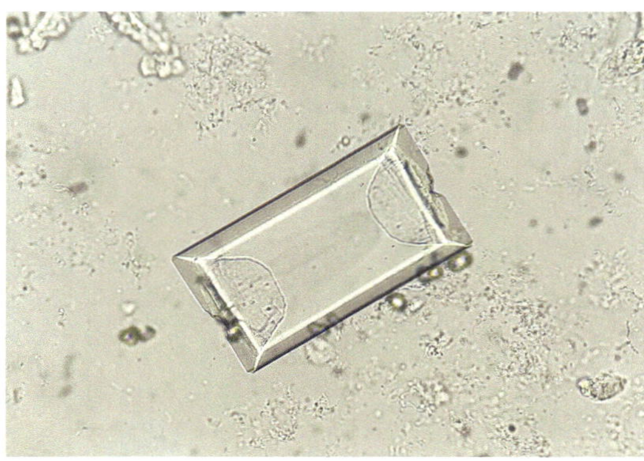

Fig. 4.89 Struvite crystals are large in size, colorless, transparent. Unstained, bright field, ×400

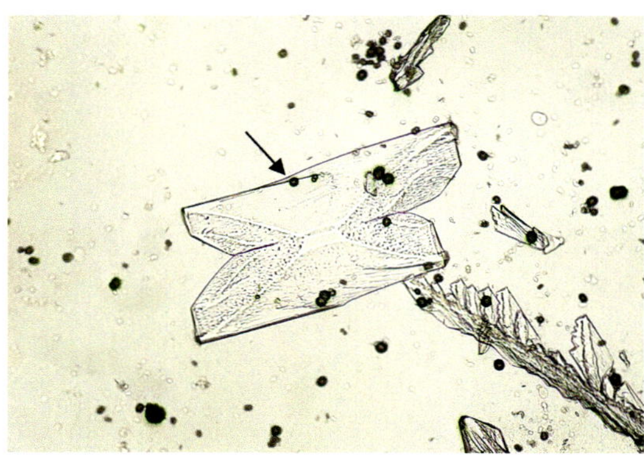

Fig. 4.90 Struvite crystals are large in size (↑), irregular. Unstained, bright field, ×200

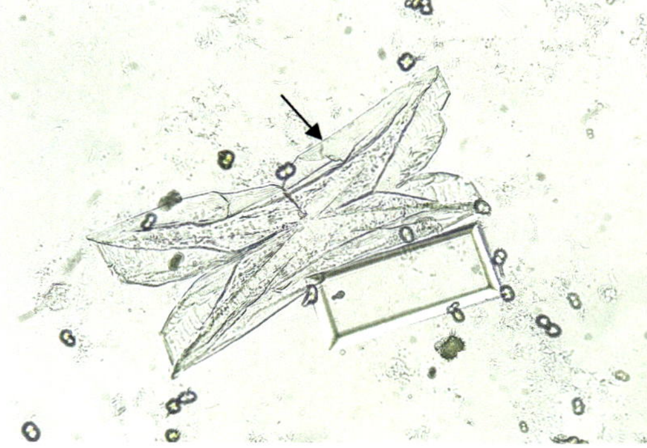

Fig. 4.91 Struvite crystals (↑), irregular. Unstained, bright field, ×400

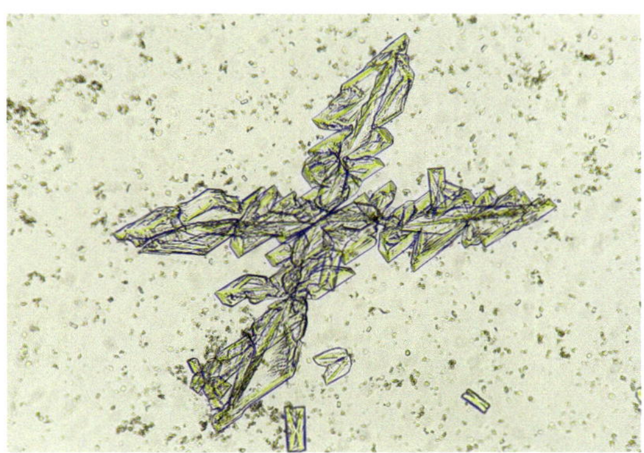

Fig. 4.92 Struvite crystals. They are large in size, irregular. Unstained, bright field, ×200

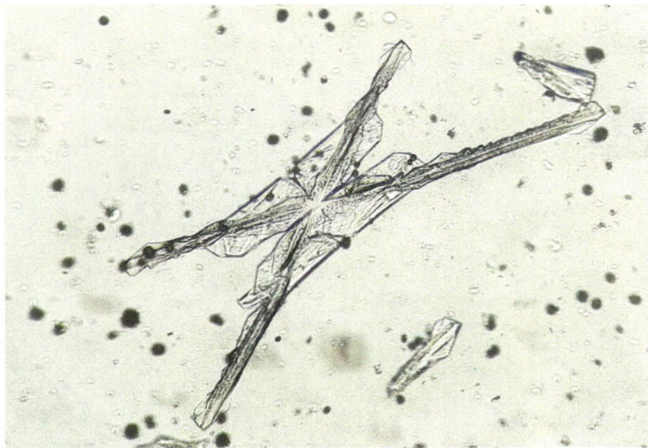

Fig. 4.93 Struvite crystals, scissor-shaped. Unstained, bright field, ×200

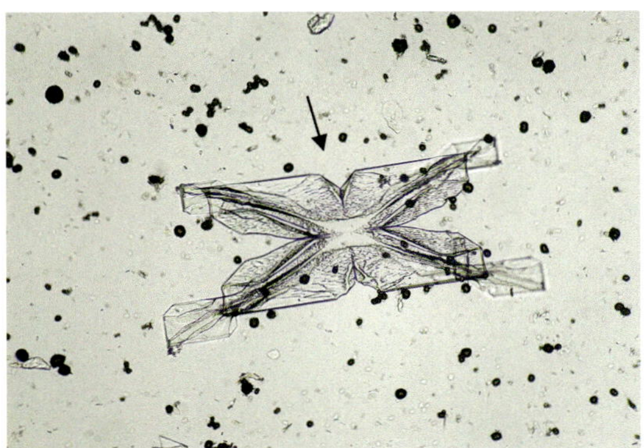

Fig. 4.94 Struvite crystals(↑), colorless, transparent. Ammonium biurate crystals are visible in the background, Unstained, bright field, ×200

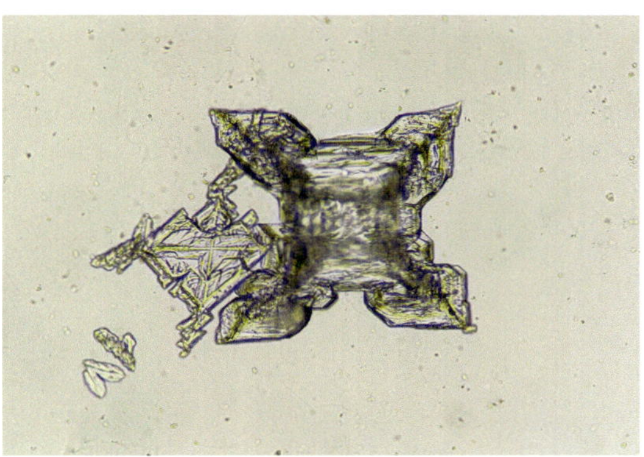

Fig. 4.95 Struvite crystals, rare morphology. Unstained, bright field, ×200

The most common struvite crystals are seen in alkaline urine and dissolved in hydrochloric acid and acetic acid, while they are insoluble in 10% KOH solution [19].

4.7.2 Clinical Significance

Struvite crystals can be found in the urine of healthy people, but they are more likely to occur in fresh urine specimen with chronic urinary tract infection or urinary retention. Struvite is well known as being the most frequent species found in infection induced stones [20]. It has been claimed that the primary cause is chronic renal infection by microorganisms capable of producing urease [21, 22].

4.8 Calcium Phosphate Crystal

4.8.1 Characteristics

Calcium phosphate crystals are flaky, firewood-like, or dumbbell-shaped, chrysanthemums-like, or form bundles (Fig. 4.96). These crystals exhibit strong refractivity when observed under both phase contrast and dark field microscopy (Fig. 4.97). They are colorless and exhibit varying sizes and diverse forms (Figs. 4.98, 4.99, 4.100, 4.101, 4.102, 4.103, 4.104, 4.105, 4.106, and 4.107). Calcium phosphate crystals are commonly seen in alkaline urine, soluble in acetic acid, hydrochloric acid, and insoluble in 10% KOH solution; the centrifugal sediments are greyish-white [16].

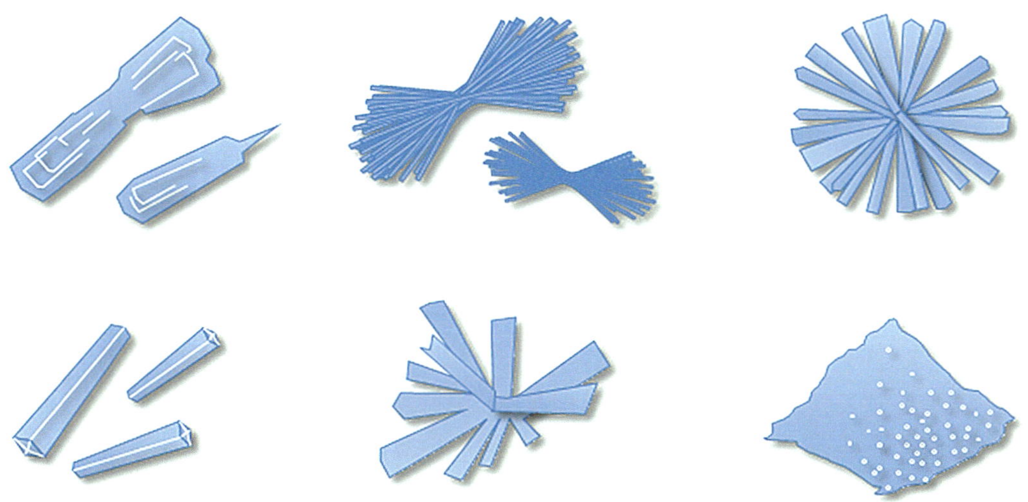

Fig. 4.96 Appearance of calcium phosphate crystals

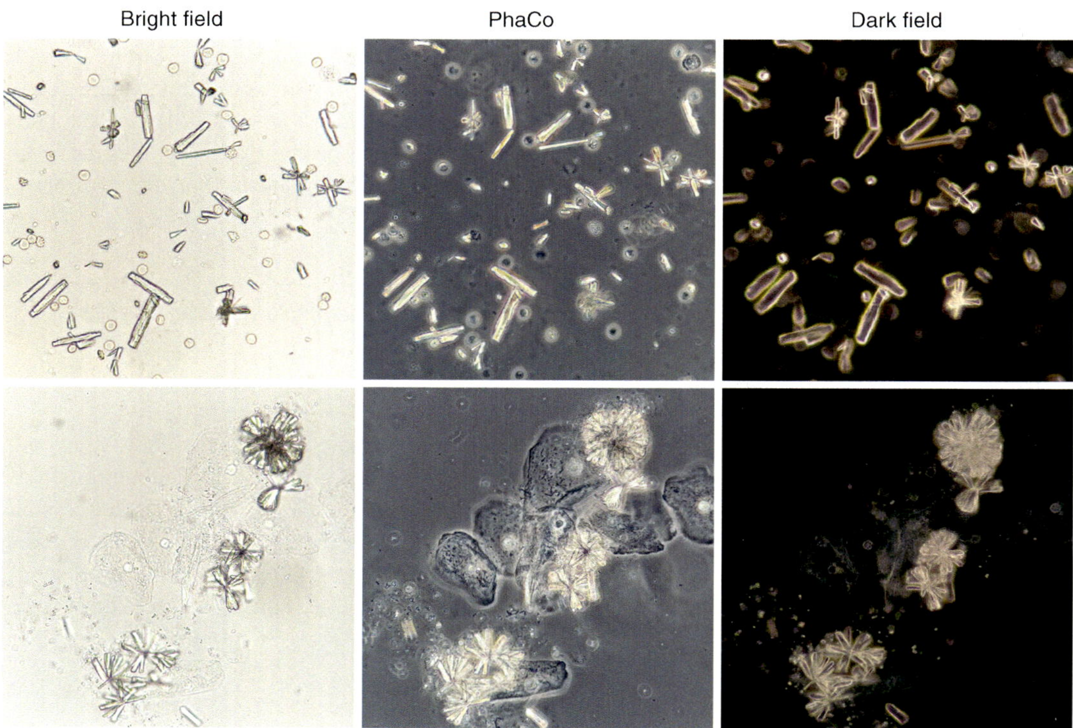

Fig. 4.97 Calcium phosphate crystals, colorless, irregular. Unstained, ×400

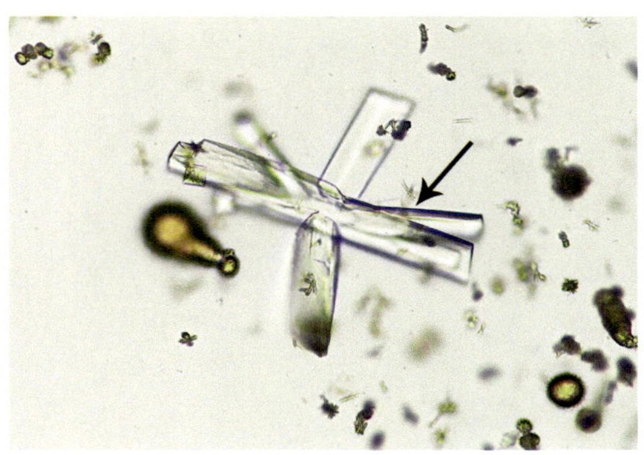

Fig. 4.98 Calcium phosphate crystals (↑), colorless, irregular. Unstained, bright field, ×400

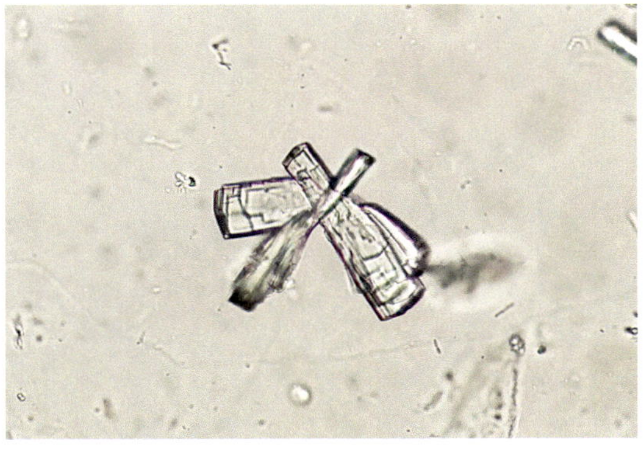

Fig. 4.99 Calcium phosphate crystals, irregular. Unstained, bright field, ×400

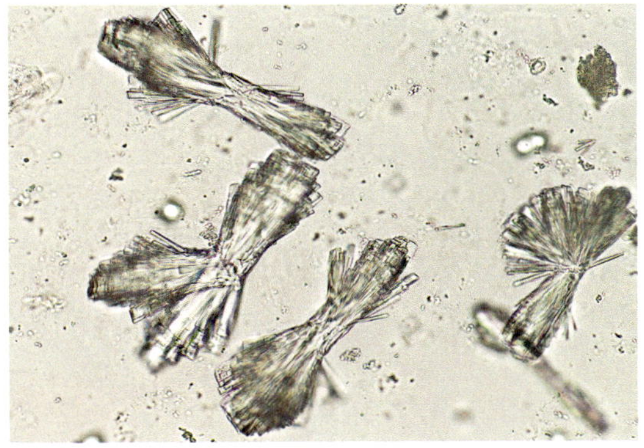

Fig. 4.100 Calcium phosphate crystals, firewood-like. Unstained, bright field, ×400

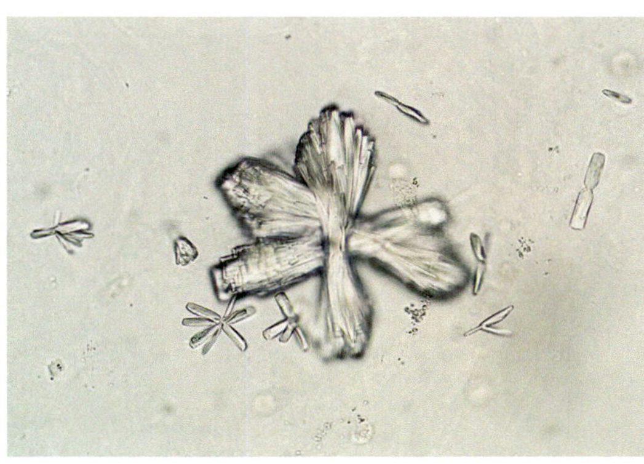

Fig. 4.101 Calcium phosphate crystals. These crystals vary in size and aggregate into bundles. Unstained, bright field, ×400

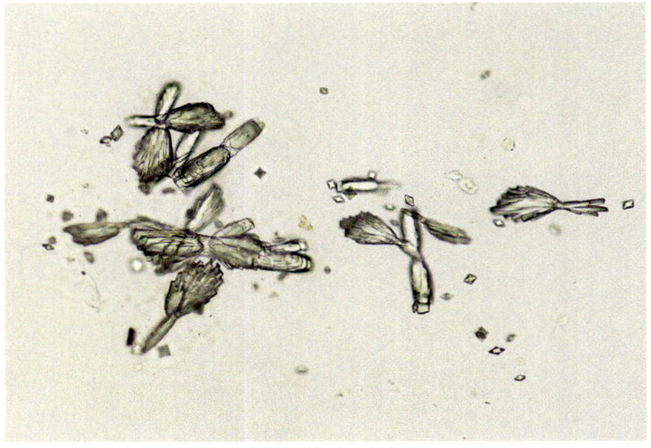

Fig. 4.102 Calcium phosphate crystals, firewood-like. Unstained, bright field, ×200

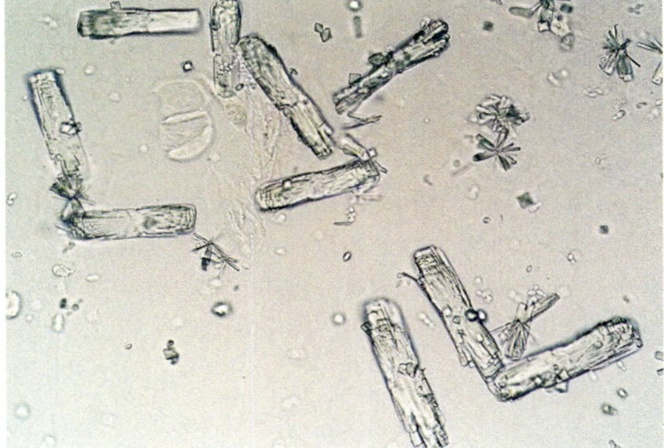

Fig. 4.103 Calcium phosphate crystals, colorless. Unstained, bright field, ×400

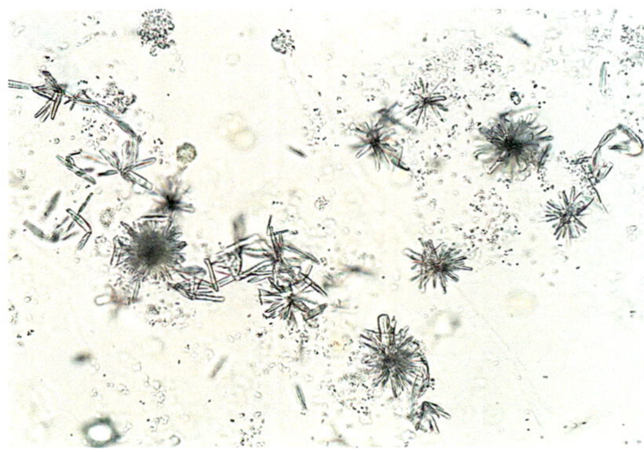

Fig. 4.104 Calcium phosphates crystals. These crystals aggregate into flower-like patterns. Unstained, bright field, ×200

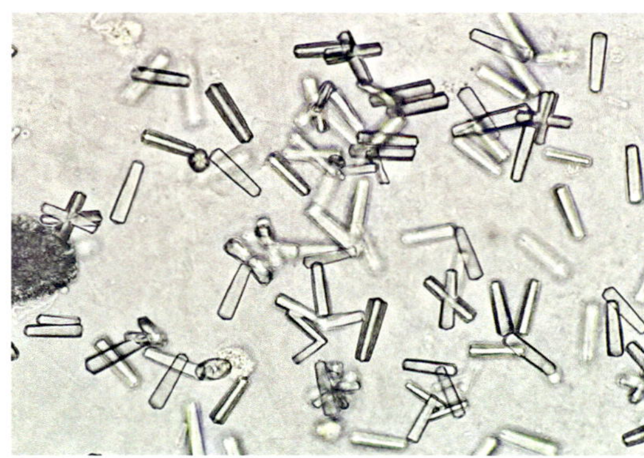

Fig. 4.106 Calcium phosphate crystals, rod-shaped. Unstained, bright field, ×400

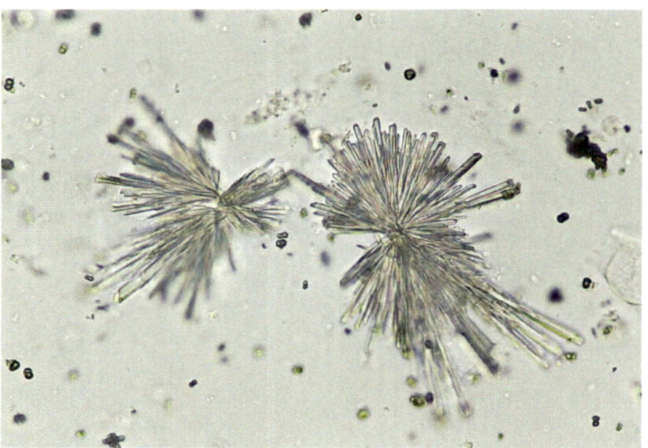

Fig. 4.105 Calcium phosphate crystals. They have atypical forms and dissolve in acetic acid, and the patient has not taken any medication. Bright field, ×200

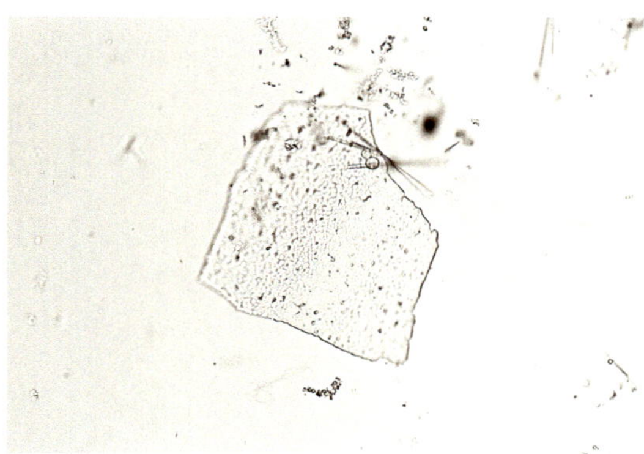

Fig. 4.107 Calcium phosphate crystals, colorless, flakey. Unstained, bright field, ×400

4.8.2 Clinical Significance

They may be observed in the urine of healthy individuals and have no clinical significance. It may also occur in chronic urinary tract infection, in renal tubular acidosis, or in diseases that result in urinary retention and may also be observed in the urine of patients with hyperparathyroidism [23]. If a large number of crystals are present for a long period of time, there is a risk of phosphate stone formation.

4.9 Amorphous Phosphates

4.9.1 Characteristics

This kind of crystals is amorphous, granular, colorless, and transparent under high power microscope (Fig. 4.108). Amorphous phosphates are seen in neutral urine and alkaline urine, soluble in HCl and acetic acid, and insoluble in 10% KOH solution; centrifugal precipitation is grayish white (Fig. 4.109). Amorphous phosphates exhibit strong refractivity under phase contrast and dark field microscopy (Fig. 4.110).

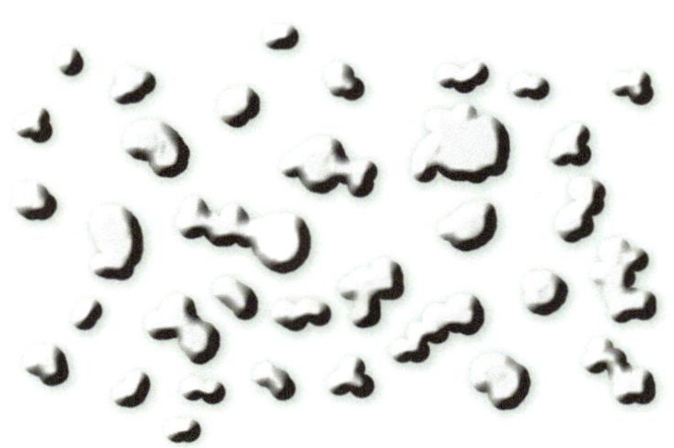

Fig. 4.108 Appearance of amorphous phosphates

4.9.2 Clinical Significance

These crystals often occur when urine is stored for a long time, when the urine is concentrated, or when the external environmental temperature is low. Generally, they have no clinical significance. However, if these crystals persist in fresh urine for an extended period, they may contribute to the formation of urinary calculi. Additionally, they can be observed in the urine of patients with urinary tract infections.

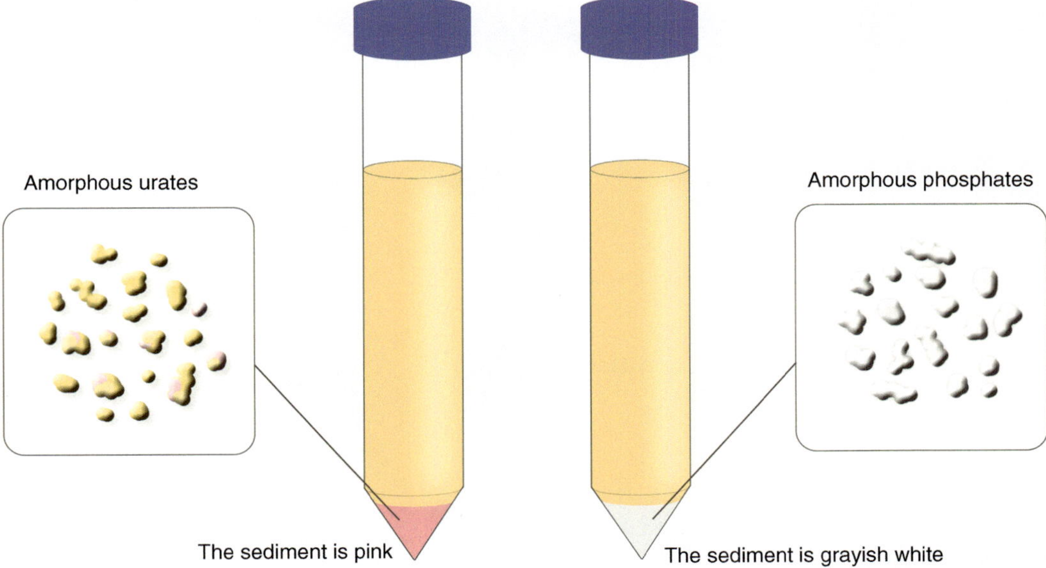

Fig. 4.109 The color of the amorphous salt sediment after centrifugation

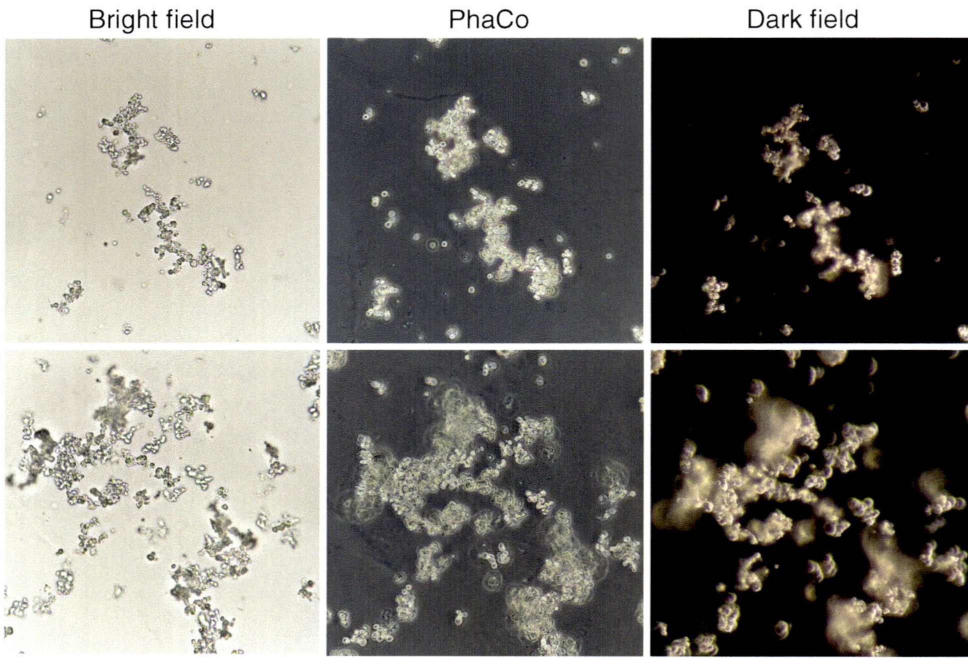

Fig. 4.110 Amorphous phosphates. These crystals consist of granules of various sizes. Unstained, ×400

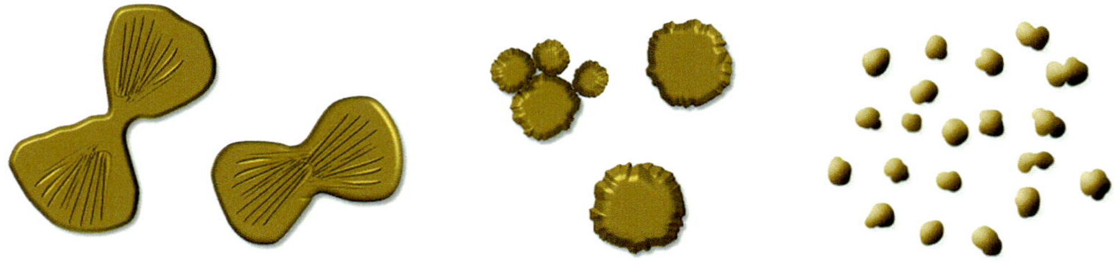

Fig. 4.111 Appearance of calcium carbonate crystals

4.10 Calcium Carbonate Crystals

4.10.1 Characteristics

Calcium carbonate crystals are primarily small spherical particles and dumbbell-shaped or amorphous in appearance (Fig. 4.111). They have a brown-yellow color (Figs. 4.112 and 4.113). These crystals are commonly found in weakly to alkaline urine. They share similarities with amorphous urates and ammonium urates. Calcium carbonate crystals dissolve and release CO_2 gas when acetic acid or HCl is added [21].

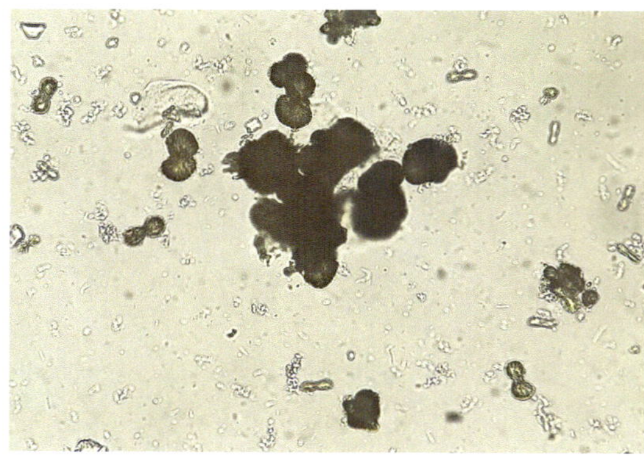

Fig. 4.112 Calcium carbonate crystals, brown, dumbbell shaped, scattered, or clustered in heaps. Unstained, bright field, ×400

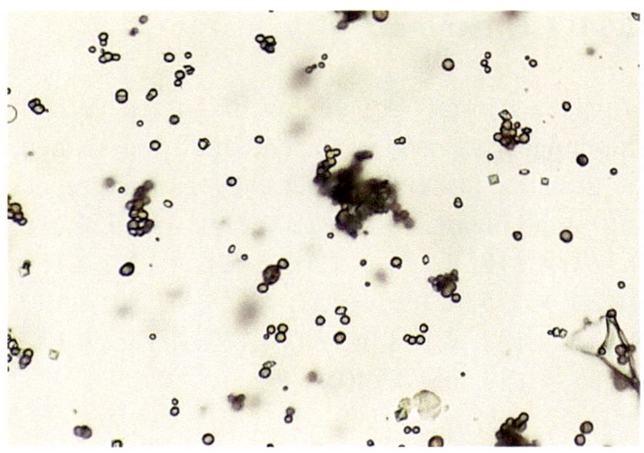

Fig. 4.113 Calcium carbonate crystals, brown, small spherical. Unstained, bright field, ×200

4.10.2 Clinical Significance

Calcium carbonate crystals typically have no clinical significance [19]. They can be found in the urine of healthy individuals and often coexist with phosphate crystals. Some individuals with urine containing daisy-like crystals have been hypothesized to have a possible association with a diet rich in vegetables [24, 25].

In addition to some common normal crystals, bilirubin crystals, cholesterol crystals, cystine crystals, tyrosine crystals, and leucine crystals can also be found in urine (Table 4.2). These crystals are closely associated with diseases and have important clinical significance.

Table 4.2 Characteristics of abnormal urine crystals

Types	Characteristics	Diagram
Bilirubin crystals	• Needle-like, granular, irregular, or precipitate within the cells • Yellow or yellow-brown • Soluble in alkali	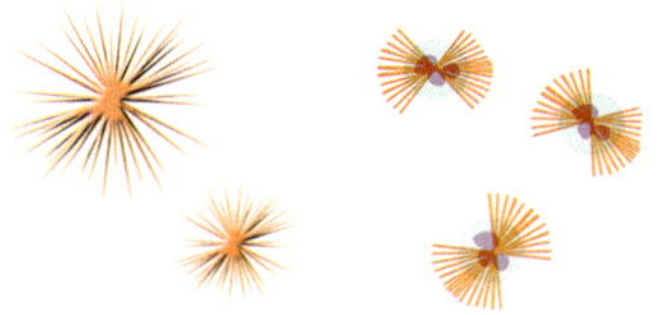
Cystine crystals	• Hexagonal, thin, and overlapping plate-like structures • Colorless and transparent • Soluble in alkali	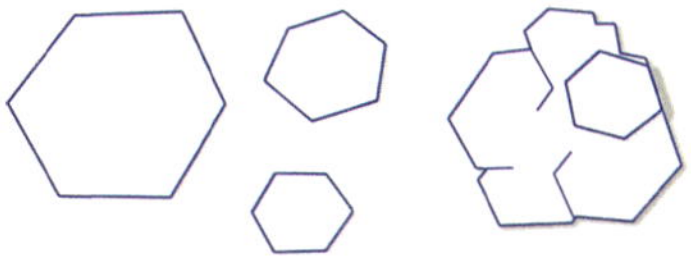
Cholesterol crystals	• Colorless and transparent • Thin, plate-like • Soluble in chloroform and ether	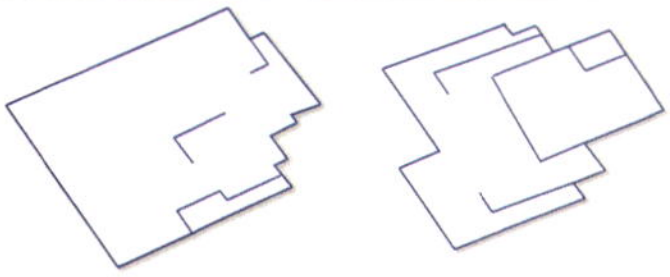
Tyrosine crystals	• Colorless • Needle-like bundles • Soluble in alkali	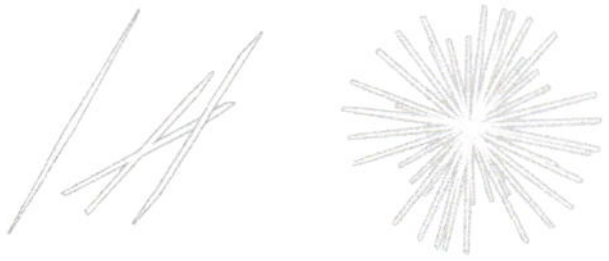
Leucine crystals	• Yellow or brown-yellow • Circular with concentric patterns, striped appearance, or droplet-shaped • Soluble in alkali	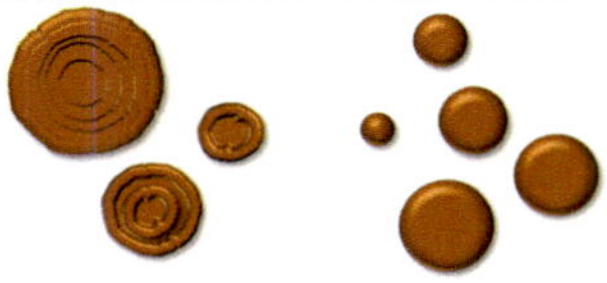

4.11 Bilirubin Crystals

4.11.1 Characteristics

Bilirubin crystals are typically yellow or orange-yellow. They appear as clumped needle, filamentous, rod-like, granular, fine sand-like, or cube-like shapes (Fig. 4.114). Some bilirubin crystals can be found in epithelial cells or leukocytes in bilirubinuria [26].

4.11.2 Unstained

Bilirubin crystals are yellow or golden yellow; they appear as needle-shaped, small rod-shaped, or granular structures, and they can aggregate into small bundles or clusters (Figs. 4.115, 4.116, 4.117, 4.118, 4.119, 4.120, 4.121, 4.122, 4.123, 4.124, 4.125, 4.126, 4.127, 4.128, 4.129, 4.130, 4.131, 4.132, 4.133, 4.134, 4.135, 4.136, 4.137, 4.138, 4.139, and 4.140).

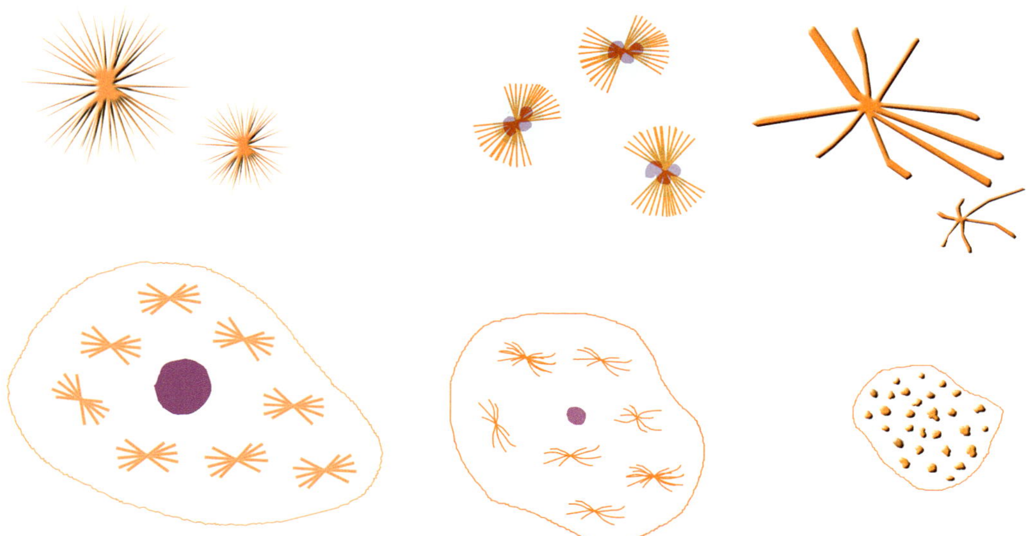

Fig. 4.114 Appearance of bilirubin crystals

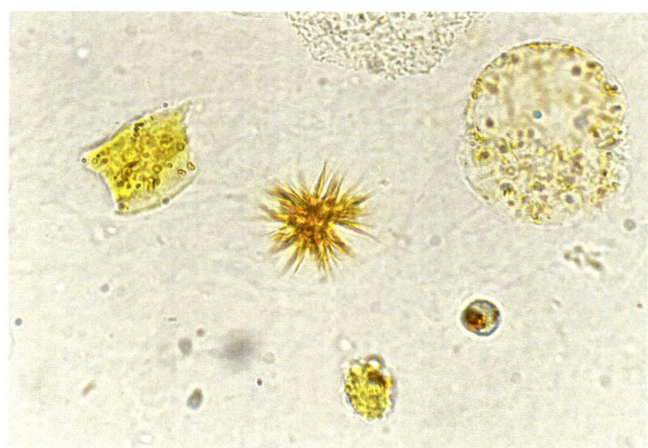

Fig. 4.115 Bilirubin crystals, yellow, needle-like bundle. Unstained, bright field, ×1000

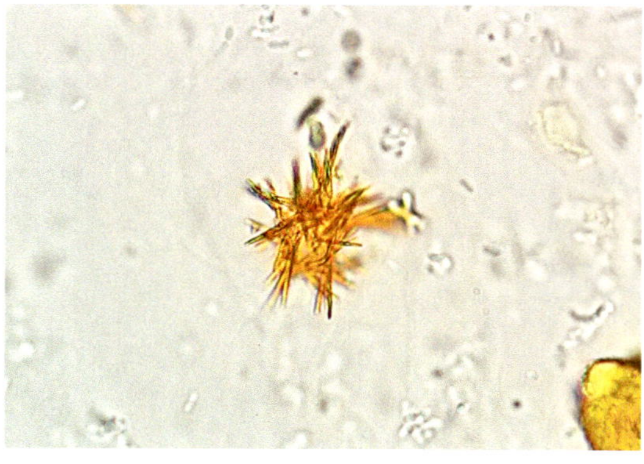

Fig. 4.116 Bilirubin crystals, orange, small bundles. Unstained, bright field, ×1000

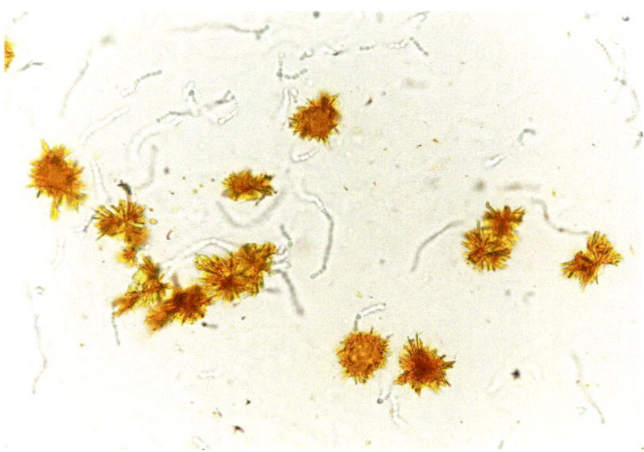

Fig. 4.117 Bilirubin crystals. Unstained, they cluster together, with streptococcus visible in the background. Bright field, ×1000

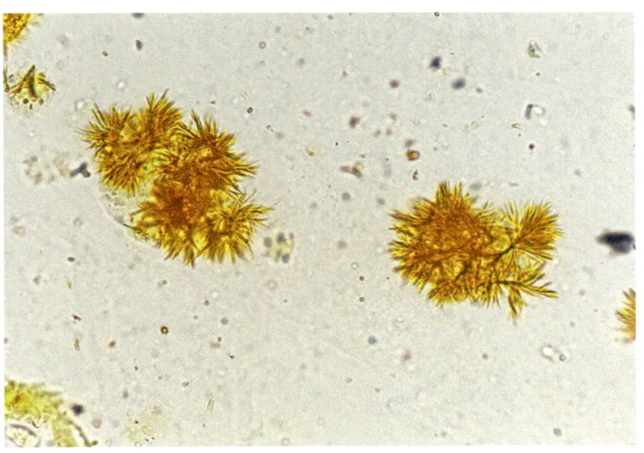

Fig. 4.118 Bilirubin crystals. Unstained, golden yellow, bright field, ×1000

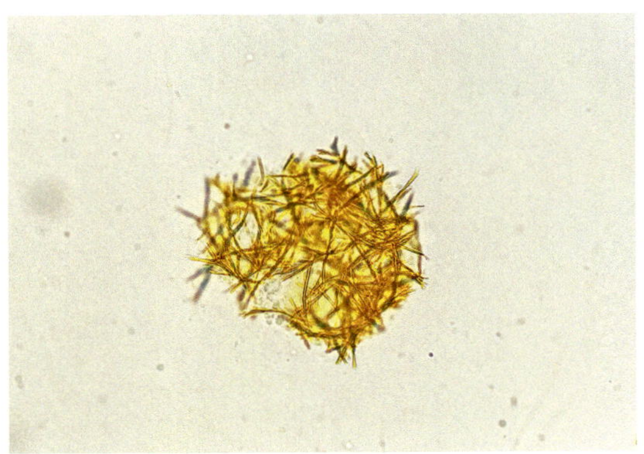

Fig. 4.119 Bilirubin crystals, disorganized arrangement. Unstained, bright field, ×1000

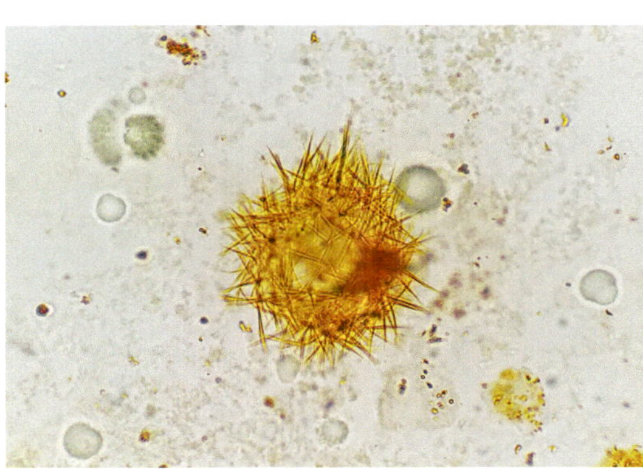

Fig. 4.120 Bilirubin crystals, needle-shaped bundles. Unstained, bright field, ×1000

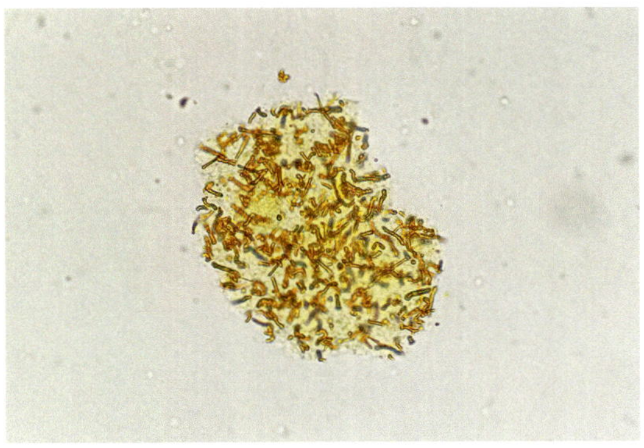

Fig. 4.121 Bilirubin crystals. These crystals are numerous and rod-like shape. Unstained, bright field, ×1000

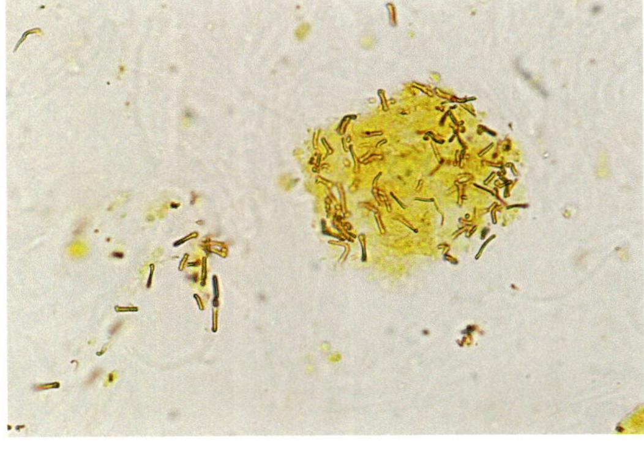

Fig. 4.122 Bilirubin crystals, rod-like. Unstained, bright field, ×1000

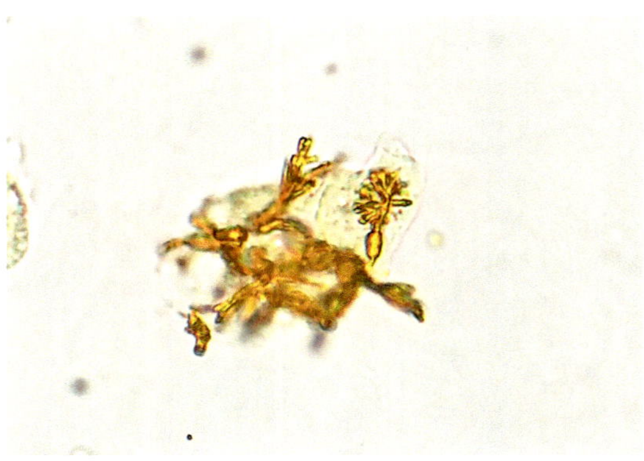

Fig. 4.123 Bilirubin crystals, irregular. Unstained, bright field, ×1000

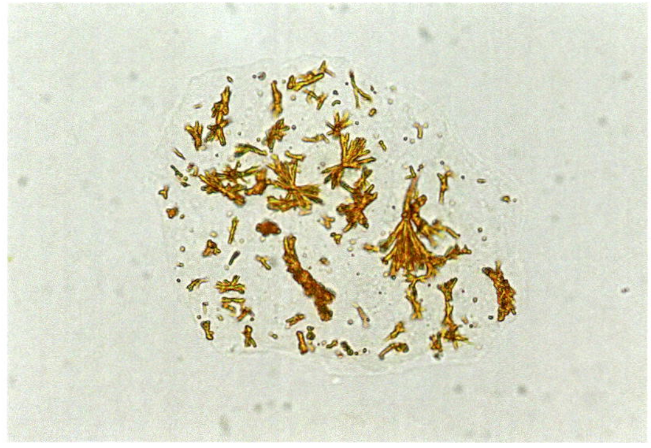

Fig. 4.124 Bilirubin crystals vary in size and do not have a fixed shape. Unstained, bright field, ×1000

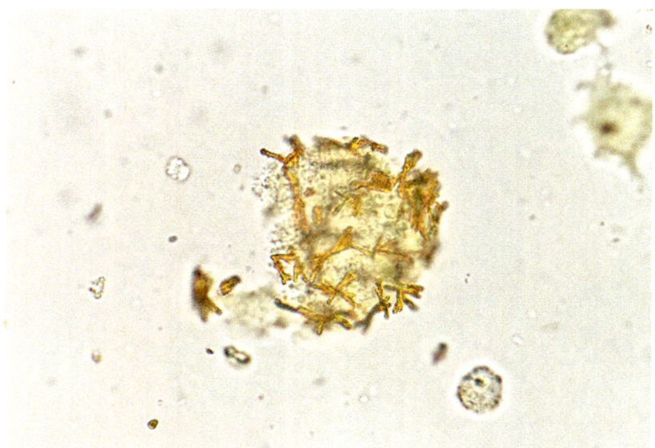

Fig. 4.125 Bilirubin crystals, firewood bundle shape. Unstained, bright field, ×1000

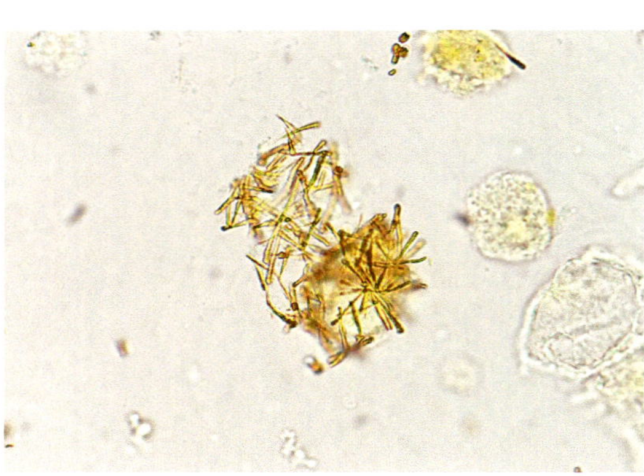

Fig. 4.126 Bilirubin crystals, rod-shaped. Unstained, bright field, ×1000

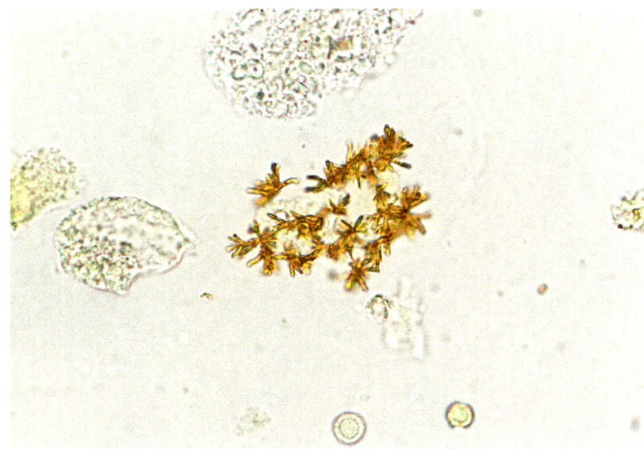

Fig. 4.127 Bilirubin crystals, arranged in bundles. Unstained, bright field, ×1000

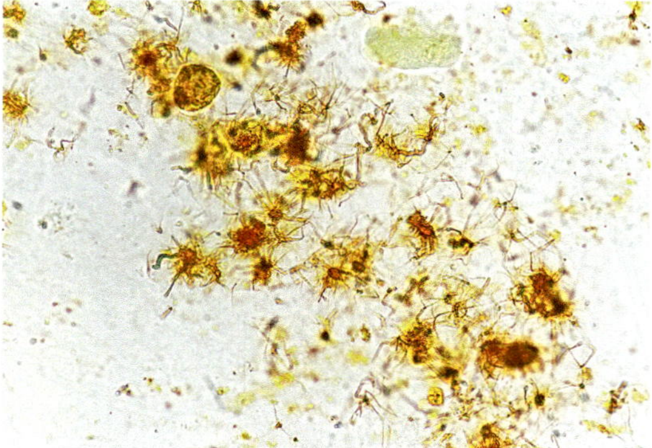

Fig. 4.128 Bilirubin crystals, golden yellow, irregular. Unstained, bright field, ×1000

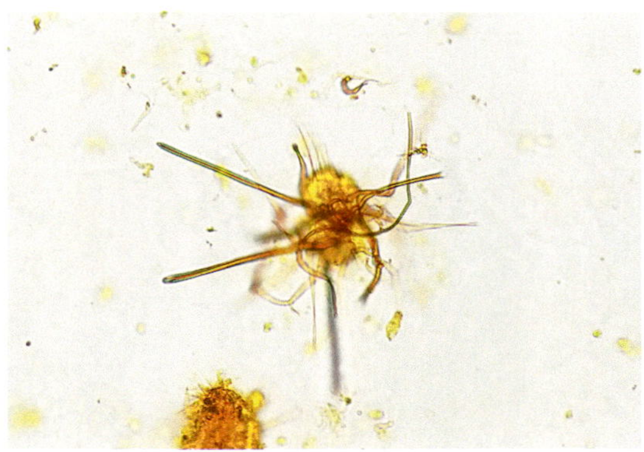

Fig. 4.129 Bilirubin crystals. These crystals have a slender, rod-like shape. Unstained, bright field, ×1000

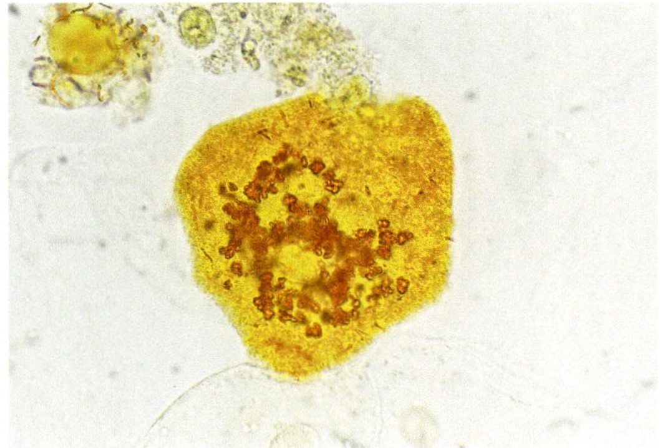

Fig. 4.130 Bilirubin crystals, granular crystals precipitated within the cells. Unstained, bright field, ×1000

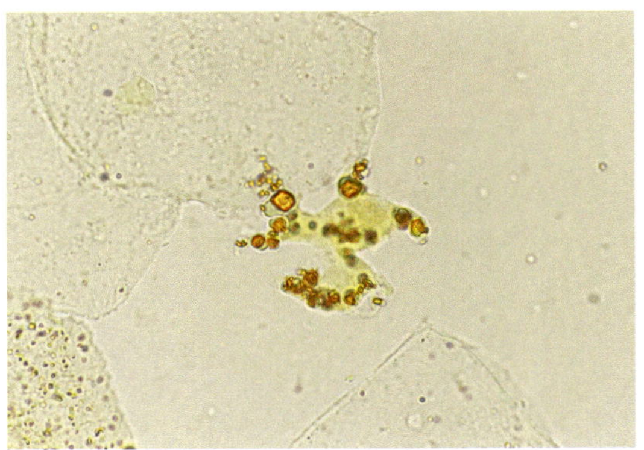

Fig. 4.131 Bilirubin crystals, golden yellow, granular, of different sizes. Unstained, bright field, ×1000

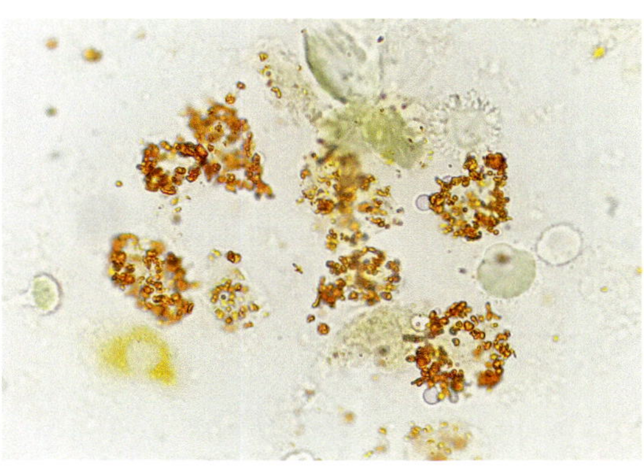

Fig. 4.132 Bilirubin crystals, small granular shape. Unstained, bright field, ×1000

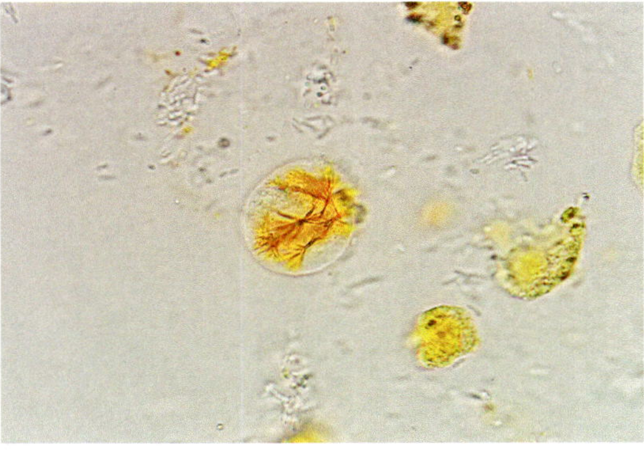

Fig. 4.133 Bilirubin crystals, filamentous, distributed in cells. Unstained, bright field, ×1000

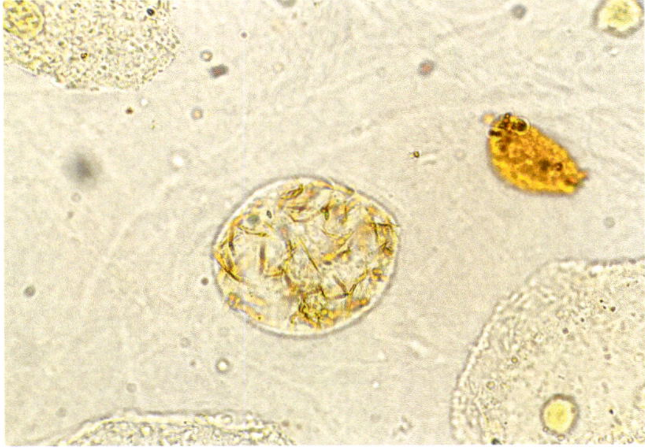

Fig. 4.134 Bilirubin crystals, filamentous. Unstained, bright field, ×1000

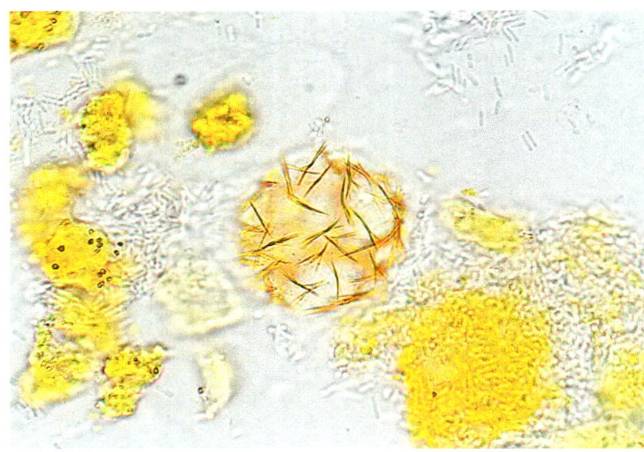

Fig. 4.135 Bilirubin crystals, fine needle-like crystals within the cells. Unstained, bright field, ×1000

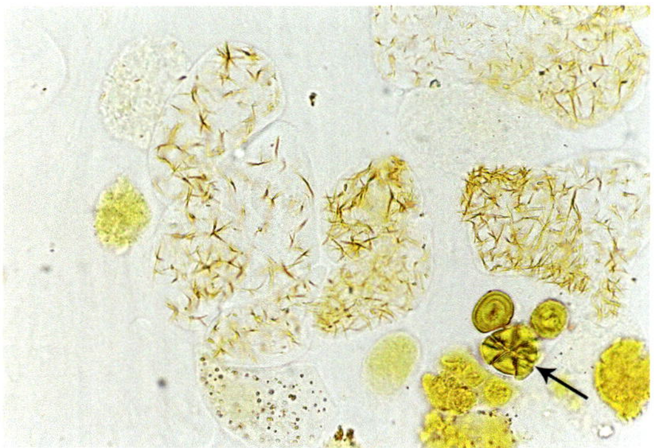

Fig. 4.136 Bilirubin crystals, filamentous, distributed in cells. Calcium oxalate crystal (↑). Unstained, bright field, ×1000

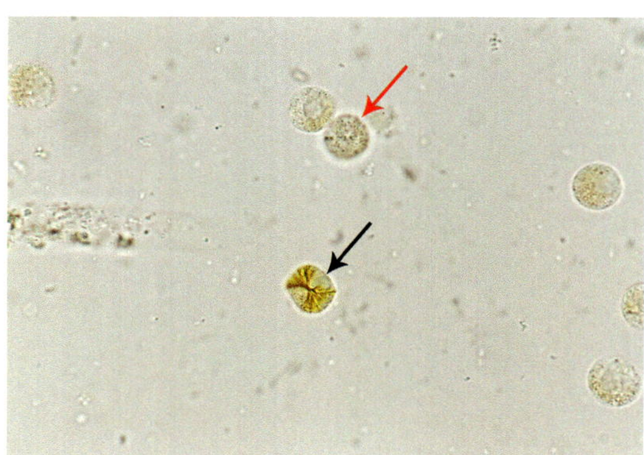

Fig. 4.137 Bilirubin crystals (↑), distributed in leukocytes, WBC (↑). Unstained, bright field, ×1000

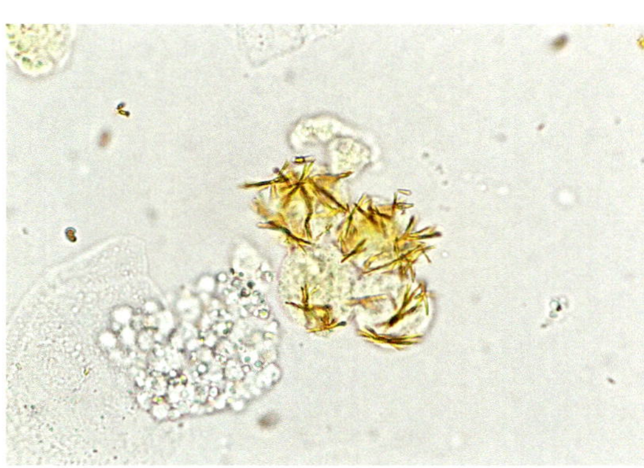

Fig. 4.138 Bilirubin crystals, distributed in cells. Unstained, bright field, ×1000

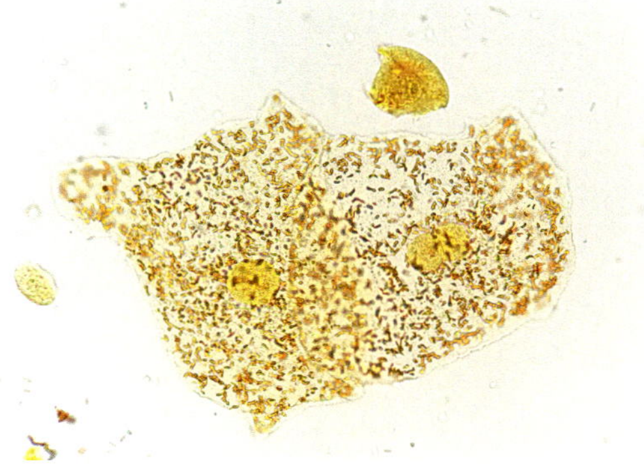

Fig. 4.139 Bilirubin crystals, fine granular crystals precipitated within the cells. Unstained, bright field, ×1000

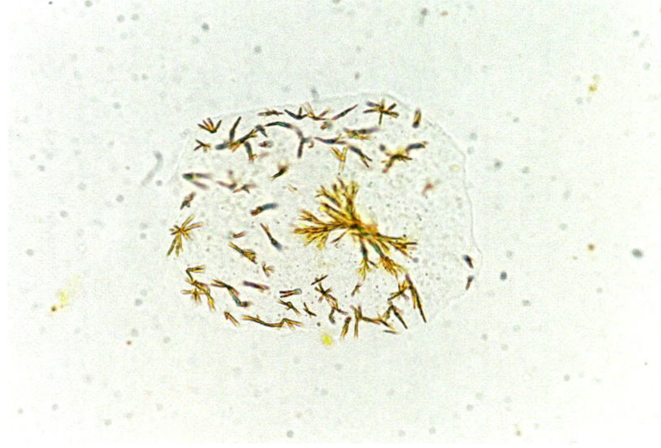

Fig. 4.140 Bilirubin crystals, needle-like crystals precipitated within the cells. Unstained, bright field, ×1000

4.11.3 Wright's Stain

The cellular distribution can be observed within the cells under Wright's stain, while the crystals remain unstained. The cell nuclei appear purplish-red (Figs. 4.141, 4.142, 4.143, 4.144, 4.145, 4.146, 4.147, 4.148, 4.149, 4.150, 4.151, and 4.152).

4.11.4 Clinical Significance

Bilirubin crystals are pathological crystals, which are common in the urine of patients with hepatobiliary diseases, such as obstructive jaundice, liver cirrhosis, and liver cancer, as well as in the urine of patients with acute severe hepatitis, acute organophosphorus poisoning, and multiple organ failure [27].

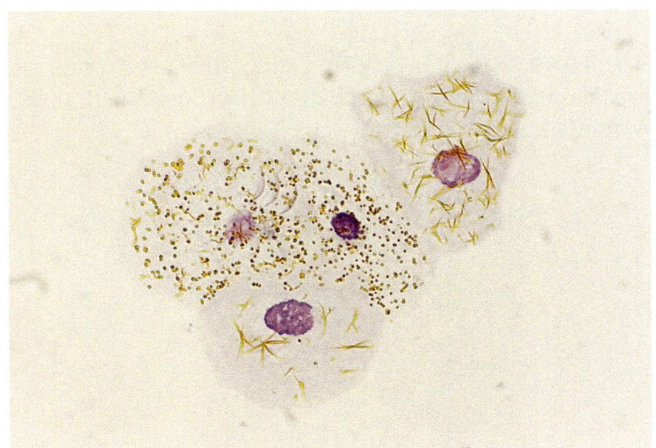

Fig. 4.141 Bilirubin crystals, fine needle-like and small granular crystals within the cells. Wright's stain, ×1000

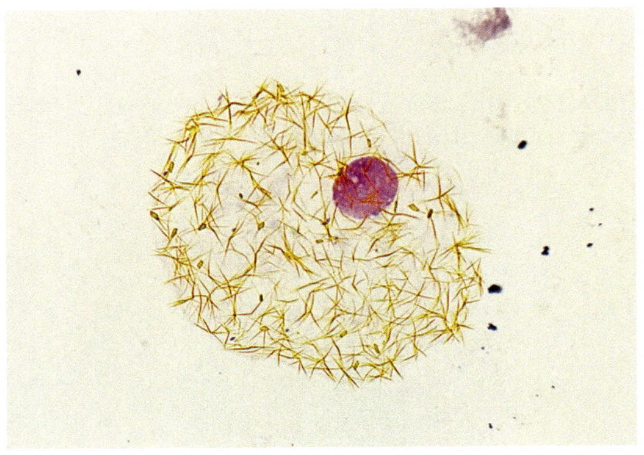

Fig. 4.142 Bilirubin crystals, fine needle-like crystals within the cells. Wright's stain, ×1000

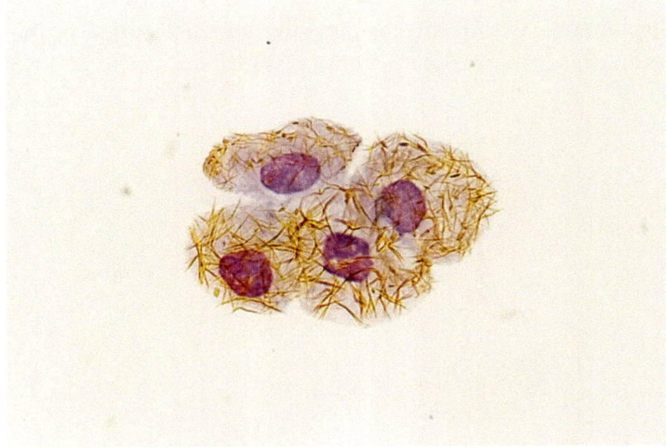

Fig. 4.143 Bilirubin crystals, needle-like crystals within the urinary epithelial cells. Wright's stain, ×1000

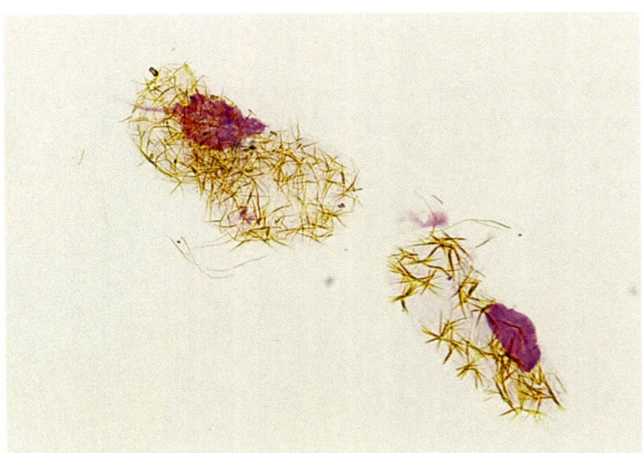

Fig. 4.144 Bilirubin crystals, distributed in cells. Wright's stain, ×1000

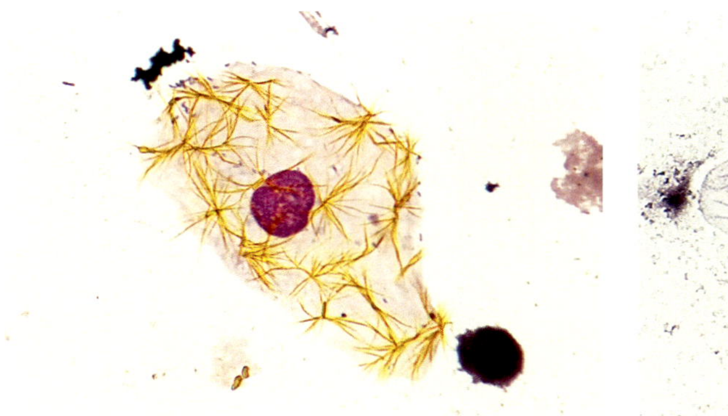

Fig. 4.145 Bilirubin crystals, bundles, distributed in the urothelial cells. Wright's stain, ×1000

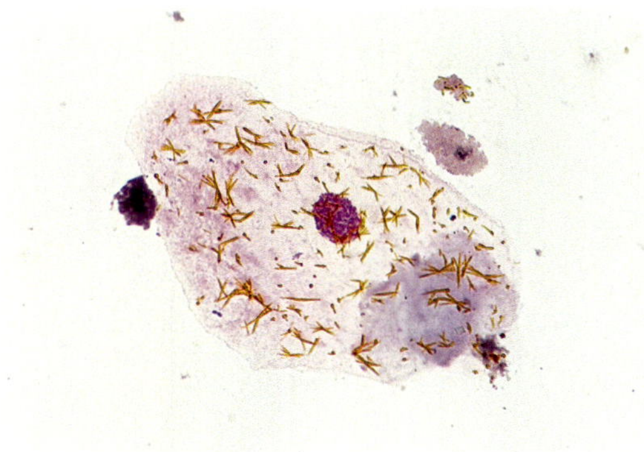

Fig. 4.146 Bilirubin crystals, the crystals within the cells vary in size. Wright's stain, ×1000

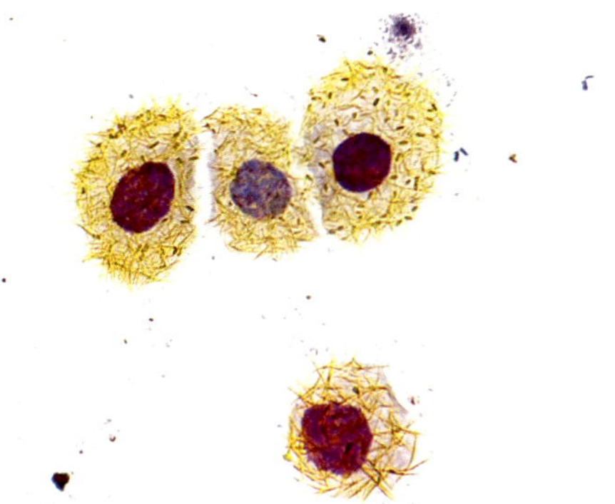

Fig. 4.147 Bilirubin crystals, needle bundle, evenly distributed in squamous epithelial cells. Wright's stain, ×1000

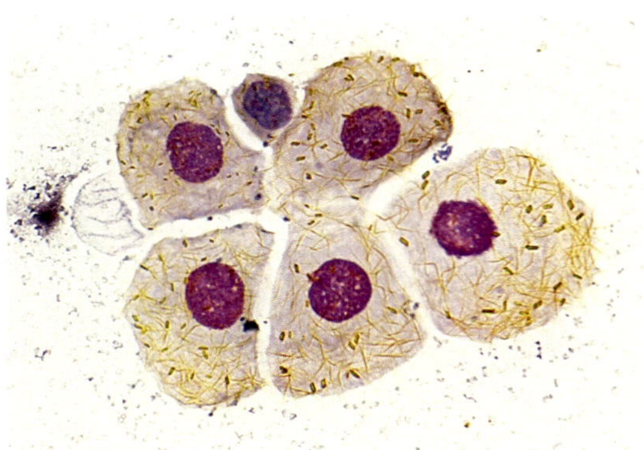

Fig. 4.148 Bilirubin crystals, two different forms of crystals within the superficial urinary epithelial cells. Wright's stain, ×1000

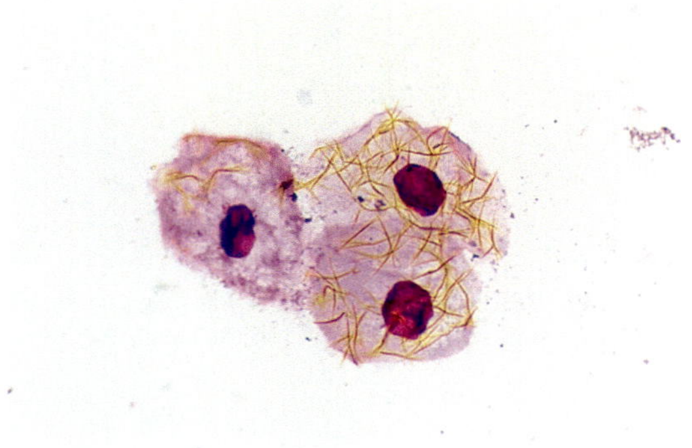

Fig. 4.149 Bilirubin crystals, filamentous crystals within urinary epithelial cells. Wright's stain, ×1000

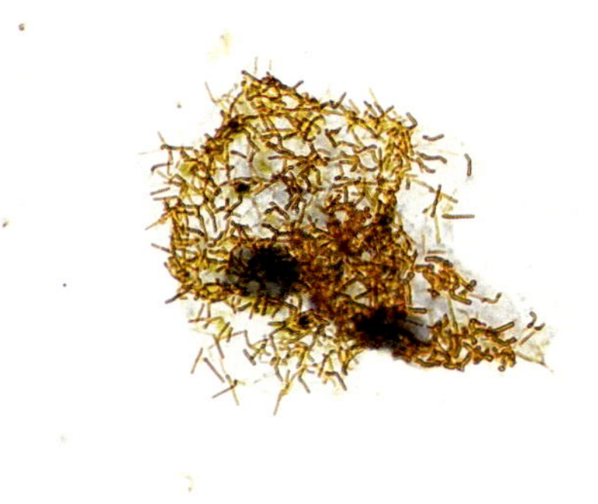

Fig. 4.150 Bilirubin crystals, a large number of rod-shaped crystals within the cells. Wright's stain, ×1000

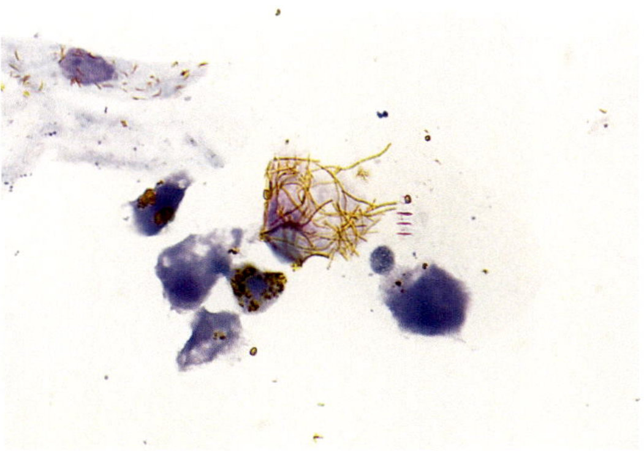

Fig. 4.151 Bilirubin crystals, long filamentous crystals within the cells. Wright's stain, ×1000

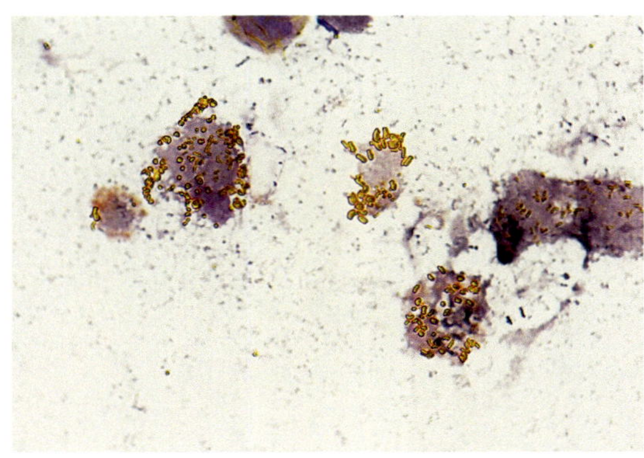

Fig. 4.152 Bilirubin crystals, granular crystals within the renal tubular epithelial cells. Wright's stain, ×1000

4.12 Cystine Crystals

4.12.1 Characteristics

Cystine crystals are colorless, transparent, hexagonal, or multilayered flake structure [28] (Figs. 4.153, 4.154, 4.155, 4.156, 4.157, and 4.158). Cystine crystals occur in acidic urine and can be dissolved in 10% KOH solution. Cystine assay: Add 1 drop of Lugol iodine and dilute sulfuric acid solution to the sediment, mix well, and if it appears blue or blue green, it suggests that there are the cystine crystals.

4.12.2 Clinical Significance

Cystine crystals are observed in the urine of persons with inherited cystinuria. Cystinuria is an inherited disorder characterized by the impaired reabsorption of cystine in the proximal tubule of the nephron and the gastrointestinal epithelium [29]. Persons with cystinuria have a tendency to form cystine calculi, which may also be seen in patients with severe hepatic disease [30].

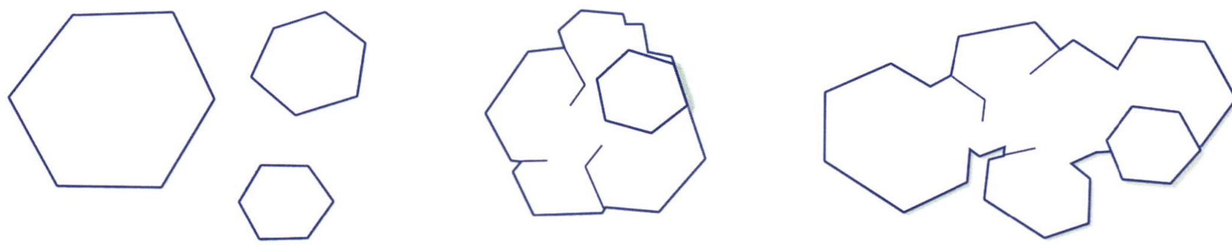

Fig. 4.153 Appearance of cystine crystals

Fig. 4.154 Cystine crystals, colorless, transparent, hexagonal. Unstained, bright field, ×400

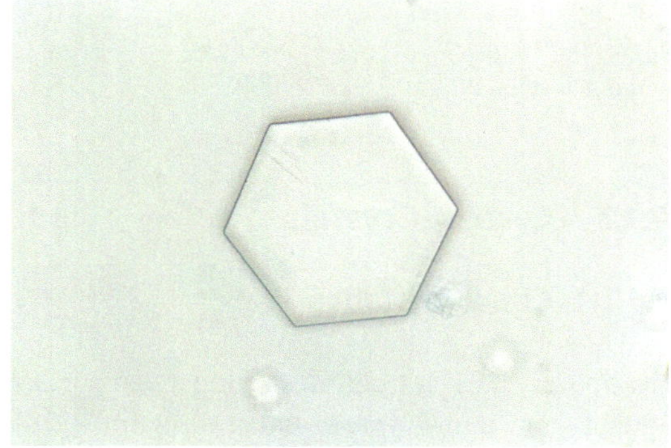

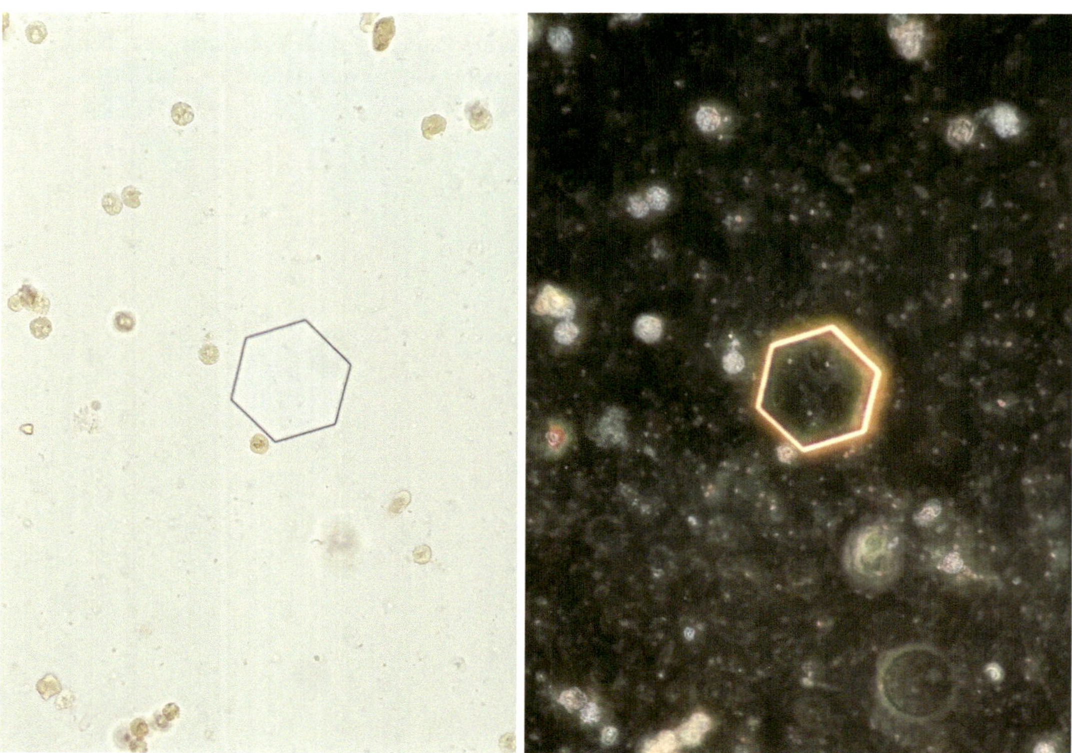

Fig. 4.155 Cystine crystals, hexagonal. Unstained, bright field and dark field, ×400

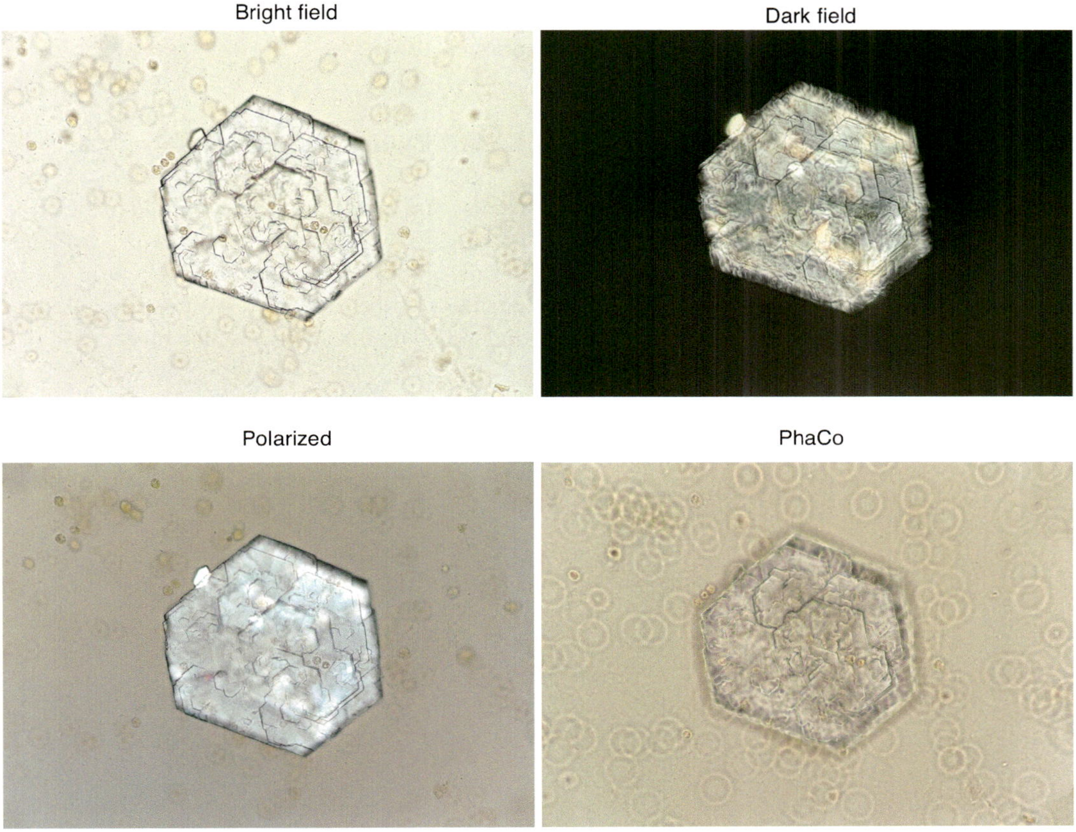

Bright field

Dark field

Polarized

PhaCo

Fig. 4.156 Cystine crystals, colorless, large in size, with multiple layers overlapping. Unstained, ×400

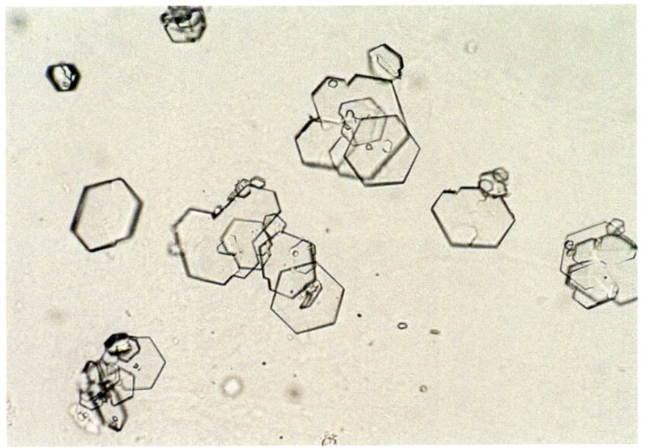

Fig. 4.157 Cystine crystals, colorless, transparent, hexagonal, flaky. Unstained, ×400

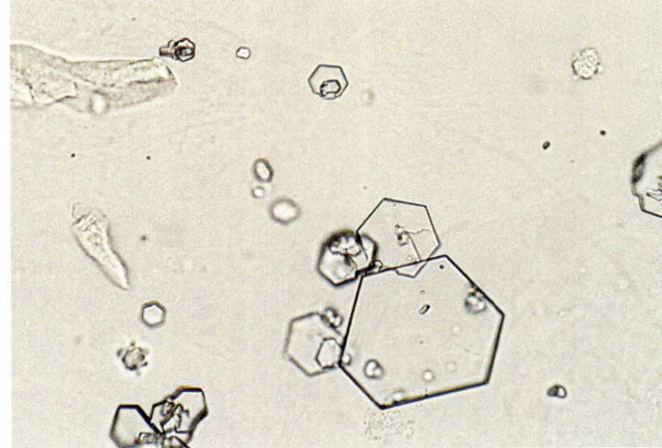

Fig. 4.158 Cystine crystals, hexagonal, vary in size. Unstained, ×400

4.13 Cholesterol Crystals

4.13.1 Characteristics

Cholesterol crystals are colorless and transparent, squares or angular layers of flakes (Figs. 4.159 and 4.160), sometimes with variably sized fat droplets attached to the crystal surface. Cholesterol crystals are dissolved in chloroform and ether. Some cholesterol crystals are similar in appearance to colorless uric acid crystals. The former can be confirmed by the cyanide nitroprusside test.

4.13.2 Clinical Significance

Cholesterol crystals may be observed in the urine of patients with nephrotic syndrome, pyelonephritis, and cystitis, as well as in chyluria due to dilatation of the abdominal lymphatics caused by abdominal tumors, filariasis, and others [31].

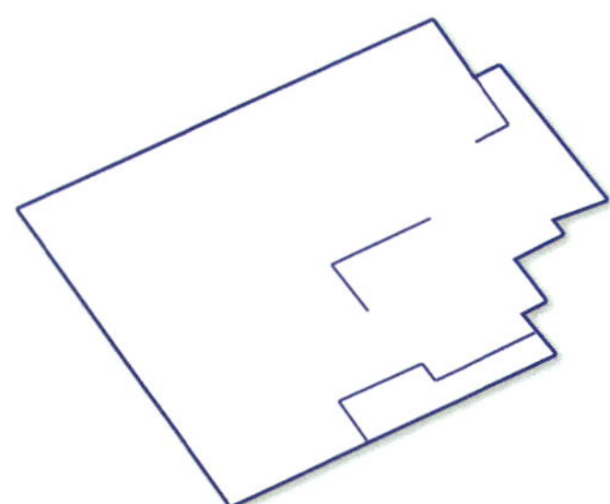
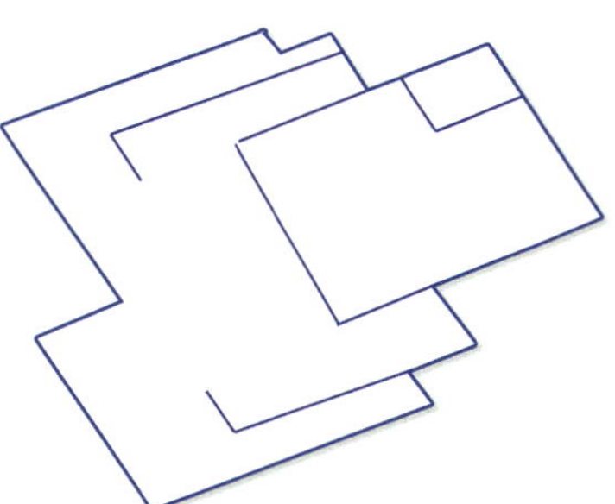

Fig. 4.159 Appearance of cholesterol crystals

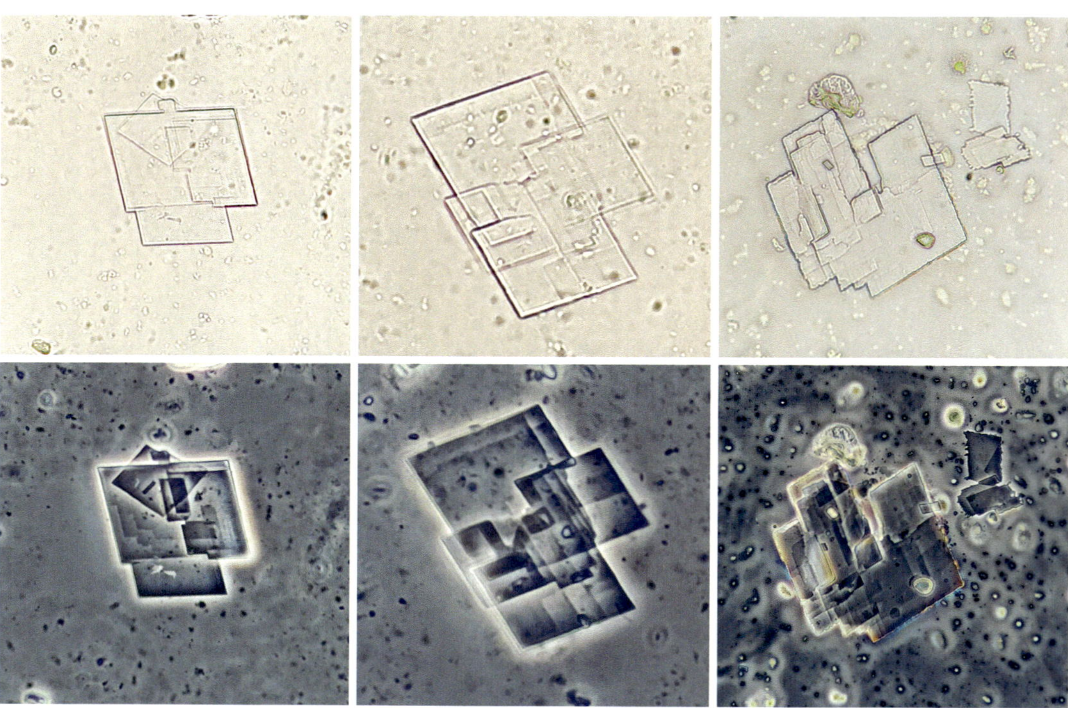

Fig. 4.160 Cholesterol crystals, colorless, plate-like, and varied in size. Unstained, ×400

4.14 Tyrosine Crystals

4.14.1 Characteristics

Tyrosine crystals are slightly black needle-like, which may be aggregated into bundles (Figs. 4.161 and 4.162). They are soluble in 10% KOH solution but insoluble in acetic acid. Tyrosine test: formaldehyde, distilled water, concentrated hydrochloric acid mixed at 1:45:55, 2–3 mL, mixed with urine sediment, and heated; the positive reaction was green.

4.14.2 Clinical Significance

Tyrosine crystals are the products of protein breakdown, and the occurrence of this type of crystal indicates a poor prognosis, which is more common in the urine of persons with acute hepatic necrosis, organophosphate poisoning, cirrhosis of the liver, and the like. It can also be seen in a large number of tissue-necrotizing diseases, diabetic nephropathy, and metabolic disorders [32].

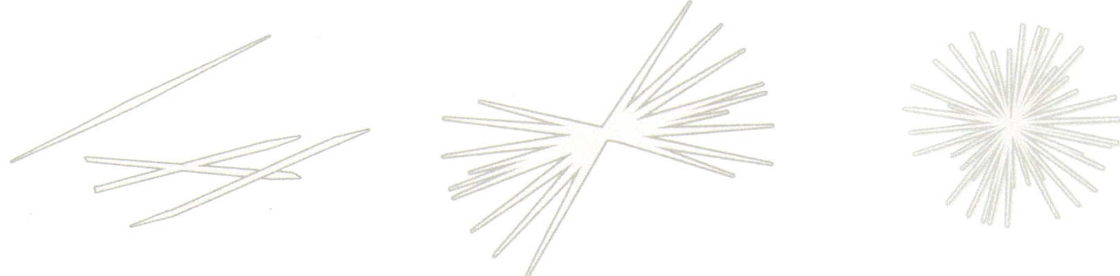

Fig. 4.161 Appearance of tyrosine crystals

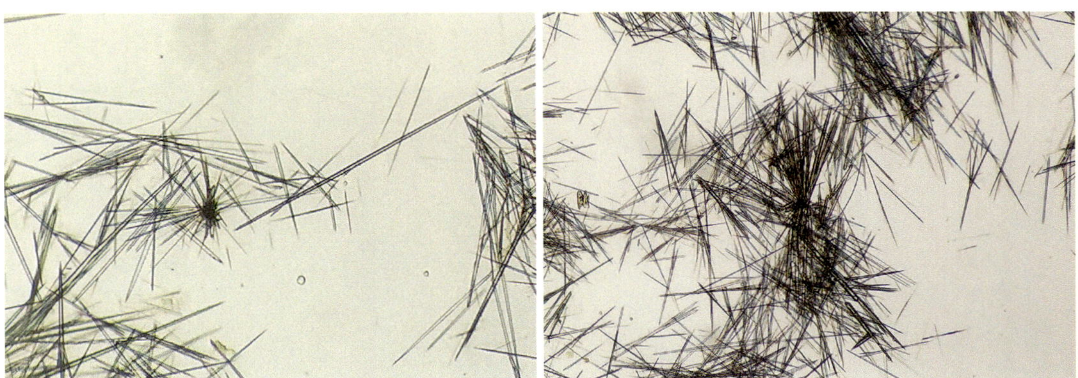

Fig. 4.162 Tyrosine crystals, needle-like bundles, scattered or aggregated into bundles. Unstained, ×400

4.15 Leucine Crystals

4.15.1 Characteristics

Leucine crystals are brown-yellow or brown, disc-shaped, spherical, oil drop-shaped, or irregular (Fig. 4.163). The crystals have concentric rings, radial stripes, or annual rings (Figs. 4.164, 4.165, 4.166, 4.167, 4.168, and 4.169). Leucine crystals dissolve in warm acetic acid, alcohol, which is insoluble in hydrochloric acid. They will turn blue-green after adding 10% CuSO4 solution, and the color does not disappear after heating (Fig. 4.170).

4.15.2 Clinical Significance

Leucine crystals are metabolites of some protein breakdown, which can be observed in the urine of patients with severe liver disease, acute liver necrosis, tissue necrotic diseases, acute phosphorus poisoning, diabetic coma, leukemia, typhoid, metabolic disorders, etc. [33].

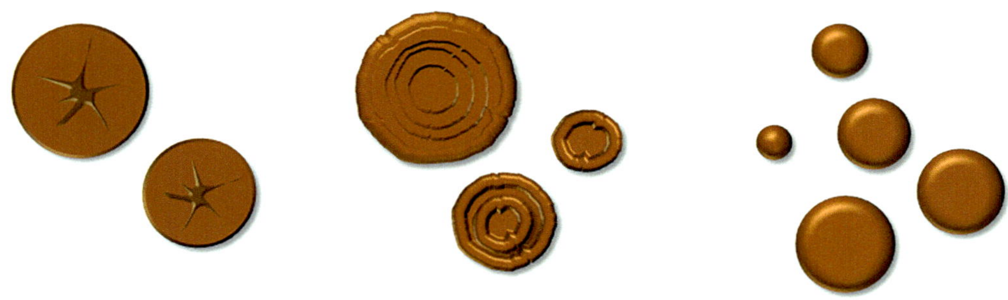

Fig. 4.163 Appearance of leucine crystals

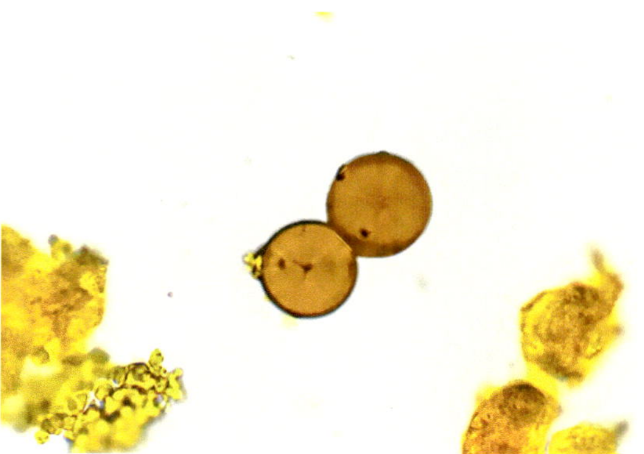

Fig. 4.164 Leucine crystals, brown-yellow, spherical, bilirubinuria, ×1000

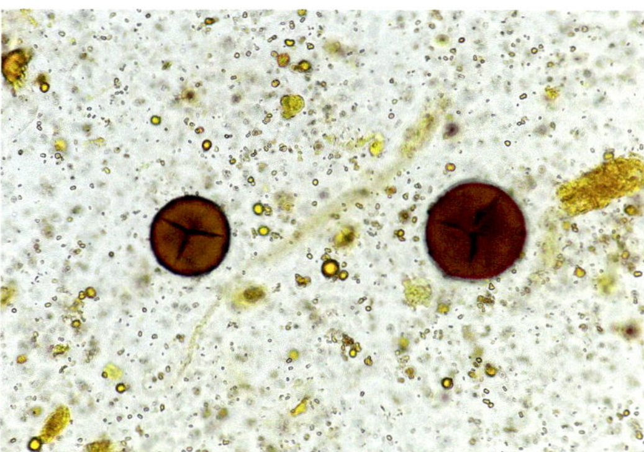

Fig. 4.165 Leucine crystals, brown, cracks can be seen in the central area, bilirubinuria, ×1000

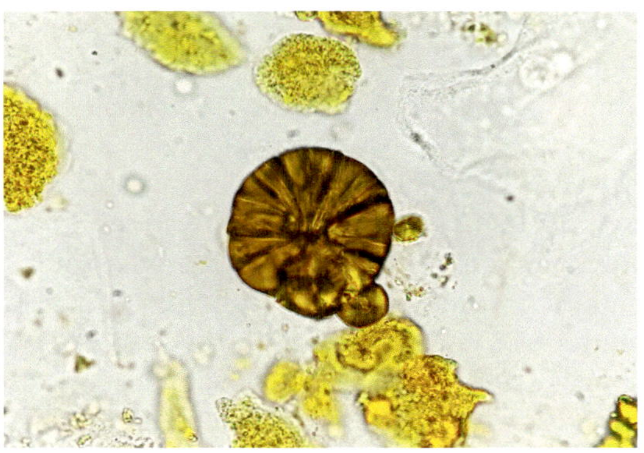

Fig. 4.166 Leucine crystals, fragmentation, bilirubinuria, ×1000

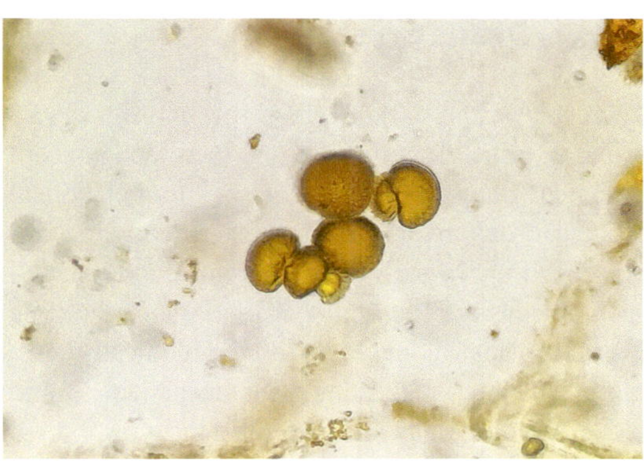

Fig. 4.167 Leucine crystals, mushroom-like, bilirubinuria, ×1000

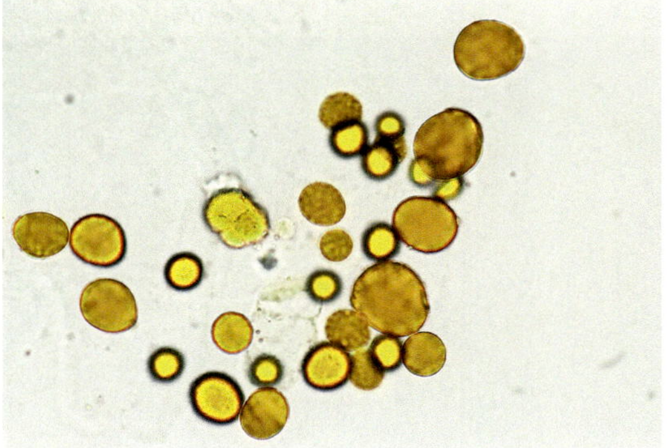

Fig. 4.168 Leucine crystals, oil droplet-shaped, vary in size, bilirubinuria, ×1000

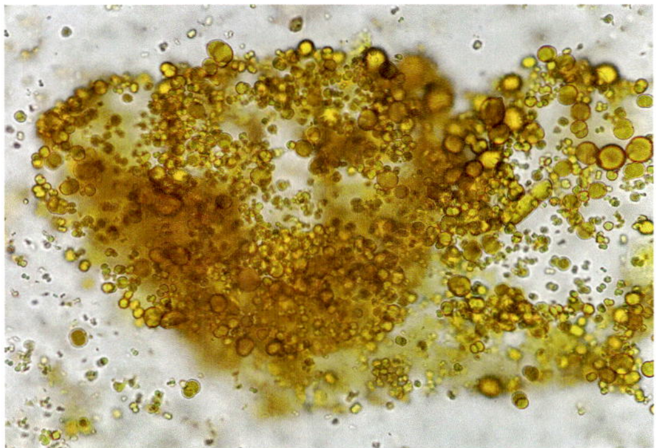

Fig. 4.169 Leucine crystals, small granular oil droplet-shaped, bilirubinuria, ×400

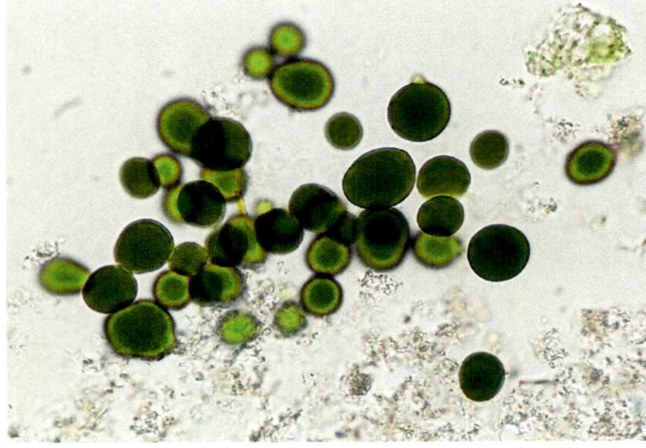

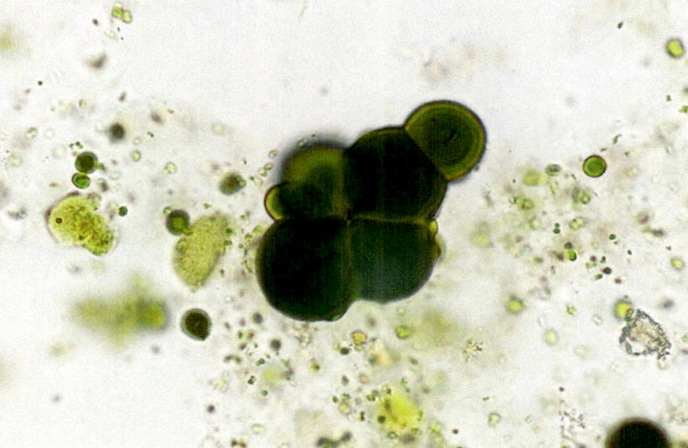

Fig. 4.170 Leucine crystals. They turn green upon the addition of a CuSO4 solution, ×1000

4.16 Drugs Crystals

There are various of types and forms of drug crystals found in urine. As a result of the increased concentration of unmetabolized drugs in the metabolism process, drugs are excreted via the urine and precipitate the drug crystals under certain conditions. If such crystals are found in the urine indicating drug overdose, this should be reported clinically in a timely manner, suggesting that the patient should reduce the dose of the drug or adjust the type of drug, so as not to cause renal damage.

Many drug crystals are not differentiated from pathological crystal due to the variety of drugs, which brings difficulty in judging crystal. A comprehensive analysis can be made based on the combination of patients' medication history and other investigations [34]. Commonly used drug crystals include sulfonamides crystals [35, 36] (Figs. 4.171, 4.172, and 4.173), amoxicillin crystals [34] (Figs. 4.174 and 4.175), acyclovir crystals [37] (Figs. 4.176 and 4.177), and other cephalosporin crystals.

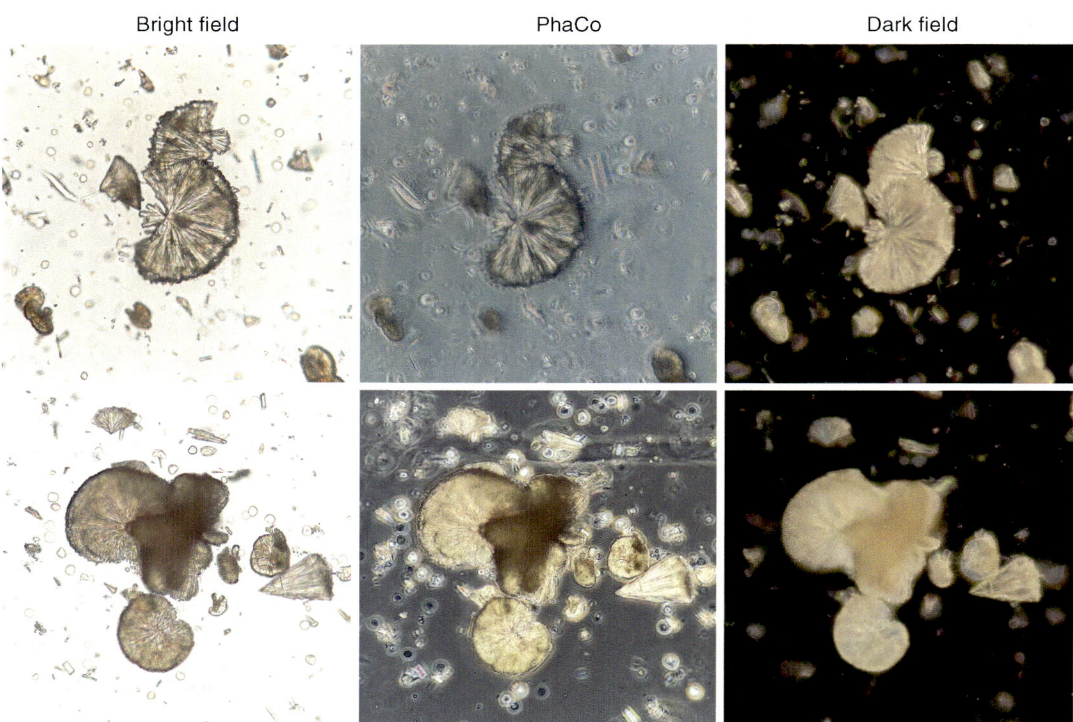

Fig. 4.171 Sulfonamides crystals, brown-yellow, ×400

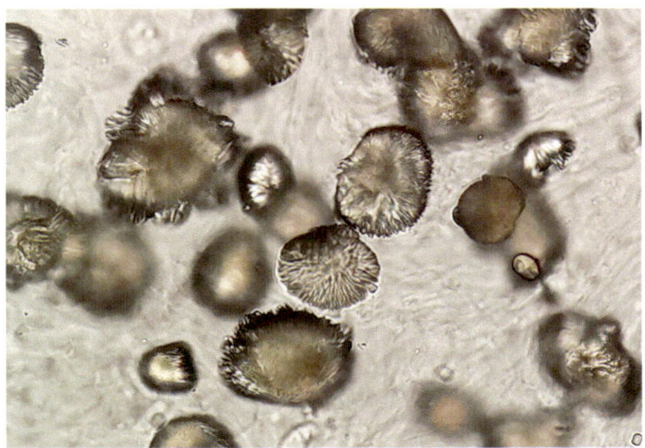

Fig. 4.172 Sulfonamides crystals. Unstained, ×400

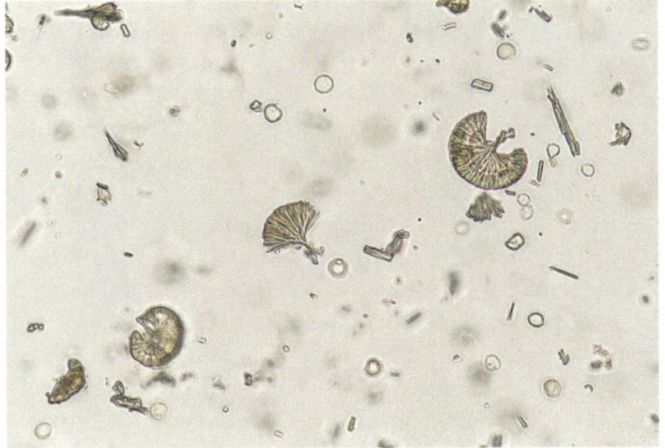

Fig. 4.173 Sulfonamides crystals. Fan-shaped, ×400

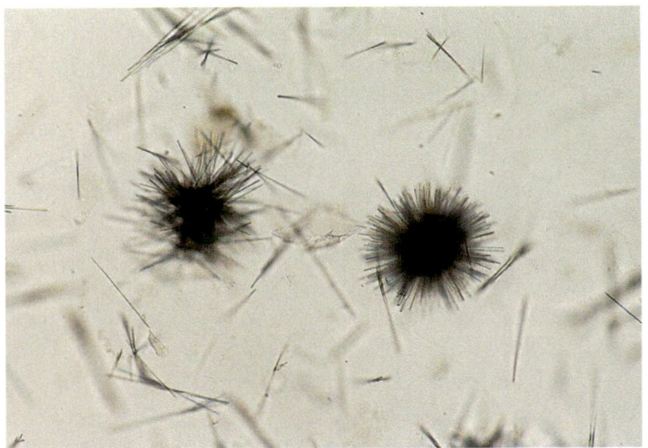

Fig. 4.174 Amoxicillin clavulanate potassium crystals. Unstained, ×400

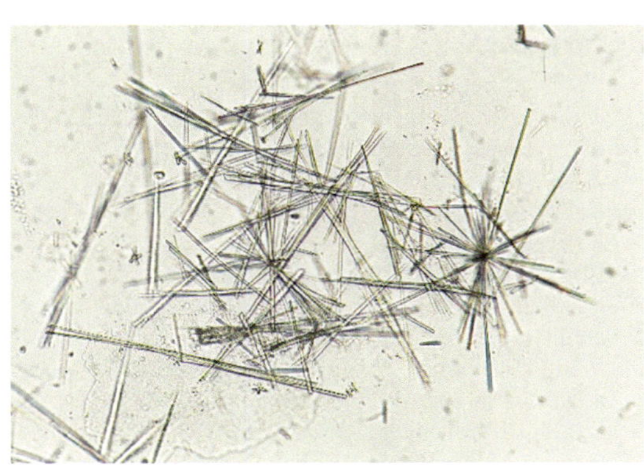

Fig. 4.175 Amoxicillin clavulanate potassium crystals. Needle-like bundles, ×1000

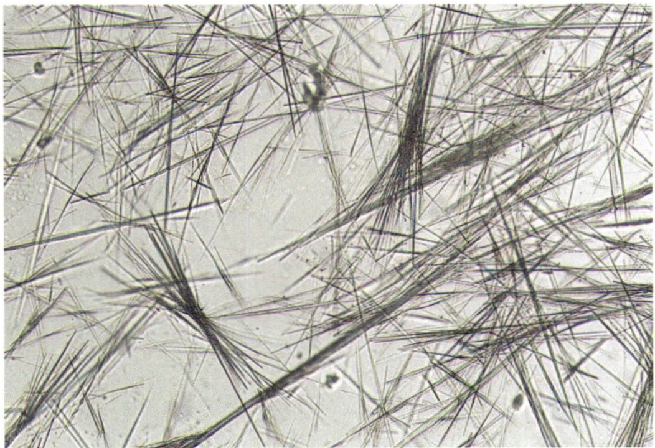

Fig. 4.176 Acyclovir crystals with morphology similar to tyrosine crystals. Unstained, ×400

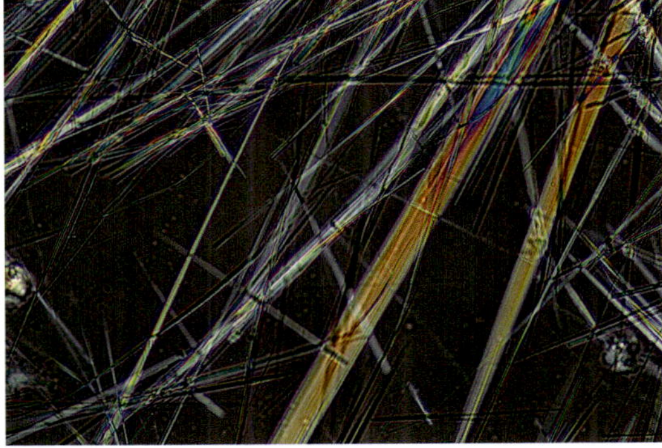

Fig. 4.177 Acyclovir crystals, polarizing microscopy, ×400

References

1. Miller NL, Evan AP, Lingeman JE. Pathogenesis of renal calculi. Urol Clin North Am. 2007;34(3):295–313.
2. Caleffi A, Lippi G. Cylindruria. Clin Chem Lab Med. 2015;53(s2):s1471–7.
3. Romero V, Akpinar H, Assimos DG. Kidney stones: a global picture of prevalence, incidence, and associated risk factors. Rev Urol. 2010;12(2–3):e86–96.
4. Wang Z, Zhang Y, Zhang J, Deng Q, Liang H. Recent advances on the mechanisms of kidney stone formation. Int J Mol Med. 2021;48(2):1–10.
5. Daudon M, Frochot V, Bazin D, Jungers P. Crystalluria analysis improves significantly etiologic diagnosis and therapeutic monitoring of nephrolithiasis. C R Chim. 2016;19(11–12):1514–26.
6. Clark B, Baqdunes MW, Kunkel GM. Diet-induced oxalate nephropathy. BMJ Case Rep. 2019;12(9):e231284.
7. Efe O, Verma A, Waikar SS. Urinary oxalate as a potential mediator of kidney disease in diabetes mellitus and obesity. Curr Opin Nephrol Hypertens. 2019;28(4):316–20.
8. Ng G, Chau EM, Shi Y. Recent developments in immune activation by uric acid crystals. Arch Immunol Ther Exp. 2010;58:273–7.
9. Shirasu A, Ashida A, Matsumura H, Nakakura H, Tamai H. Clinical characteristics of rotavirus gastroenteritis with urinary crystals. Pediatr Int. 2015;57(5):917–21.
10. Trinchieri A, Montanari E. Biochemical and dietary factors of uric acid stone formation. Urolithiasis. 2018;46:167–72.
11. Trinchieri A, Montanari E. Prevalence of renal uric acid stones in the adult. Urolithiasis. 2017;45:553–62.
12. Martillo MA, Nazzal L, Crittenden DB. The crystallization of monosodium urate. Curr Rheumatol Rep. 2013;16(2):400.
13. Shi Y, Mucsi AD, Ng G. Monosodium urate crystals in inflammation and immunity. Immunol Rev. 2010;233(1):203–17.
14. Fogazzi G. Crystalluria: a neglected aspect of urinary sediment analysis. Nephrol Dial Transplant. 1996;11(2):379–87.
15. Behan KJ, Johnston MA. Protocols to dissolve amorphous urate crystals in urine. Lab Med. 2022;53(3):e63–8.
16. Lee AJ, Yoo EH, Bae YC, Jung SB, Jeon CH. Differential identification of urine crystals with morphologic characteristics and solubility test. J Clin Lab Anal. 2022;36(11):e24707.
17. Dick WH, Lingeman JE, Preminger GM, Smith LH, Wilson DM, Shirrell WL. Laxative abuse as a cause for ammonium urate renal calculi. J Urol. 1990;143(2):244–7.
18. Pak CY, Poindexter JR, Adams-Huet B, Pearle MS. Predictive value of kidney stone composition in the detection of metabolic abnormalities. Am J Med. 2003;115(1):26–32.
19. Strasinger SK, Di Lorenzo MS. Urinalysis and body fluids. FA Davis; 2014.
20. Rosenstein IJ, Hamilton-Miller JM, Brumfitt W. Role of urease in the formation of infection stones: comparison of ureases from different sources. Infect Immun. 1981;32(1):32–7.
21. Brunzel NA. Fundamentals of urine and body fluid analysis. Elsevier Health Sciences; 2021.
22. Griffith DP. Struvite stones. Kidney Int. 1978;13(5):372–82.
23. Daudon M, Doré J-C, Jungers P, Lacour B. Changes in stone composition according to age and gender of patients: a multivariate epidemiological approach. Urol Res. 2004;32(3):241–7.
24. Fogazzi G, Anderlini R, Canovi S, Covarelli C, Gras J, Kučera J, Fusarini CF. "Daisy-like" crystals: a rare and unknown type of urinary crystal. Clin Chim Acta. 2017;471:154–7.
25. Frochot V, Castiglione V, Lucas IT, Haymann J-P, Letavernier E, Bazin D, Daudon M. Advances in the identification of calcium carbonate urinary crystals. Clin Chim Acta. 2021;515:1–4.
26. Basu D, Solo S, Nilkund J. Bilirubin crystals in peripheral blood neutrophils in neonatal hyperbilirubinaemia. Br J Haematol. 2005;131(2):141.
27. Ridley JW. Fundamentals of the study of urine and body fluids. Berlin/Heidelberg: Springer; 2018.
28. Ahmed K, Dasgupta P, Khan MS. Cystine calculi: challenging group of stones. Postgrad Med J. 2006;82(974):799–801.
29. Mattoo A, Goldfarb DS. Cystinuria. Semin Nephrol. 2008;28(2):181–91.
30. Trivedi DJ, Patil VP, Kamble PS. CYSTINURIA: crystals that make a baby cry. Indian J Clin Biochem. 2017;32:364–6.
31. Baumer Y, McCurdy SG, Boisvert WA. Formation and cellular impact of cholesterol crystals in health and disease. Adv Biol. 2021;5(11):2100638.
32. Torous VF, Dodd LG, McIntire PJ, Jiang XS. Crystals and crystalloids in cytopathology: incidence and importance. Cancer Cytopathol. 2022;130(10):759–70.
33. Perazella MA. The urine sediment as a biomarker of kidney disease. Am J Kidney Dis. 2015;66(5):748–55.
34. Hentzien M, Lambert D, Limelette A, N'Guyen Y, Robbins A, Lebrun D, Jaussaud R, Bani-Sadr F. Macroscopic amoxicillin crystalluria. Lancet. 2015;385(9984):2296.
35. Thammavaranucupt K, Spanuchart I. Sulfonamide crystals. N Engl J Med. 2021;384(11):1053.
36. Shrishrimal K, Wesson J. Sulfamethoxazole crystalluria. Am J Kidney Dis. 2011;58(3):492–3.
37. Mason WJ, Nickols HH. Crystalluria from acyclovir use. N Engl J Med. 2008;358(13):e14.

5 Other Formed Elements in Urine

Bo Situ, Dehua Sun, Rui Li, Xiufeng Gan, Shengjun Liao, Zhixin Chen, Hongying Zhao, Nannan Cao, Yuhong Luo, Xiaohe Zhang, and Yi Tian

In urine sediment, in addition to various cells, casts, and crystals, there may also exist substances such as mucus threads, bacteria, fungi and parasites. These substances can be observed using bright field microscopy or phase-contrast microscopy, and they can be identified with appropriate staining methods. It is important to note that while some of these substances have clinical significance, others may be contaminants from the external environment or fecal matter. Therefore, when analyzing urine sediment, it is crucial to recognize these substances and carefully determine their origin.

B. Situ (✉) · D. Sun · X. Gan · Y. Luo · X. Zhang
Department of Laboratory Medicine, Nanfang Hospital, Southern Medical University, Guangzhou, Guangdong, China

R. Li
Department of Laboratory Medicine, Shenyang Fifth People's Hospital, Shenyang, Liaoning, China

S. Liao
Department of Clinical Laboratory, Zhongnan Hospital of Wuhan University, Wuhan, Hubei, China

Z. Chen
Department of Laboratory Medicine, Fujian Medical University Affiliated Union Hospital, Fuzhou, Fujian, China

H. Zhao
Department of Laboratory Medicine, Guangxi District People's Hospital, Nanning, China

N. Cao
Department of Laboratory Medicine, The Second Affiliated Hospital of Guangzhou University of Chinese Medicine, Guangzhou, Guangdong, China

Y. Tian
Department of Neurosurgery, The First Affiliated Hospital Of Zhengzhou University, Zhengzhou, Henan, China

5.1 Bacteria

5.1.1 Common Uropathogens

Common bacteria include Gram-negative and Gram-positive bacteria in urine. Among them, Gram-negative bacteria are quite common in urinary tract infections [1]. Common Gram-negative bacteria include *Escherichia coli*, *Klebsiella pneumoniae*, and *Proteus mirabilis*, among others. *Escherichia coli* is the most common pathogen causing urinary tract infections. Common Gram-positive bacteria in urine include *Staphylococcus*, *Enterococcus*, and *Streptococcus*. Among them, *Staphylococcus aureus* and *Enterococcus faecalis* are common pathogens [2].

Anaerobic bacteria are relatively less common in urine but may be present under certain conditions. For instance, urinary tract obstructions or the formation of stones may lead to anaerobic bacterial infections. Common anaerobic bacteria found in urine include *Bacteroides* genus, *Clostridium perfringens*, etc.

Microscopic examination of urine sediment can reveal bacteria of various shapes, com-

L. Zheng et al. (eds.), *Urine Formed Elements*, https://doi.org/10.1007/978-981-99-7739-0_5

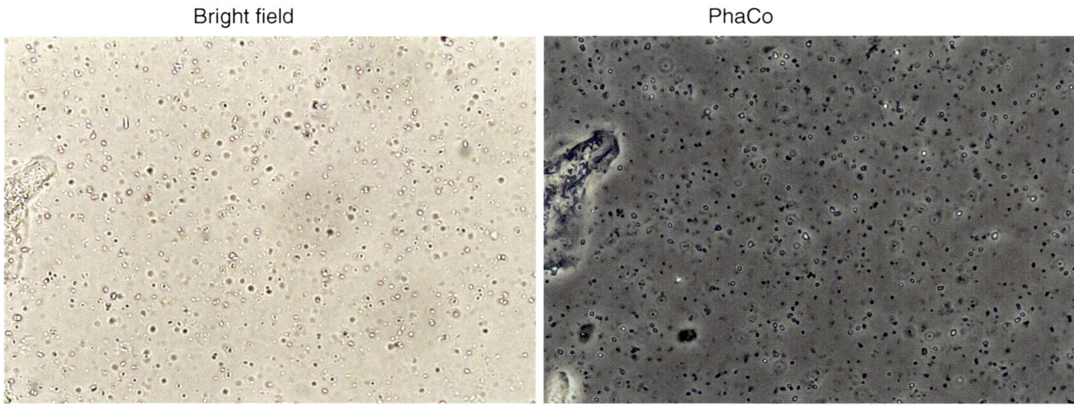

Fig. 5.1 Cocci. Unstained, ×400

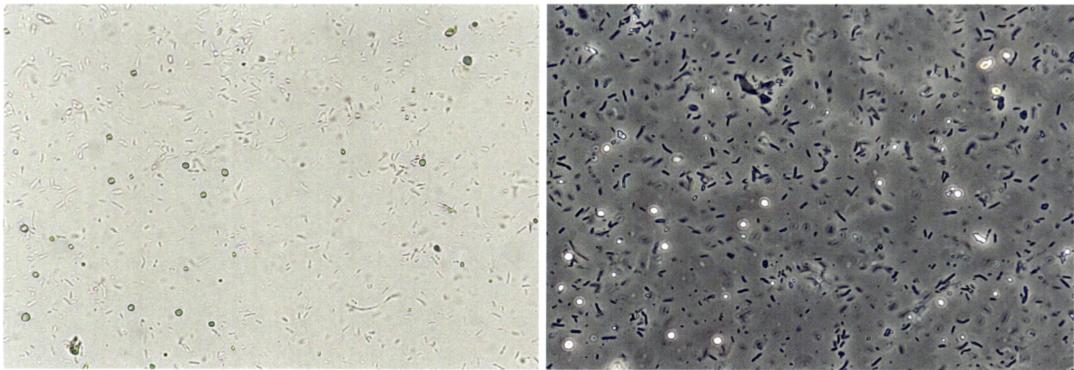

Fig. 5.2 Bacilli. Unstained, ×400

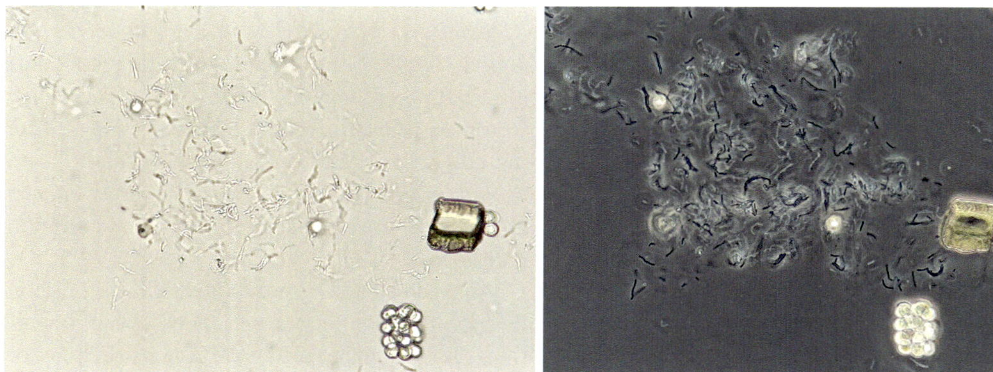

Fig. 5.3 Streptococcus. Unstained, ×400

monly including cocci and bacilli (Figs. 5.1, 5.2, and 5.3). However, it is impossible to determine the type of bacteria and distinguish pathogenic bacteria when unstained or uncultured.

5.1.2 Clinical Significance

Some bacteria are pathogenic in urine, while others may be contaminants. The type of bacteria is usually determined through urine culture and identification. The identification of pathogenic bacteria in urine holds a significant clinical value in the diagnosis of urinary tract infections, the selection of antibiotics, guiding treatment, monitoring treatment efficacy, observing drug resistance, and other aspects [3].

5.2 Fungi

A variety of fungi may be found in urine, and the most common of which include *Candida*, *Cryptococcus*, *Aspergillus*, and *Fusarium* [4].

Cryptococcus typically exhibits a spherical shape and can cause urinary tract infections, kidney infections, or systemic infections. Among them, *Cryptococcus neoformans* is the most common species [5]. *Aspergillus* form branched hyphae and produce conidia. It can cause urinary tract infections or kidney infections, particularly in immunocompromised patients.

Candida is the most common type of fungi found in urine, with prevalent species including *Candida albicans* and *Candida glabrata*, among others. *Candida* may present in yeast form and hyphal form. The yeast cell form is round or oval, similar to yeast, with a diameter of 3–6 μm (Fig. 5.4). They reproduce by budding and often produce pseudohyphae of varying lengths (Fig. 5.5). Due to the nature of the infectious process, leukocytes are easily observed in the urine sediment where fungal structures are found. They can be observed in small numbers or in large amounts. Sometimes, they can be observed trying to perform phagocytosis of fungal spores or pseudohyphae. They can reflect an infectious/inflammatory process [6]. If fungi are found in the urine, adding a 10% KOH solution can destroy the red blood cells, white blood cells, and epithelial cells, making the yeasts cells and fungal hyphae in the field of view clearer and easier to identify (Fig. 5.6).

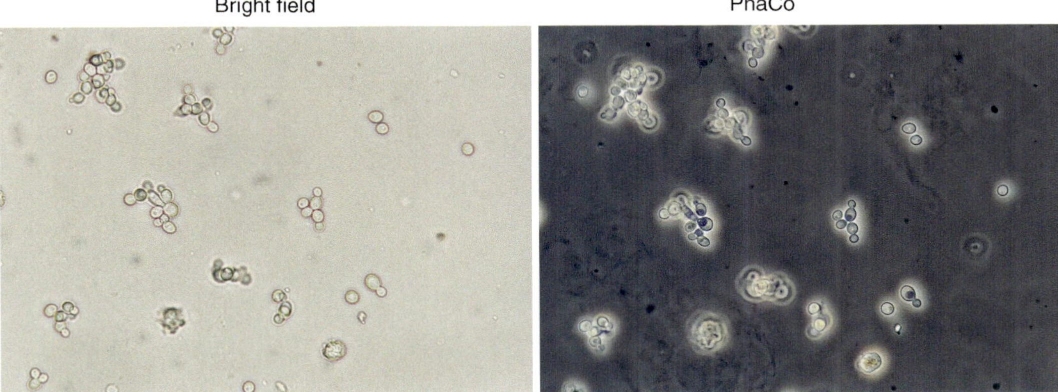

Fig. 5.4 Yeast cells. Unstained, ×400

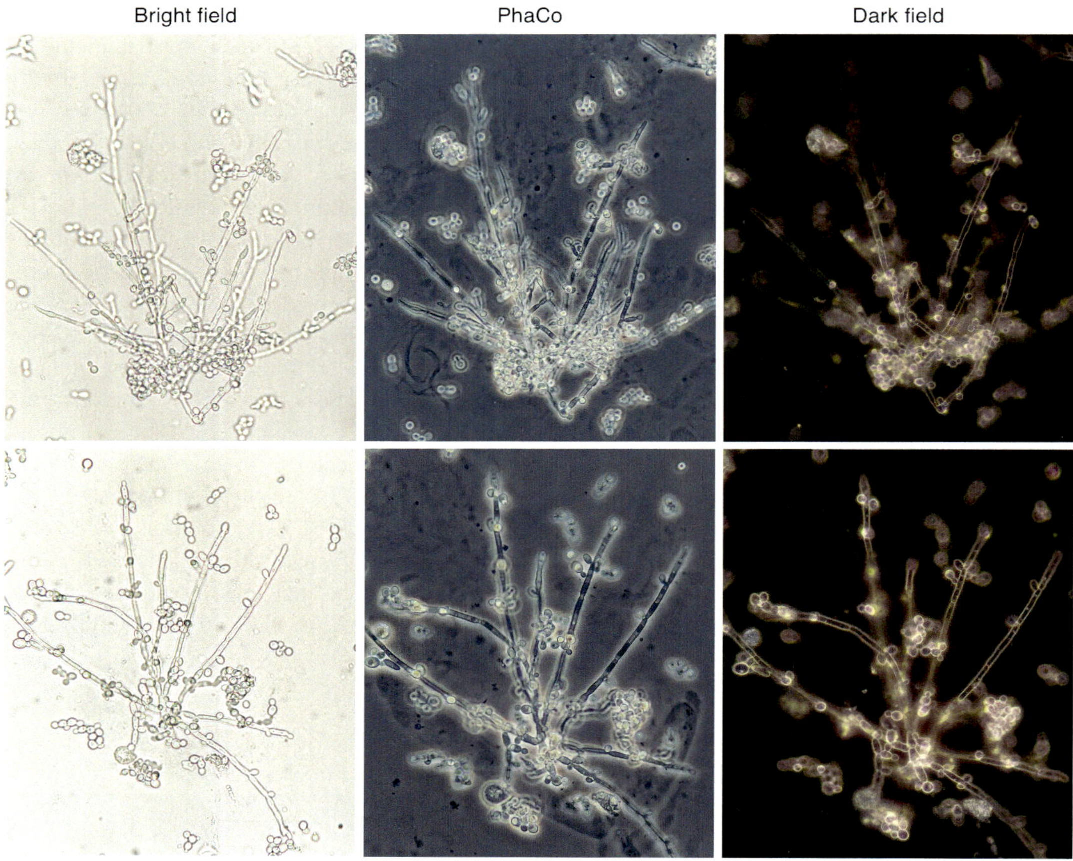

Fig. 5.5 Yeast cells and fungal hyphae. Unstained, ×400

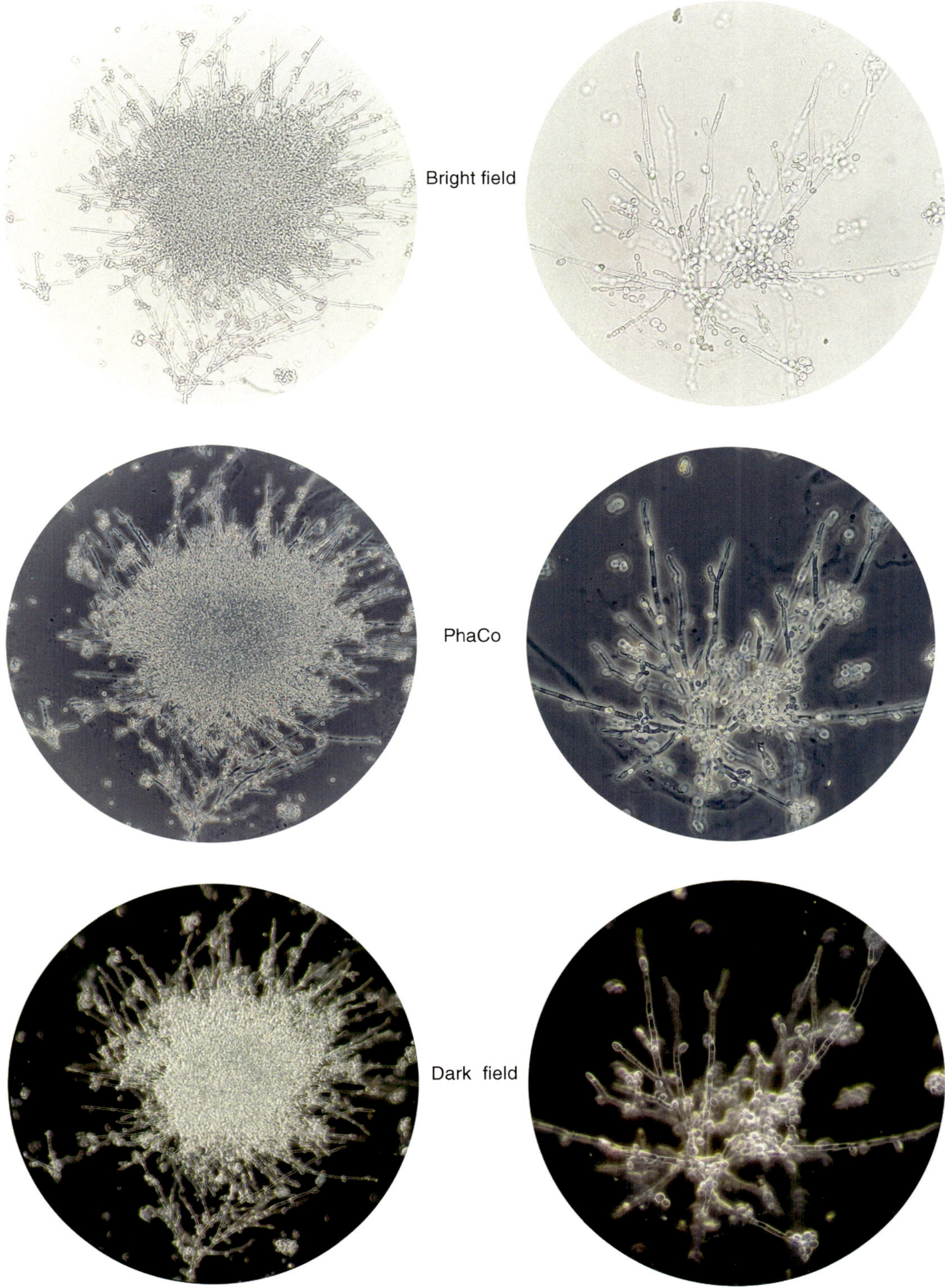

Fig. 5.6 Fungal hyphae. Unstained, ×400

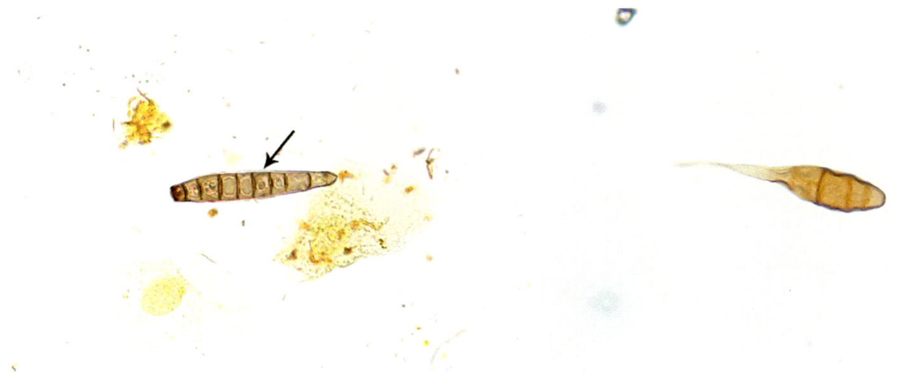

Fig. 5.7 Conidium. Unstained, ×400

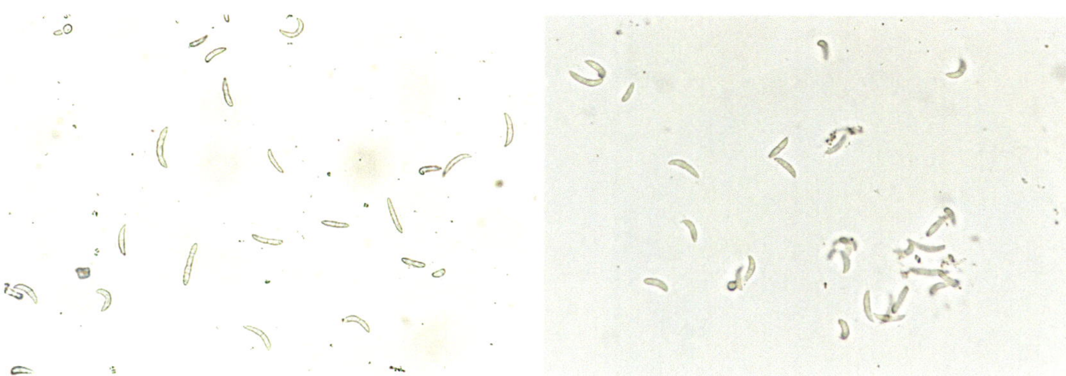

Fig. 5.8 Fusarium. Unstained, ×200

Sometimes, airborne fungi such as *Aspergillus*, *Conidium* (Fig. 5.7), and *Fusarium* (Fig. 5.8) may be mixed into the urine.

5.3 Parasites

5.3.1 *Trichomonas vaginalis*

5.3.1.1 Characteristics

Trichomonas vaginalis typically takes on an inverted pear shape, oval shape, or circular shape, about twice the size of a WBC, measuring 9 × 7 μm. A spindle-shaped nucleus can often be seen in the center, though it may sometimes be off-center or along the edge. The organism has four flagella at the top and one flagellum at the rear [7], with the latter extending backward and connecting to the outer edge of the undulating membrane without freeing itself from the membrane (Fig. 5.9). The undulating membrane is a very thin membranous structure formed by the extension of cytoplasm, located on one side of the anterior half of the organism, not exceeding half of the body length. Under the microscope, the organisms move in a spiraling motion (Fig. 5.10).

The body of the trichomonas appears grey-purple with deep purple granules. A purple-red spindle-shaped nucleus can be seen at the front of the body, and the flagella can also observable under Wright's staining (Fig. 5.11).

5.3.1.2 Clinical Significance

Trichomonas vaginalis mainly parasitizes the urinary and reproductive systems, with the posterior fornix of the vagina in females being the most common site. The infection is often seen in

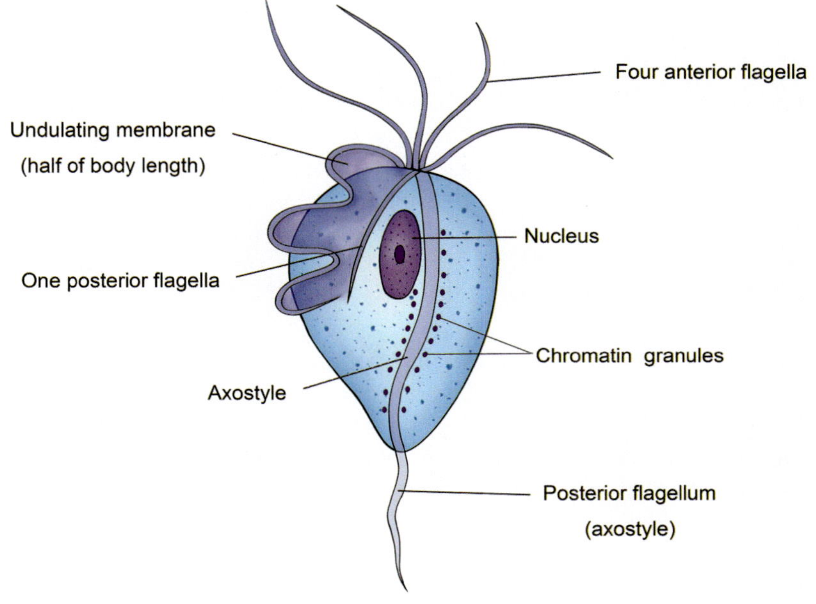

Fig. 5.9 The diagram of *Trichomonas vaginalis* [8]

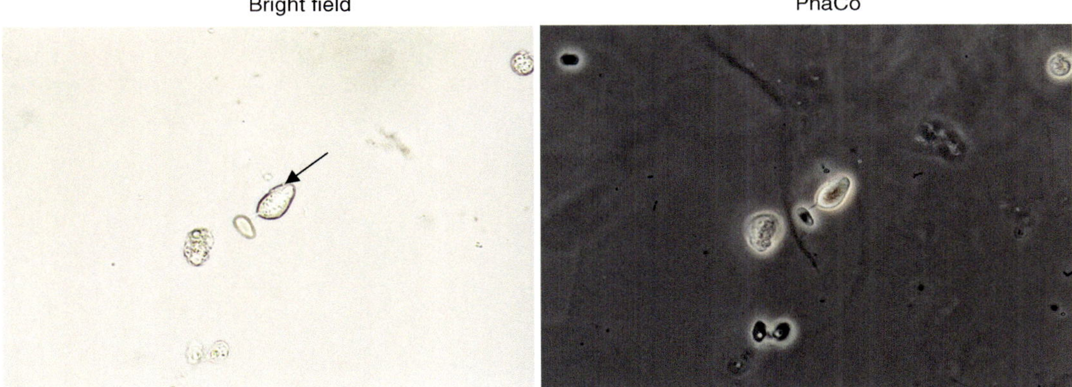

Fig. 5.10 *Trichomonas vaginalis*. Unstained, ×400

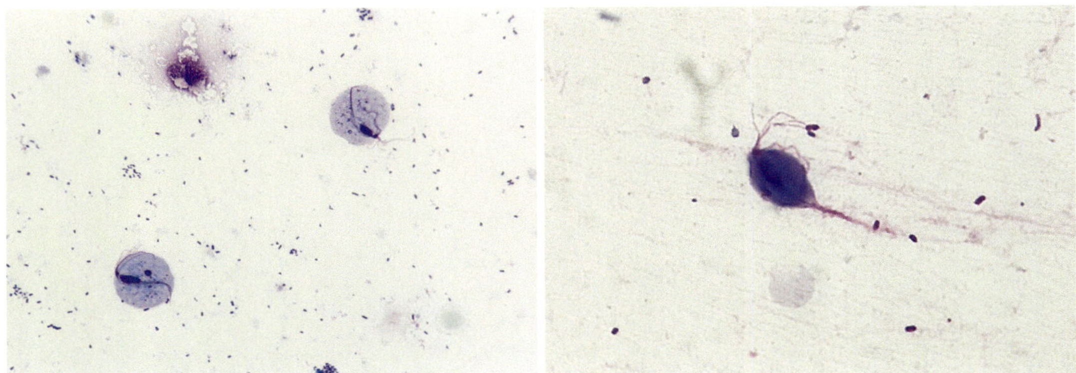

Fig. 5.11 *Trichomonas vaginalis*. Wright's staining, ×1000

the urethra or prostate [9] but can also affect the testicles, epididymis, or tissues under the foreskin in males. *Trichomonas vaginalis* is mainly transmitted between humans through sexual contact, and human beings are its only known host, so it is classified as a sexually transmitted disease.

5.3.2 *Giardia lamblia*

Giardia lamblia, a common intestinal parasite, has two stages in its life cycle: the cyst stage and the trophozoite stage. They may be observed in urine sediment as the result of fecal contamination from infected individuals. Giardiasis is most often acquired by drinking contaminated water—from inadequate sanitation of city water supplies or from contaminated freshwater lakes and streams.

The cysts of *Giardia lamblia* are oval and measure 8–14 μm in length. They have a thick, protective wall and contain four nuclei, fibrils, and granules in the cytoplasm. These features allow them to survive harsh environmental conditions outside the host. They also have two parabasal bodies and a curved median body visible under a microscope (Fig. 5.12).

The trophozoite of *Giardia lamblia* is the active, feeding stage of the parasite. Trophozoites are pear-shaped and measure about 12–15 μm long and 5–9 μm wide. They have a distinctive symmetrical appearance, with two nuclei that resemble "owl's eyes." They also feature four pairs of flagella, which allow for their motility, and a ventral adhesive disc that helps the organism attach to the host's intestinal wall (Fig. 5.13). Additionally, they contain fibrils and granules in their cytoplasm. Unlike the cyst stage, trophozoites are very fragile and can't survive for a long time outside the host's intestines.

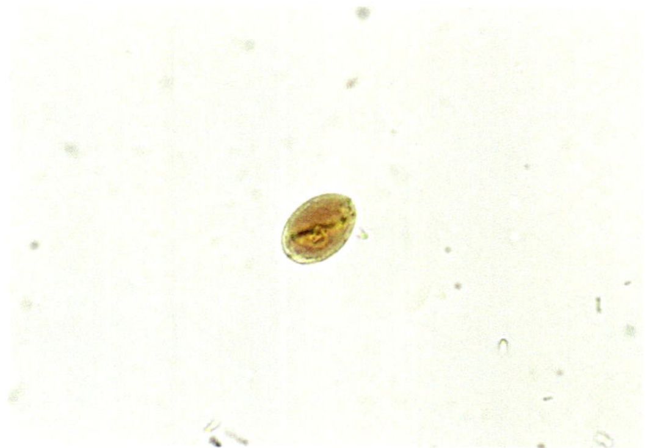

Fig. 5.12 The cysts of *Giardia lamblia*. Iodine stain, ×1000

5.3.3 Other Parasites or Parasitic Eggs

5.3.3.1 Pinworm Eggs

Pinworm eggs are asymmetrical, with one side being flat and the other slightly convex, measuring between 50–60 and 20–30 μm in size. The eggshell is thick and transparent (Fig. 5.14). When the eggs are expelled from the body of the worm, they contain a tadpole stage embryo. After several hours of exposure to the air, they develop

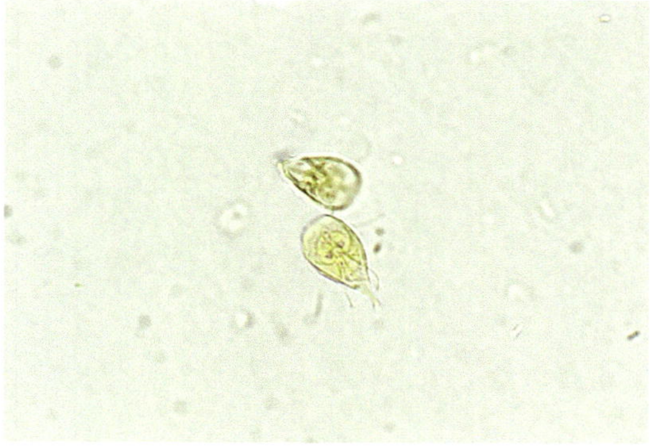

Fig. 5.13 The trophozoite of *Giardia lamblia*. Iodine stain, ×1000

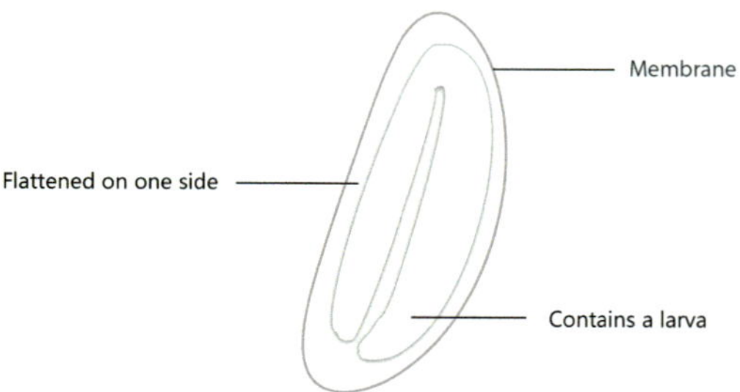

Fig. 5.14 The diagram of pinworm eggs [8]

into infectious eggs that contain curled larvae [10] (Fig. 5.15).

5.3.3.2 *Ascaris lumbricoides* Eggs

Ascaris lumbricoides eggs in urine may originate from fecal contamination and can be classified into fertilized *Ascaris* eggs and unfertilized *Ascaris* eggs [11] (Fig. 5.16).

The fertilized eggs are laid by females after being inseminated through mating with a male. These eggs undergo embryonation and develop into infective eggs. They measure approximately 50–70 × 40–50 μm. The eggs contain a large unsegmented ovum with a granular mass and clear space at both ends. They have an outer coarsely mamillated albuminoid coat, a thick transparent middle layer, and an inner lipoidal vitelline membrane. Some eggs may be found in feces without the outer mamillated albuminous coat (Fig. 5.17).

The unfertilized eggs are laid by the female. These eggs are non-embryonated and cannot become infective. They measure approximately 90 μm × 45 μm. The albuminous coat is thin, distorted, and scanty. The egg contains an unsegmented, small, atrophied ovum with a mass of disorganized, highly refractile granules (Fig. 5.18).

5.3.3.3 Egg of *Schistosoma haematobium*

Schistosoma haematobium is also known as the urinary blood fluke. It is the only blood fluke that infects the urinary tract, causing urinary schistosomiasis, and is the leading cause of bladder cancer [13, 14]. Adults are found in the venous plexuses around the urinary bladder, and the released eggs travels to the wall of the urine bladder causing hematuria and fibrosis of the bladder. The bladder becomes calcified,

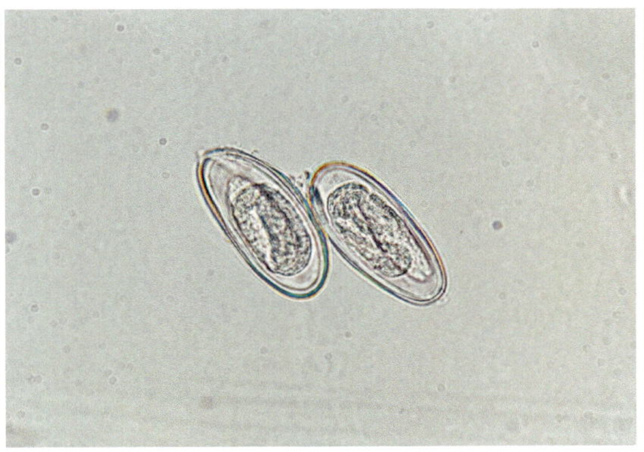

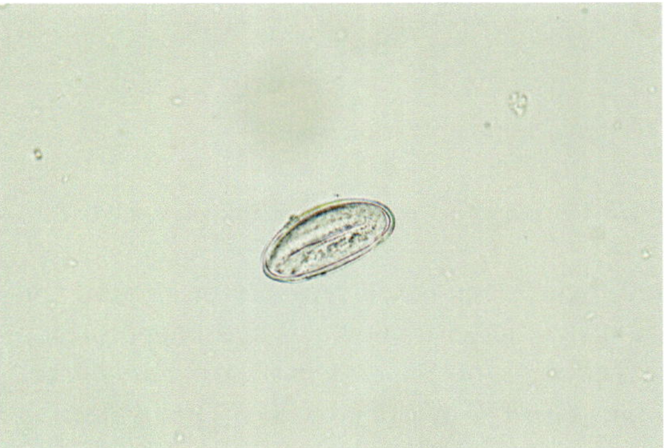

Fig. 5.15 Pinworm eggs. Unstained, ×1000

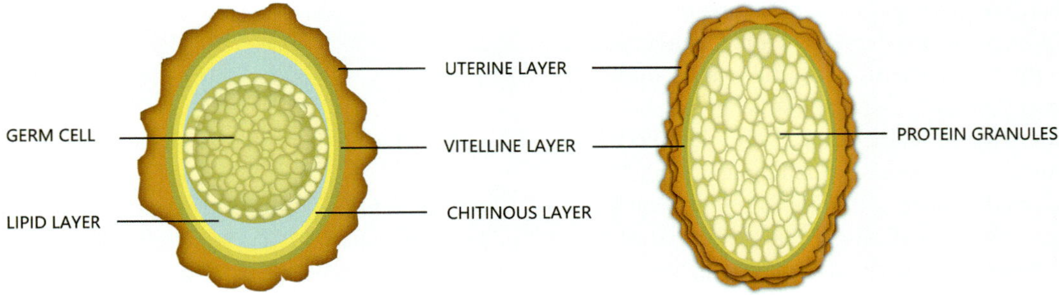

Fig. 5.16 The diagram of *Ascaris lumbricoides* egg [12]

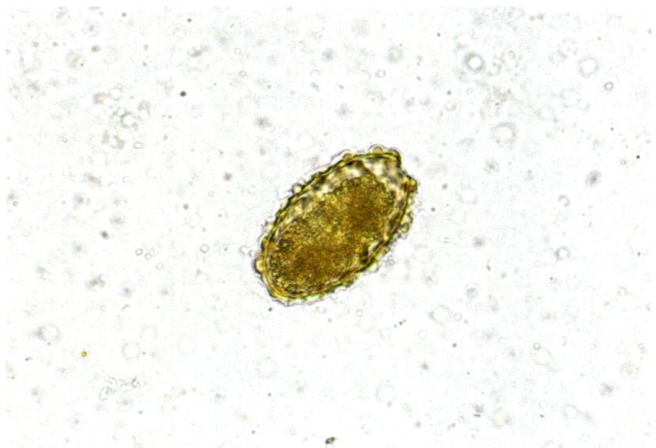

Fig. 5.17 The unfertilized eggs. Unstained, ×1000

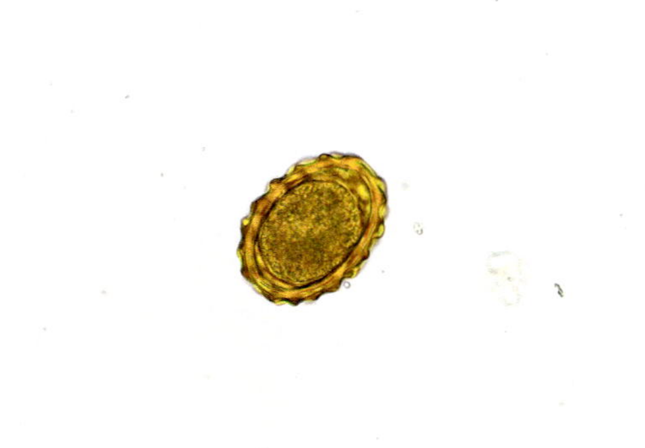

Fig. 5.18 The fertilized eggs. Unstained, ×1000

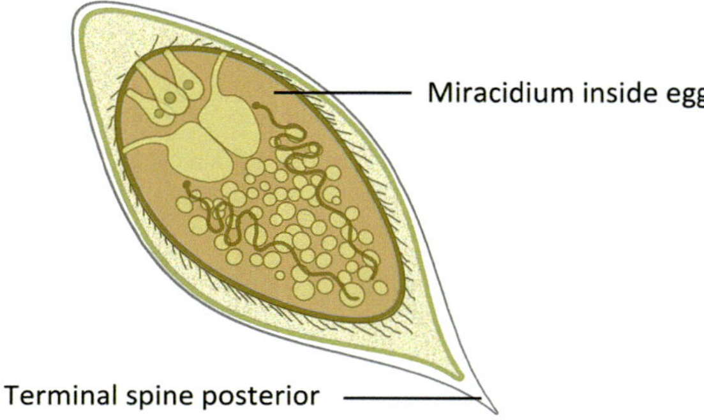

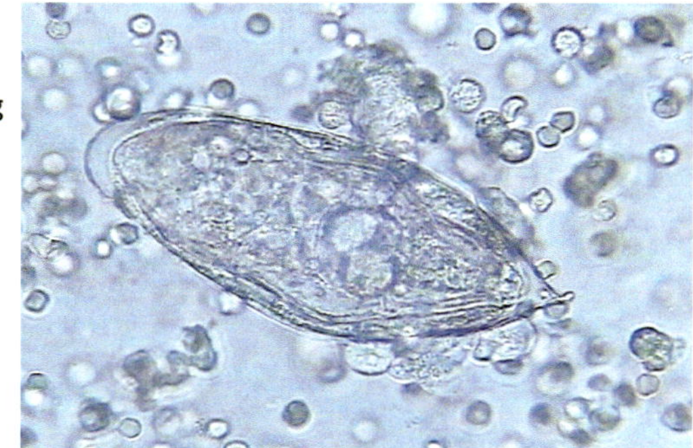

Fig. 5.19 Egg of *Schistosoma haematobium*, ×400 [8]

and there is increased pressure on ureters and kidneys otherwise known as hydronephrosis.

The eggs of *Schistosoma haematobium* are large (110–170 μm long by 40–70 μm wide) and bear a conspicuous terminal spine (Fig. 5.19). Eggs contain a mature miracidium when shed in urine.

5.3.3.4 *Strongyloides stercoralis*

Strongyloides stercoralis is a facultative parasite. During the parasitic generation, adult worms primarily reside in the host's small intestine. Larvae, however, have the capacity to invade various organs and tissues including the lungs, brain, liver, and kidneys leading to a condition known as strongyloidiasis. The life stages of *Strongyloides stercoralis* within the host include adults, eggs, rhabditiform larvae and filariform larvae [15]. Rhabditiform larvae are 0.2–0.45 mm in length, with a rounded head and a tapering tail. A double-bulb pharynx is discernible (Fig. 5.20).

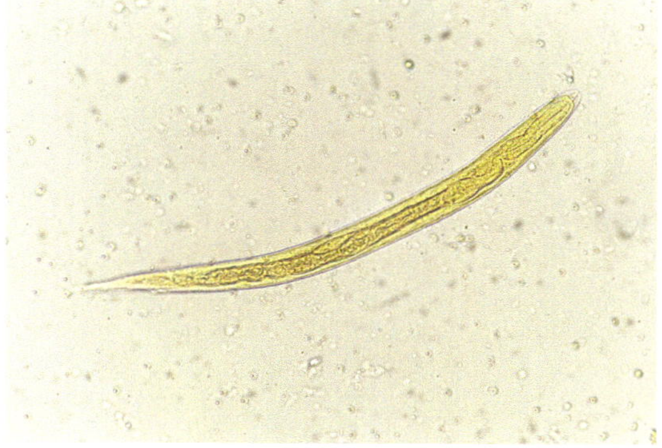

Fig. 5.20 Rhabditiform larvae. Iodine stain, ×400

Filariform larvae, on the other hand, are slender and approximately 0.6–0.7 mm long with a tapering, bifurcated tail end. A primordial reproductive system can be observed toward the rear (Fig. 5.21). The presence of rhabditiform and filariform larvae in urine may likely result from fecal contamination.

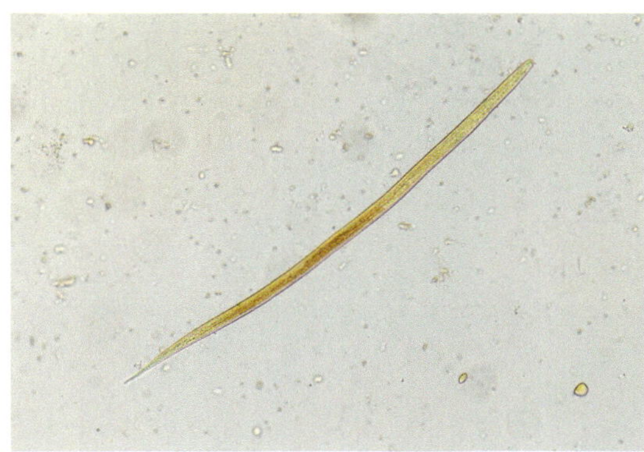

Fig. 5.21 Filariform larvae. Iodine stain, ×400

5.4 Sperm

A normal sperm has an oval-shaped head, an intact midpiece, and an uncoiled single tail (Fig. 5.22). Sperms with normal morphology are able to swim well and in a straight line. Normal sperm will also contain healthy genetic information, rather than too many or too few chromosomes, which are common in abnormally shaped sperm.

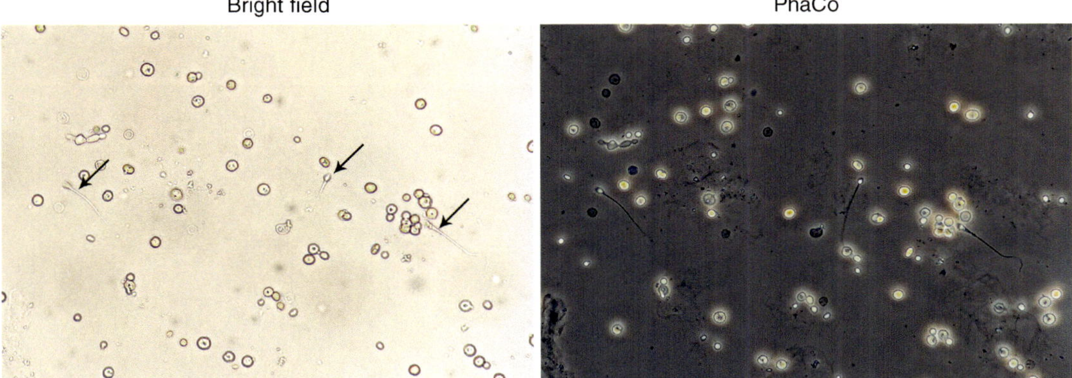

Fig. 5.22 Sperm. Unstained, ×400

5.5 Glass Fragments

During microscopic examination of urine sediment, one can often observe glass fragments. These substances bear a resemblance to some forms of urinary crystals due to their strong refractivity. However, glass fragments typically lack a consistent shape and vary in size (Fig. 5.23).

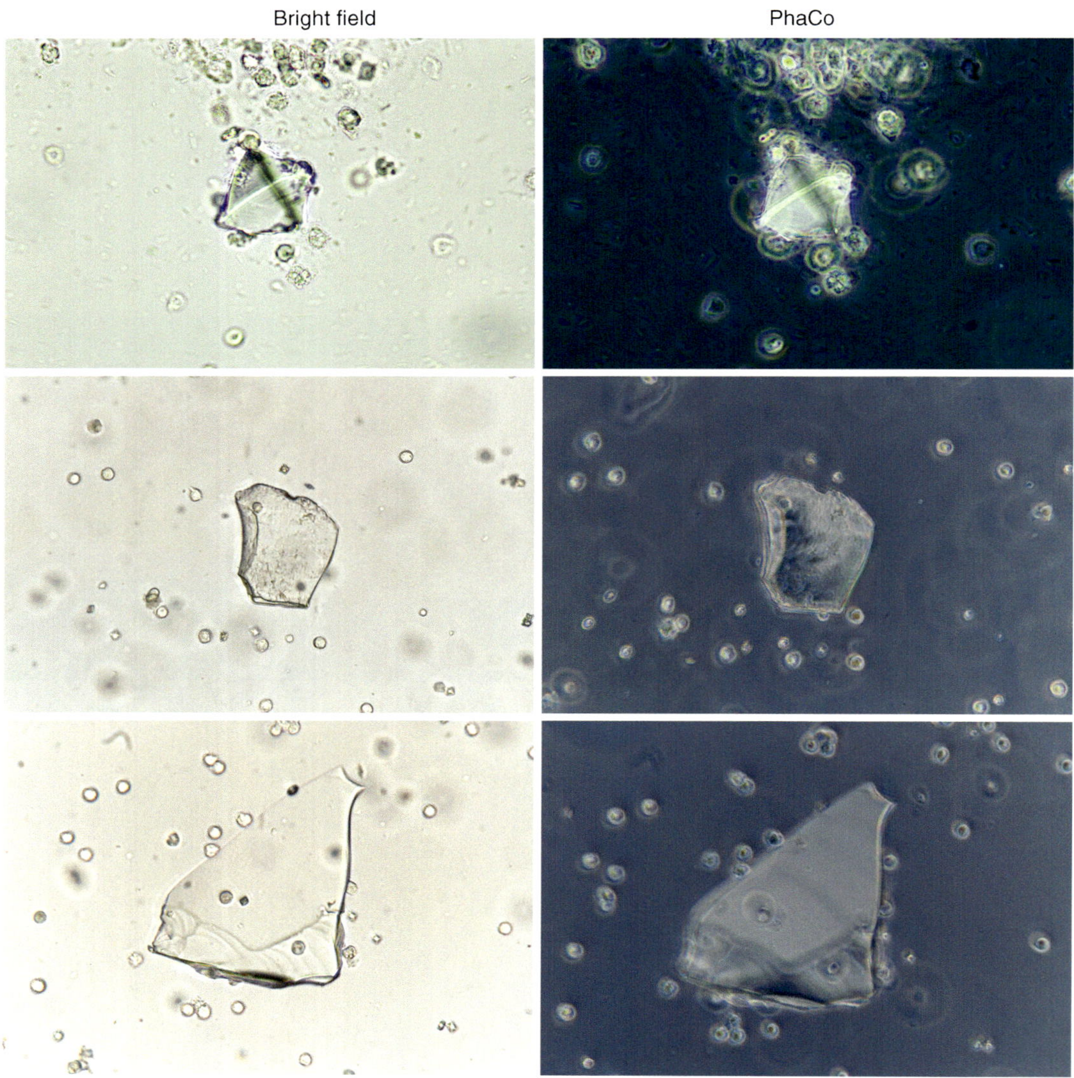

Fig. 5.23 Glass fragments, ×400

5.6 Fibers

Fibers originate from external environmental contamination. They are coarse, vary in length, and closely resemble certain types of casts (Fig. 5.24). Their specific structures can be observed using bright field or phase-contrast microscopy. These substances lack the matrix of casts and exhibit various forms (Fig. 5.25).

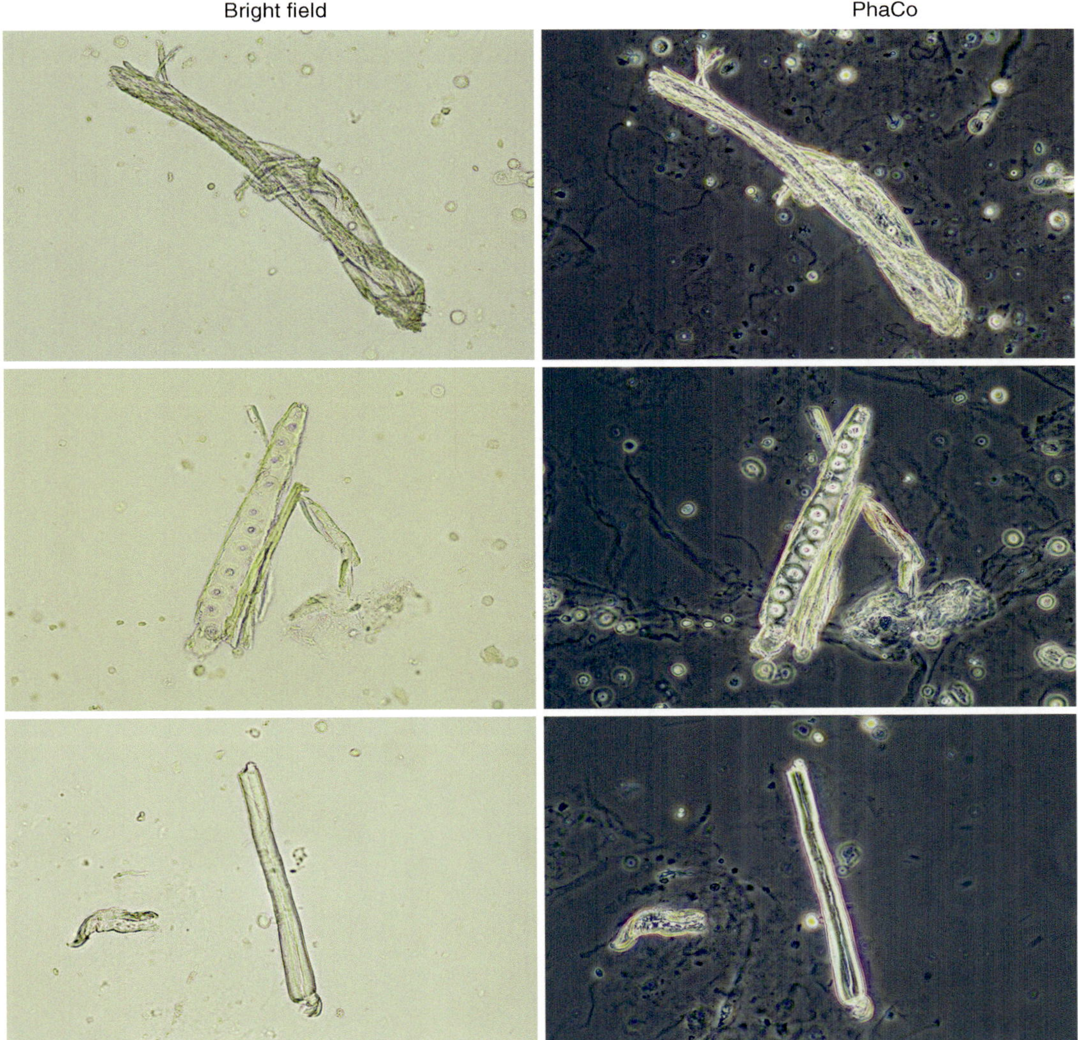

Fig. 5.24 Fibers. They vary in length and thickness, and some of them resemble cast. Unstained, ×400

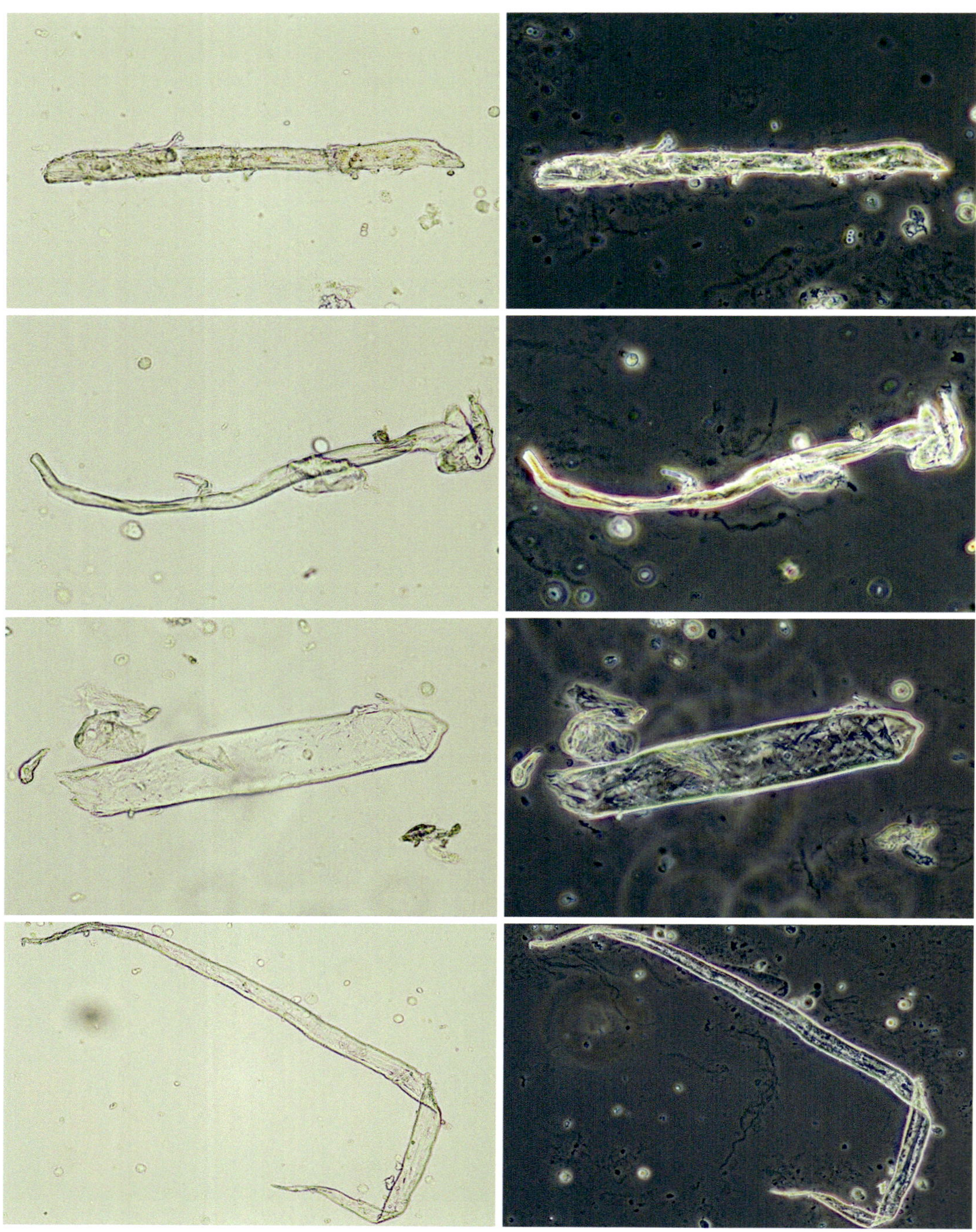

Fig. 5.25 Fibers. Unstained, ×400

5.7 Mucus Threads

Mucus threads in urine are elongated, fibrous structures that are typically transparent but may be influenced by the color of the urine. These structures resemble the morphology of hyaline casts and can be observed under phase-contrast microscopy. Some of the mucus threads can adhere to crystals, cells, or other substances (Fig. 5.26).

The presence of mucus threads in urine can be normal in certain situations, particularly when the urine contains higher levels of mucous secretions, such as after excessive water intake or the use of certain medications. The number of mucus threads in urine might increase during urinary tract infections (such as urethritis or cystitis). Additionally, irritation of the urinary tract mucosa by stones may lead to an increase in mucus threads.

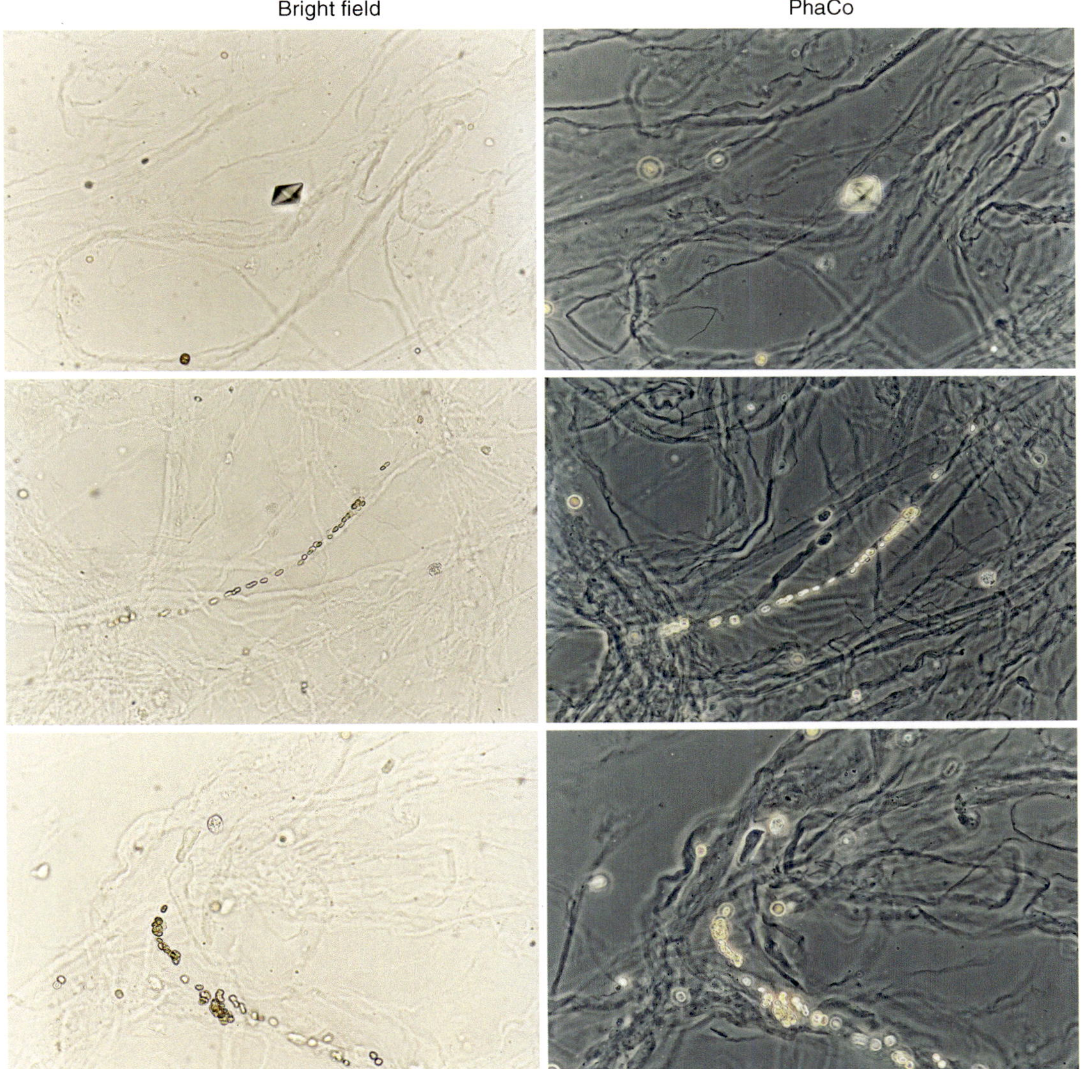

Fig. 5.26 Mucus threads vary in thickness and length and can adhere to cells. Unstained, ×400

5.8 Pollen

Pollen in urine originates from external environmental contamination. Some of this pollen resembles the morphology of macrophages or parasitic eggs. Care should be taken to distinguish them when observing under a microscope (Fig. 5.27).

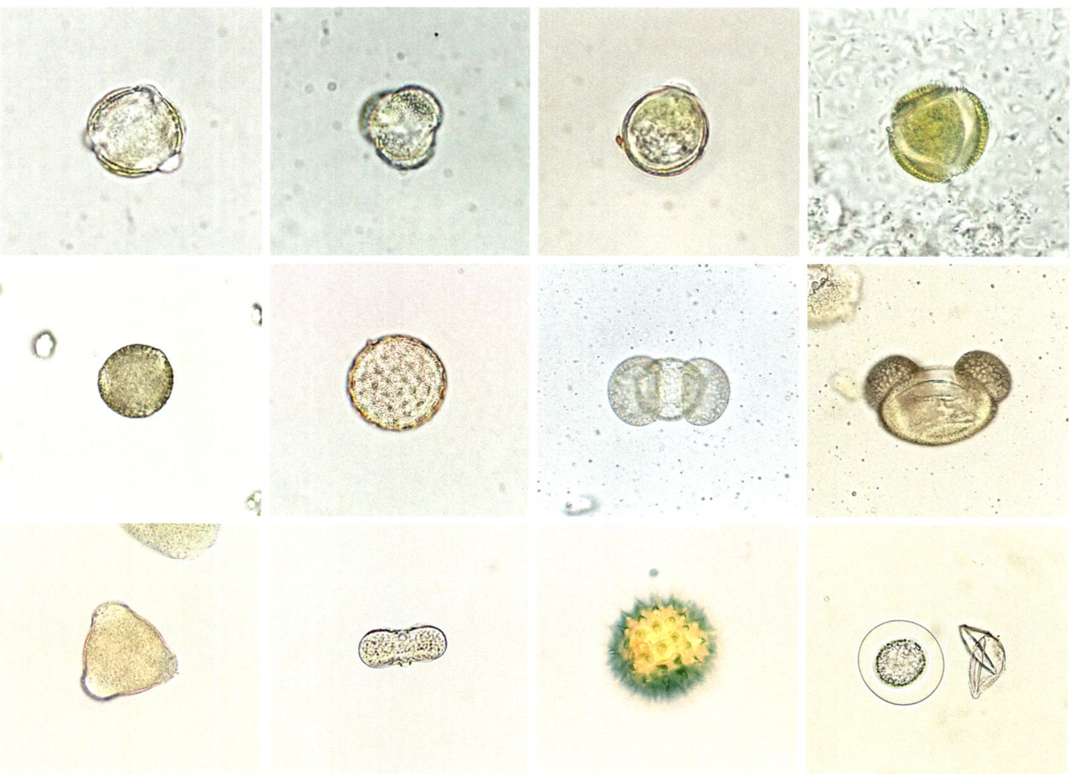

Fig. 5.27 Pollen exhibits diverse forms. Unstained, bright field, ×400

5.9 Corpora Amylacea and Prostatic Secretory Granules

Corpora amylacea and prostatic secretory granules originate from contamination by prostatic fluid. Corpora amylacea is usually composed of glycoproteins and calcium salts, their size varies, and their shape is irregular, characterized by an annular or concentric circular structure (Fig. 5.28). They are common in the prostatic fluid of elderly males. The prostatic fluid also contains prostatic secretory granules (Prostatic bodies). These granules are rich in phosphatidylcholine, a normal component of the prostate. They are grayish in color, vary in size, and have slight refractivity. Their presence decreases during prostatic inflammation.

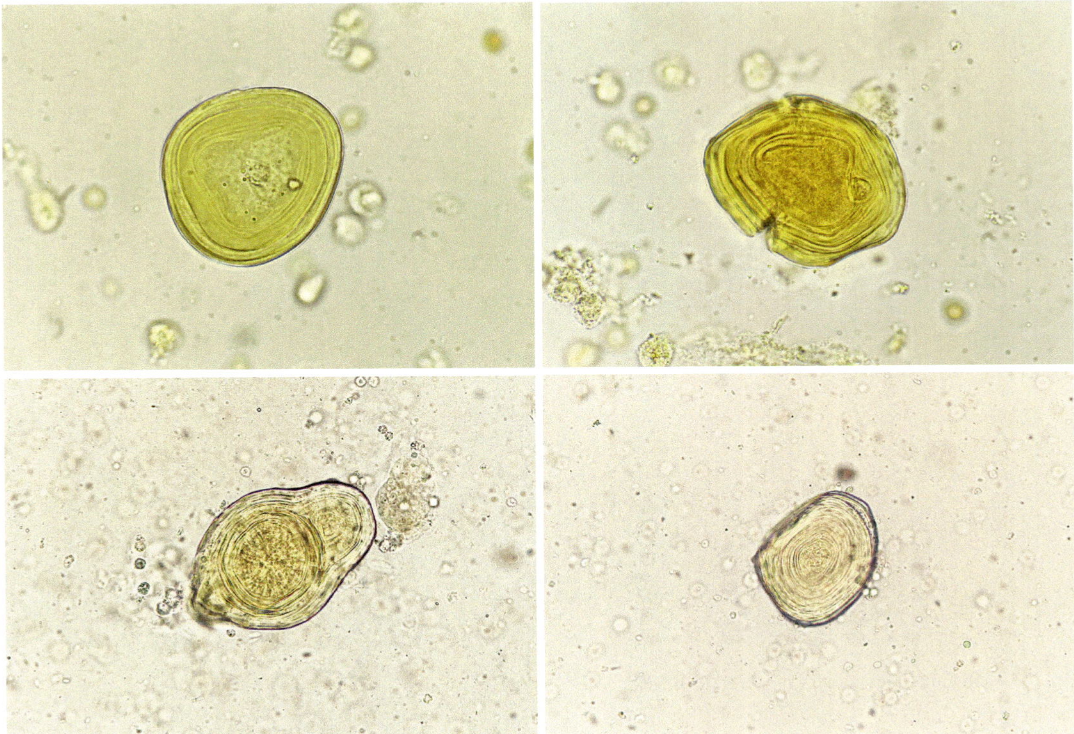

Fig. 5.28 Corpora amylacea. Unstained, bright field, ×1000

5.10 Rotifers

Rotifers are a small phylum of about 2000 species of tiny, bilaterally symmetrical. Because they are among the smallest of freshwater metazoans—most are between 50 and 2000 μm. They exhibit diverse morphologies, possess varied life history strategies, and occupy a wide range of habitats. The presence of rotifers in urine indicates contamination, primarily due to improper specimen collection procedures not being followed (Fig. 5.29).

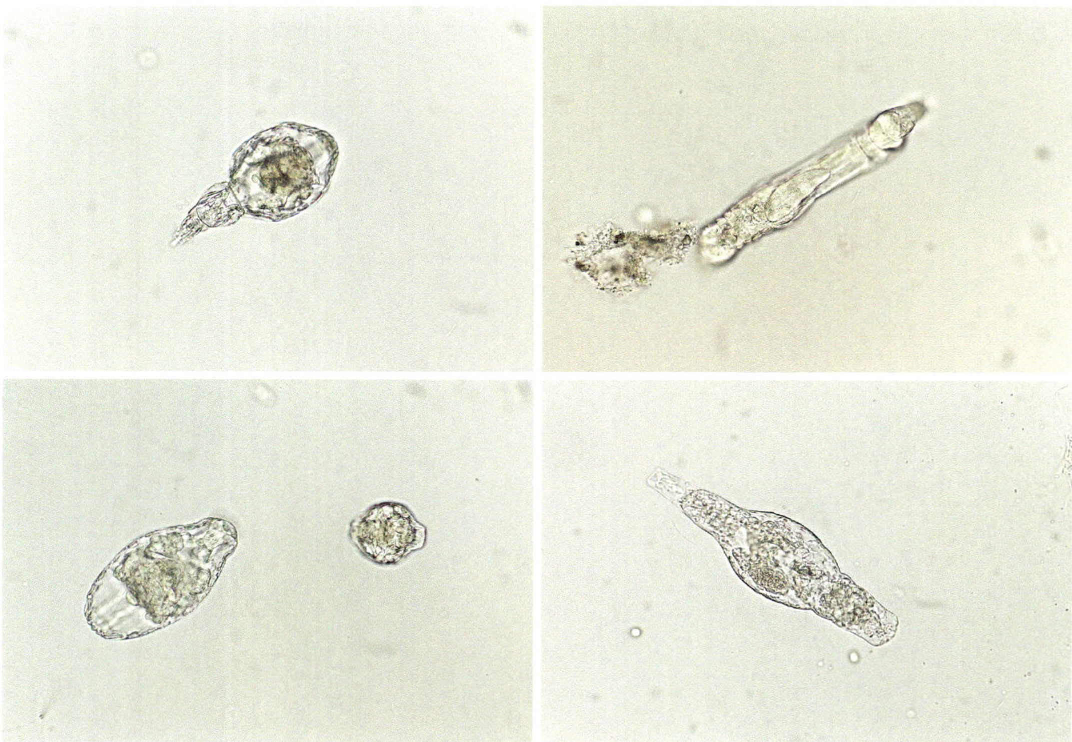

Fig. 5.29 Rotifers. Unstained, bright field, ×1000

References

1. Mattoo TK, Shaikh N, Nelson CP. Contemporary management of urinary tract infection in children. Pediatrics. 2021;147(2):e2020012138.
2. Ronald A. The etiology of urinary tract infection: traditional and emerging pathogens. Dis Mon. 2003;49(2):71–82.
3. Olin SJ, Bartges JW. Urinary tract infections: treatment/comparative therapeutics. Vet Clin North Am Small Anim Pract. 2015;45(4):721–46.
4. Sobel JD, Vazquez JA. Fungal infections of the urinary tract. World J Urol. 1999;17(6):410–4.
5. Agrawal C, Sood V, Kumar A, Raghavan V. Cryptococcal infection in transplant kidney manifesting as chronic allograft dysfunction. Indian J Nephrol. 2017;27(5):392–4.
6. Poloni JAT, Rotta LN. Urine sediment findings and the immune response to pathologies in fungal urinary tract infections caused by Candida spp. J Fungi. 2020;6(4):245.
7. Schwebke JR, Burgess D. Trichomoniasis. Clin Microbiol Rev. 2004;17(4):794–803.
8. Brunzel NA. Fundamentals of urine and body fluid analysis. Amsterdam: Elsevier Health Sciences; 2021.
9. Leitsch D. Recent advances in the molecular biology of the protist parasite Trichomonas vaginalis. Fac Rev. 2021;10:26.
10. Cook GC. Enterobius vermicularis infection. Gut. 1994;35(9):1159–62.
11. Rogers RA. A study of eggs of Ascaris lumbricoides var. suum with the electron microscope. J Parasitol. 1956;42(2):97–108.
12. Holland C. Ascaris: the neglected parasite. Newnes; 2013.
13. Antoni S, Ferlay J, Soerjomataram I, Znaor A, Jemal A, Bray F. Bladder cancer incidence and mortality: a global overview and recent trends. Eur Urol. 2017;71(1):96–108.
14. Khurana S, Dubey ML, Malla N. Association of parasitic infections and cancers. Indian J Med Microbiol. 2005;23(2):74–9.
15. Czeresnia JM, Weiss LM. Strongyloides stercoralis. Lung. 2022;200(2):141–8.

GPSR Compliance

The European Union's (EU) General Product Safety Regulation (GPSR) is a set of rules that requires consumer products to be safe and our obligations to ensure this.

If you have any concerns about our products, you can contact us on ProductSafety@springernature.com

In case Publisher is established outside the EU, the EU authorized representative is:

Springer Nature Customer Service Center GmbH
Europaplatz 3
69115 Heidelberg, Germany

Batch number: 10372211

Printed by Printforce, the Netherlands